Neonatal Haematology: A Practical Guide

Neonatal Haematology: A Practical Guide

Irene Roberts

Department of Paediatrics and
MRC Weatherall Institute of Molecular Medicine
John Radcliffe Hospital
University of Oxford
UK

Barbara J. Bain

Imperial College Faculty of Medicine
St Mary's Hospital
London
UK

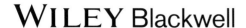

Registered Offices
John Wiley & Sons, Inc., 111 River Street, Hoboken, NJ 07030, USA
9600 Garsington Road, Oxford, OX4 2DQ, UK

Editorial Office
John Wiley & Sons Ltd, The Atrium, Southern Gate, Chichester, West Sussex, PO19 8SQ, UK

For details of our global editorial offices, customer services, and more information about Wiley products visit us at www.wiley.com.

Wiley also publishes its books in a variety of electronic formats and by print-on-demand. Some content that appears in standard print versions of this book may not be available in other formats.

Library of Congress Cataloging-in-Publication Data applied for

Hardback ISBN: 9781119371588

Cover Design: Wiley
Cover Image: Courtesy of Irene Roberts

Set in 9.5/12.5pt STIXTwoText by Straive, Pondicherry, India

Printed in Singapore
M075700_260522

Contents

Preface

This neonatal haematology guide aims to fill a gap in an important, but often poorly understood, area of diagnostic haematology by focusing particularly on common blood problems in this unique group of patients, although not neglecting the rarities that can also be important. We specifically chose to use a text-atlas format because the starting point for so many haematological problems in neonates is the information to be found through careful evaluation of a blood film in conjunction with an automated blood count. Given that many neonates with haematological abnormalities weigh less than 1000 g at birth and have an estimated blood volume at birth of 40–80 ml with very precarious vascular access, there is huge practical value in being able to extract the maximum amount of diagnostic information from a single drop of blood.

The book has been organised into four chapters based on the most frequently occurring clinical problems: interpretation of normal results and blood film appearances (Chapter 1); anaemias and haematological causes of jaundice (Chapter 2); diagnosis of systemic disorders, such as infection, and less common leucocyte disorders, such as leukaemia and storage disorders (Chapter 3); and disorders of coagulation and thrombosis, including common causes of thrombocytopenia and their investigation (Chapter 4). We hope that this handbook will be a core resource for haematologists on call in any hospital with a maternity unit who may not be neonatal experts, and that it will act as a core text for neonatal and paediatric haematologists. It is very much aimed to be a practical resource, based on real-life experience of neonatal haematology in large teaching hospitals and contains algorithms, tables and illustrative cases with full colour images. While the focus is on common problems, we also describe when to look for, and how to spot, rare haematological disorders presenting in the neonatal period.

Almost all the images and cases described in this book derive from more than 25 years' experience as a 'neonatal haematologist', which involved daily examination of blood films from neonates in a number of neonatal intensive care units and special care baby units and daily conversations with the clinical teams responsible for their care. This was only possible with the support, open-mindedness and enthusiasm of the neonatalogists on the one hand and the dedication and rigour of the highly skilled biomedical scientists of the diagnostic haematology labs on the other. Particular thanks go to David Roper, Andrew Osei-Bimpong and the late Corinne Jury of the Hammersmith and Queen Charlotte's Hospitals Haematology Laboratories, who made possible the delivery of a daily 'baby films' service in the face of increasing NHS demands; to David Roper and the late Dr David Swirsky, former consultant haematologist at Hammersmith Hospital, for their help with the photomicrographs in the earliest years of the neonatal haematology service; to countless biomedical scientists whose pride in delivering the highest quality 'baby films' on a daily basis was an inspiration to me; to paediatric haematology colleagues in London and Oxford who posed fascinating questions to keep me on my toes; and to the long-suffering haematology trainees who usually managed to look interested in this niche subject and helped to deliver the clinical advice.

This book would never have been written without the help and support of a number of other people. Above all, I am hugely indebted to my co-author, Professor Barbara Bain. She brought to the book her 50 years' experience of diagnostic haematology. Her expertise, experience, diligence and patience, as well as her friendly advice, were invaluable. I am similarly hugely grateful to Mandy Collison at Wiley who never gave up on the project despite repeated delays on my part. Finally, I have to thank my family (Allan, Duncan and Ewan), who accepted the neonatal haematology geek in their midst, and supported the whole project from the beginning.

Irene Roberts

Abbreviations

2,3-DPG	2,3-diphosphoglycerate
ADA	adenosine deaminase
ADP	adenosine diphosphate
AGM	aorto-gonado-mesonephros
aHUS	atypical haemolytic uraemic syndrome
AIHA	autoimmune haemolytic anaemia
ALL	acute lymphoblastic leukaemia
ALPS	autoimmune lymphoproliferative syndrome
AML	acute myeloid leukaemia
APTT	activated partial thromboplastin time
ATD	asphyxiating thoracic dystrophy
ATRUS	amegakaryocytic thrombocytopenia and radio-ulnar synostosis
BCG	bacille Calmette–Guérin
BCSH	British Committee for Standards in Haematology
BHFS	Bart's hydrops fetalis syndrome
BPI	bactericidal/permeability-increasing protein
BSS	Bernard–Soulier syndrome
CAMT	congenital amegakaryocytic thrombocytopenia
CDA	congenital dyserythropoietic anaemia
CHS	Chédiak–Higashi syndrome
CMV	cytomegalovirus
CNS	central nervous system
COVID-19	coronavirus disease 19
DAT	direct antiglobulin test
DBA	Diamond–Blackfan anaemia
DIC	disseminated intravascular coagulation
DNA	deoxyribonucleic acid
ECMO	extracorporeal membrane oxygenation
EDTA	ethylene diaminetetra-acetic acid
ELP	early lymphoid progenitor
EMA	eosin-5-maleimide
EOS	early-onset sepsis

EPO	erythropoietin
ERFE	erythroferrone
FFP	fresh frozen plasma
FNAIT	fetal/neonatal alloimmune thrombocytopenia
FPD/AML	familial platelet disorder with propensity to acute myeloid leukaemia
FRC	fragmented red cell
G6PD	glucose-6-phosphate dehydrogenase
G6PT1	glucose-6-phosphate transporter 1
G-CSF	granulocyte colony-stimulating factor
Gp	glycoprotein
GPI	glucose phosphate isomerase
Hb	haemoglobin concentration
HDFN	haemolytic disease of the fetus and newborn
HELLP	haemolysis, elevated liver enzymes and low platelets
HIE	hypoxic ischaemic encephalopathy
HIV	human immunodeficiency virus
HK	hexokinase
HLH	haemophagocytic lymphohistiocytosis
HNA	human neutrophil antigen
HPA	human platelet antigen
HPFH	hereditary persistence of fetal haemoglobin
HPLC	high performance liquid chromatography
HPP	hereditary pyropoikilocytosis
HS	hereditary spherocytosis
HSC	haemopoietic stem cell
HUS	haemolytic uraemic syndrome
IBMFS	inherited bone marrow failure syndromes
ICH	intracranial haemorrhage
IG%	immature granulocyte percentage
IGF	insulin-like growth factor
IgG	immunoglobulin G
IgH	immunoglobulin heavy chain
IgM	immunoglobulin M
IL-6	interleukin-6
IPF	immature platelet fraction
IRF	interferon regulatory factor
ITP	autoimmune thrombocytopenia
IUGR	intrauterine growth restriction
IUT	intrauterine transfusion
IVH	intraventricular haemorrhage
IVIg	intravenous immunoglobulin
JAK2	Janus kinase 2
JMML	juvenile myelomonocytic leukaemia
KHE	Kaposiform haemangioendothelioma
KMP	Kasabach–Merritt phenomenon

LAD	leucocyte adhesion deficiency
LDH	lactate dehydrogenase
LOS	late-onset sepsis
MAHA	microangiopathic haemolytic anaemia
MAIPA	monoclonal antibody-specific immobilisation of platelet antigens
MCA	middle cerebral artery
MCH	mean cell haemoglobin
MCHC	mean cell haemoglobin concentration
MCV	mean cell volume
MDSC	myeloid-derived suppressor cell
ML-DS	myeloid leukaemia of Down syndrome
MPAL	mixed phenotype acute leukaemia
MPV	mean platelet volume
NA	not applicable
NADPH	nicotinamide adenine dinucleotide phosphate
NEC	necrotising enterocolitis
NETs	neutrophil extracellular traps
NICE	National Institute for Health and Care Excellence
NICU	neonatal intensive care unit
NLR	neonatal leukaemoid reaction
NRBC	nucleated red blood cell
NS/MPD	Noonan syndrome-associated myeloproliferative disorder
PCC	prothrombin complex concentrate
PCR	polymerase chain reaction
PFK	phosphofructokinase
PGK	phosphoglycerate kinase
PK	pyruvate kinase
PMN	polymorphonuclear
PT	prothrombin time
RNA	ribonucleic acid
RP	ribosomal proteins
RSV	respiratory syncytial virus
RUSAT1	radio-ulnar synostosis with amegakaryocytic thrombocytopenia
SARS-CoV-2	severe acute respiratory syndrome coronavirus-2
SCN	severe congenital neutropenia
SGA	small for gestational age
SIFD	sideroblastic anaemia, B-cell immunodeficiency, periodic fevers, and developmental delay
SLE	systemic lupus erythematosus
TACO	transfusion-associated circulatory overload
TA-GvHD	transfusion-associated graft-versus-host disease
TAM	transient abnormal myelopoiesis
TAPS	twin anaemia–polycythaemia sequence
TAR	thrombocytopenia with absent radii
TGFβ	transforming growth factor β

TOPs	Transfusion of Prematures trial
TPI	triosephosphate isomerase
TPO	thrombopoietin
TRALI	transfusion-related acute lung injury
TT	thrombin time
TTP	thrombotic thrombocytopenic purpura
TTTS	twin-to-twin transfusion syndrome
VKDB	vitamin K-dependent bleeding
VWD	von Willebrand disease
VWF	von Willebrand factor
WBC	white cell count
WHO	World Health Organization
XLSA	X-linked sideroblastic anaemia
XLT	X-linked thrombocytopenia

1

The full blood count and blood film in healthy term and preterm neonates

Introduction

Haemopoiesis is the process that ensures life-long production of haemopoietic cells. In newborn infants the process has many distinct features that differ from those in older children and adults. These differences reflect both the ontogeny of haemopoiesis during fetal development and the unique interaction between the fetus and mother, as well as the effects of birth itself. The sequential changes in the sites and regulation of haemopoiesis during development also help to explain the natural history of many neonatal haematological problems.

Brief outline of the ontogeny of haemopoiesis

Haemopoiesis in humans begins in the yolk sac between 2 and 3 weeks post-conception (Fig. 1.1).[1,2] This is known as primitive haemopoiesis. Studies in other species, particularly in mice, indicate that the predominant cell types produced in the yolk sac are erythroid cells and macrophages.[2,3] While megakaryocytes and lymphoid cells may also be yolk sac-derived, the current consensus of opinion is that true, long-lived haemopoietic stem cells (HSC) arise from a region of specialised endothelium ('haemogenic' endothelium), which is localised to the ventral wall of the dorsal aorta in a region known as the aorto-gonado-mesonephros (AGM).[4–6] In humans, haemopoiesis begins in the AGM at around 5 weeks post-conception and is known as definitive haemopoiesis.[6–8] Haemopoiesis in the aortic wall is only transient, presumably because this region lacks the necessary physical space and specialised microenvironment to support expansion and differentiation of the HSC and progenitor populations required to meet the needs of the growing fetus.

By 6 weeks post-conception, HSC and progenitor cells have migrated to the fetal liver,[8,9] which remains the main site of blood cell production throughout fetal life[10,11] and AGM haemopoiesis ceases. The first signs of haemopoiesis in the bone marrow are evident from around 11 weeks post-conception.[8,12] Although fetal bone marrow is able to give rise to cells of all lineages, it is becoming clear that the predominant cell types produced in the bone marrow are B lymphocytes and their progenitor cells together with granulocytes, monocytes and their progenitors. Although erythropoiesis and megakaryopoiesis take

Neonatal Haematology: A Practical Guide, First Edition. Irene Roberts and Barbara J. Bain.
© 2022 John Wiley & Sons Ltd. Published 2022 by John Wiley & Sons Ltd.

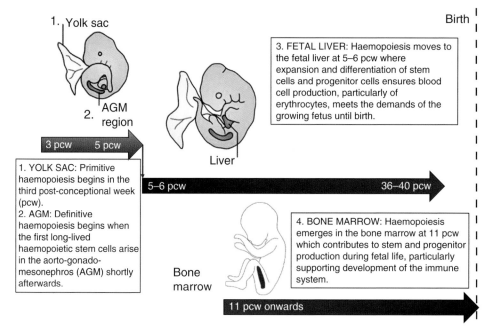

Fig. 1.1 Ontogeny of human haemopoiesis in embryonic and fetal life. AGM, aorto-gonado-mesonephros; pcw, post-conceptional week. Based on references 1 and 2.

place in the fetal bone marrow from the end of the first trimester, most red blood cell and megakaryocyte production takes place in the fetal liver until shortly before term.[8] Thus, for preterm infants, the liver is the main haemopoietic organ at and shortly after birth; this is likely to be a contributory factor in a number of disorders, including the haematological abnormalities seen in neonates with Down syndrome (see pages 154–160 and 206).

Properties of fetal haemopoietic stem and progenitor cells

Major advances in the immunological and molecular tools available to analyse haemopoietic stem and progenitor cells have allowed us to build up a much clearer picture of the process of haemopoiesis in fetal life and how this differs from adult life. Fetal HSC, like adult HSC, are the cells at the top of the haemopoietic hierarchy (Fig. 1.2). When HSC divide, they do so either through a process of 'self-renewal', where they generate more HSC (sometimes referred to 'symmetric cell division'), or through asymmetric division during which one of the two daughter cells differentiates into progenitor cells, which in turn generate the mature cells of all the haemopoietic lineages (Fig. 1.2).[9]

Fetal haemopoietic stem cells

Studies in mice, and more recently in humans, indicate that fetal HSC are markedly different from those in adult bone marrow.[9,13–16] Elucidating the nature of the differences between fetal and adult HSC, and the molecular mechanisms that underpin these differences, is likely to help our understanding of many of the haematological problems that

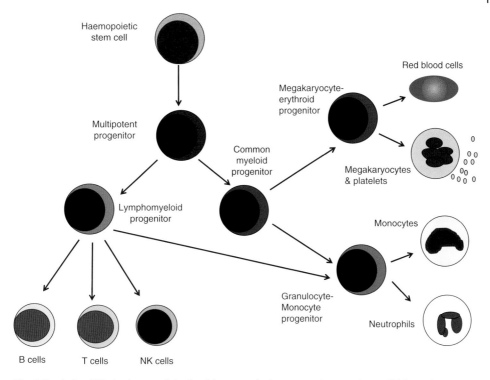

Fig. 1.2 A simplified scheme of the fetal haemopoietic stem and progenitor cell hierarchy showing the differentiation of multipotent and committed progenitor cells from haemopoietic stem cells. Details of the fetal-specific pathway of B lineage progenitor differentiation are shown in Fig. 1.3. Based on reference 9.

affect neonates and potentially open up new approaches to treatment. For example, the need for rapid expansion of haemopoietic cells to meet the needs of the growing fetus means that the numbers of fetal HSC have to increase more rapidly than at any other time of life. Furthermore, since HSC are responsible for life-long haemopoiesis, this process of HSC expansion needs to be precisely regulated to prevent either uncontrolled proliferation (and the risk of haematological malignancy) on the one hand or HSC 'exhaustion' (and the risk of bone marrow failure) on the other. These properties are thought to underlie the particular prevalence of certain haematological diseases in fetal and neonatal life, including Diamond–Blackfan anaemia and juvenile myelomonocytic leukaemia.[17]

There are differences both in the intrinsic properties of the HSC and in the regulatory signals produced by the haemopoietic microenvironment during fetal life.[16] One of the characteristic intrinsic differences in fetal HSC is the increased proportion of HSC that are actively cycling and undergoing a process of 'self-renewal' that results in expansion of the pool of long-lived HSC in fetal life.[18] This behaviour of fetal HSC contrasts dramatically with adult HSC which are largely quiescent cells that enter the cell cycle infrequently.[9,16,18] The amplification in fetal HSC numbers probably takes place mainly in fetal liver rather than in the bone marrow,[16,19] which may explain why so many haematological disorders in neonates are accompanied by hepatomegaly. A second characteristic of fetal HSC is that they are primed to give rise to a higher proportion of erythroid and megakaryocytic progenitors compared with adult HSC, reflecting the requirement of the fetus for large numbers of red blood cells and the importance of adequate numbers of platelets to maintain vascular integrity.[9,17] Finally, fetal HSC exhibit different sensitivity to and dependence upon haemopoietic growth factors, such as insulin-like growth factors, compared with adult cells[20,21] and a different pattern of mature cell output.[9,16,18] Reflecting this, fetal HSC also have unique gene expression programmes,[13,15–17,22–26] which have recently been shown to be important in the leukaemic transformation events that lead to infant acute lymphoblastic leukaemia (ALL).[27]

Fetal haemopoietic progenitor cells
The different types of haemopoietic progenitor cell present in fetal life are shown in Figs 1.2 and 1.3. The overall scheme of differentiation of HSC is similar in fetal and adult life. However, recent studies have identified fetal-specific lymphoid progenitors, including early lymphoid progenitors (ELP) and PreProB progenitors that may be important not only to rapidly boost B cell production during the second trimester, but also to act as targets of leukaemic transformation in infant and childhood ALL.[9,27–29] ELP are found very early in fetal life (from around 6 weeks post-conception in the fetal liver and from around 11 weeks post-conception in bone marrow) but are very rare in adult haemopoietic tissues.[29] They are defined both by their immunophenotype (CD34$^+$CD127$^+$CD19$^-$CD10$^-$) and their ability to generate B, T and NK cells as well as a small number of myeloid cells.[8,29] PreProB progenitors are one of two types of committed B progenitor cell in fetal life; they lack expression of the CD10 molecule and, like ELP, are very rare in adult bone marrow. By contrast, the second type of B progenitor, the ProB progenitor, is CD10$^+$ and is the main, or sole, type of B progenitor found in adult bone marrow.[29] It is likely that ProB progenitors lie downstream of PreProB in B lymphoid differentiation and, consistent with this, they have been shown to have undergone complete V_H-D_H-J_H rearrangement of their immunoglobulin heavy chain (IgH) loci, in contrast to ELP and PreProB progenitors, which show only

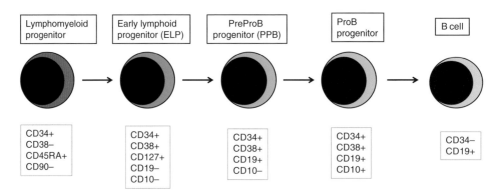

Fig. 1.3 Immunophenotypically defined progenitor populations along the B cell differentiation trajectory in the human fetus. The cell surface markers used to define these populations are shown below each cell type. Based on reference 9.

partial (D_H-J_H) IgH rearrangement.[8] The reasons for the existence of two types of B progenitor and a unique ELP cell in fetal life are unknown but it suggests that there are two pathways of fetal B cell production which may have different physiological roles.

Red blood cell production and development in the fetus and neonate

Normal erythropoiesis, the production of red blood cells, is crucial to early embryonic and fetal development. Most of our knowledge about the cells and genes involved in this process derives either from mouse models or from inherited anaemias, particularly in children. Almost all the characteristic features of red blood cells are different in the fetus and the newborn compared with their adult counterparts. These differences are even greater in preterm neonates and are directly relevant to our understanding of neonatal anaemias. The differences in erythropoiesis during fetal development are summarised in Table 1.1 and those that are important for our understanding of neonatal anaemias are discussed below.

Table 1.1 Features of fetal and neonatal red cells compared with adult red cells

Haemoglobin production	Embryonic haemoglobins (globin chains)
	Gower 1 ($\zeta_2\varepsilon_2$)
	Gower 2 ($\alpha_2\varepsilon_2$)
	Portland ($\zeta_2\gamma_2$)
	Fetal haemoglobin (globin chains)
	Fetal haemoglobin ($\alpha_2\gamma_2$)
	Adult haemoglobins (globin chains)
	Haemoglobin A ($\alpha_2\beta_2$) lower
	Haemoglobin A_2 ($\alpha_2\delta_2$) considerably lower
Red cell membrane	Gives resistance to osmotic lysis
	Altered expression of receptors (e.g. insulin)
	Increased lipid content and altered phospholipid profile
	More prone to oxidative damage
	Altered glucose transport
	Weak expression of A, B and I blood group antigens
	Increased variation in red cell shape (poikilocytosis)
	Red cell 'pocks' due to hyposplenism
Red cell metabolism	Glycolytic pathway
	Increased glucose consumption
	Altered enzyme levels, e.g. low 2,3-DPG and PFK
	Pentose phosphate pathway
	Increased susceptibility to oxidant-induced injury
	Lower level of glutathione peroxidase
	Reduced ability to generate NADPH

2,3-DPG, 2,3-diphosphoglycerate; NADPH, nicotinamide adenine dinucleotide phosphate; PFK, phosphofructokinase.

Erythropoietin production in the fetus and neonate

The principal cytokine responsible for regulating erythropoiesis in the fetus and newborn, as in adults, is erythropoietin (EPO).[30] Since EPO does not cross the placenta, EPO-mediated regulation of fetal erythropoiesis is predominantly under fetal control. The liver is the main site of EPO production in the fetus[31] and the only stimulus to production under physiological conditions is hypoxia with or without anaemia (reviewed in reference 32). Little or no EPO is produced under normoxic conditions, but hypoxia very rapidly triggers expression by up to 200-fold within 30 minutes, at least in hepatocyte cell lines.[33] This explains the high EPO levels in fetuses of mothers with diabetes mellitus or hypertension and in those with intrauterine growth restriction (IUGR) or cyanotic congenital heart disease;[34] EPO is also increased in fetal anaemia of any cause, including haemolytic disease of the fetus and newborn (HDFN). This, and the switch of EPO production from fetal liver to the neonatal kidney, may in part explain the physiological delay in triggering the production of new red blood cells, which is often not evident until the second month of life, even in healthy babies.

Haemoglobin synthesis and red blood cell production in the fetus and newborn

The rates of haemoglobin synthesis and red blood cell production fall dramatically immediately after birth and remain low for the first 2 weeks of life, probably in response to the sudden increase in tissue oxygenation at birth.[35] In healthy neonates the physiological rise in red cell production starts several weeks later, so that by 3 months of age a healthy infant, whatever the period of gestation at birth, should be able to produce up to 2 ml of packed red blood cells every day.[35] Studies in preterm neonates have estimated that over the first 2 months of life the maximal rate of red blood cell production may be closer to 1 ml/day. This is based on the observation that preterm babies receiving therapeutic EPO are unable to maintain their haemoglobin if more than 1 ml of blood per day is venesected for diagnostic purposes but can do so where sampling losses are less than this.[36]

The gestation-related changes in globin chain synthesis in the human embryo, fetus and neonate have been studied in detail and are summarised in Fig. 1.4.[37] The first haemoglobins, known as embryonic haemoglobins, are synthesised from approximately 2 or 3 weeks post-conception, predominantly in the blood islands of the yolk sac, by the erythroblasts and red blood cells generated there. There are three embryonic haemoglobins (see Table 1.1). ζ or α globin, encoded by adjacent genes in the α globin locus on chromosome 16, combine with ϵ or γ globin, encoded by genes in the β globin locus on chromosome 11, to produce haemoglobin Gower 1 ($\zeta_2\epsilon_2$), haemoglobin Gower 2 ($\alpha_2\epsilon_2$) and haemoglobin Portland ($\zeta_2\gamma_2$).

During normal human development, synthesis of embryonic haemoglobins is transient and largely restricted to yolk sac-derived erythroblasts which are larger than those generated once definitive haemopoiesis starts in the AGM and fetal liver (Figs 1.5 and 1.6) and express different transcription factor and epigenetic programmes. From 4 or 5 weeks post-conception, erythroblasts and red blood cells contain mainly haemoglobin F ($\alpha_2\gamma_2$), which remains the principal haemoglobin throughout fetal life. The factors that control the switch

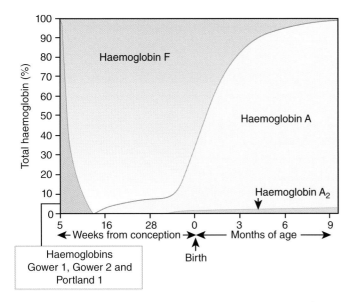

Fig. 1.4 Diagrammatic representation of the sites and rates of synthesis of different haemoglobins in the embryonic and fetal periods and during infancy. From Bain (2020)[37].

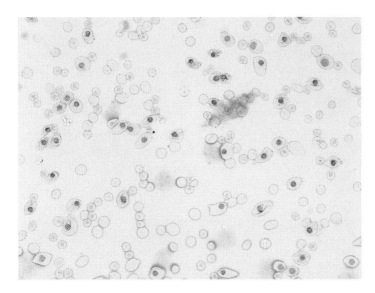

Fig. 1.5 First trimester (8 weeks) fetal blood film showing the large size of the erythroblasts (compare with Fig. 1.6) typical of those derived from the yolk sac. These erythroblasts contain mainly embryonic globins. Note the high proportion of red cells that are nucleated and the absence of white blood cells. May–Grünwald–Giemsa (MGG), ×40 objective.

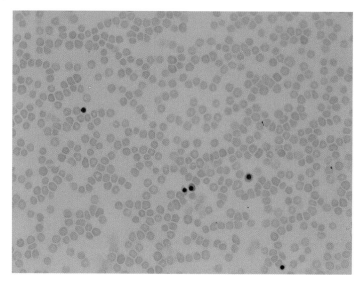

Fig. 1.6 Second trimester (14 weeks) fetal blood film showing typical erythroblasts derived from definitive haematopoiesis. These erythroblasts contain mainly fetal haemoglobin. Note the smaller size of the erythroblasts and the higher proportion of enucleated red cells compared with the first trimester (Fig. 1.5). MGG, ×40.

from primitive to definitive erythropoiesis are not yet clear due to the difficulties in studying this process at such an early stage of development. Understanding more about the mechanisms which normally silence expression of ζ globin would potentially open up new ways of treating α thalassaemia major,[38] an important cause of fetal and early neonatal death (see Chapter 2).

The production of adult haemoglobin (haemoglobin A; $α_2β_2$) begins during the second trimester and remains at low levels until 30–32 weeks post-conception, when haemoglobin A production starts to increase concomitantly with a fall in haemoglobin F production. The net result is an average haemoglobin F in term babies of 70–80% and haemoglobin A of 25–30%.[39,40] After birth, haemoglobin F falls, to approximately 2% by the age of 12 months, with a corresponding increase in haemoglobin A. The molecular control of this change from haemoglobin F to haemoglobin A is termed globin switching. In recent years, there has been considerable research into the genes involved in globin switching (e.g. *BCL11A*) in order to identify strategies to delay or reverse this physiological switch after birth and so maintain haemoglobin F production for children affected by severe β globin disorders such as sickle cell disease or thalassaemia major.[41,42]

The timing of globin switching depends on post-conceptional age rather than postnatal age. In fact, in term babies there is little change in haemoglobin F in the first 15 days after birth, but in preterm babies who are not transfused, haemoglobin F may remain at the same level for the first 6 weeks of life before haemoglobin A production starts to increase. This delay in haemoglobin A production (i.e. the switch from γ globin production to β globin production) can make the diagnosis of β globin disorders in the neonatal period difficult, particularly in preterm infants. This is in contrast to α globin disorders, which are almost invariably evident at birth since α globin chains are essential for the production of all but the very earliest embryonic haemoglobins (see Fig. 1.4 and Table 1.1).

Red blood cell lifespan and the red blood cell membrane in the fetus and neonate

Neonatal red blood cells, particularly in preterm babies, have a shorter lifespan than adult red blood cells. Red cell lifespan is inversely proportional to gestational age at birth. Studies over 50 years ago using isotopically labelled red blood cells estimated red blood cell lifespans for preterm infants at 35–50 days, compared with 60–70 days for term infants and 120 days for healthy adults.[35] More recent estimates, using mathematical modelling and transfusion of autologous cord blood cells, have also calculated the red cell lifespan in preterm neonates to be approximately 50 days.[43]

The reasons for a lower red cell lifespan in neonates, although not fully understood, are thought to include the many biochemical and functional differences in the membrane of neonatal versus adult red blood cells (see Table 1.1). Known differences between neonatal and adult red blood cells include increased resistance to osmotic lysis, increased mechanical fragility, increased total lipid content with an altered lipid profile, increased insulin-binding sites and reduced expression of blood group antigens such as A, B and I.[35] Together these differences translate into the characteristic morphological differences seen in neonatal blood films, particularly in preterm neonates (Figs 1.7–1.9), and are associated with accelerated red cell membrane loss[44] leading to reduced red cell lifespan. Indeed, the distinctive geometry of neonatal red blood cells and the membrane deformability of some of the irregularly shaped cells have been compared to the properties of red blood cells in the inherited red cell membrane disorders.[45]

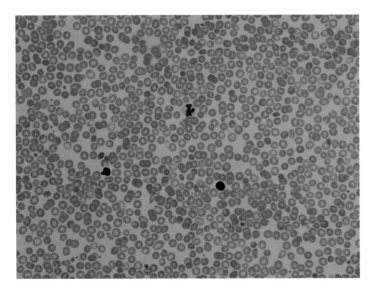

Fig. 1.7 Normal blood film at term. MGG, ×40.

(a)   (b)

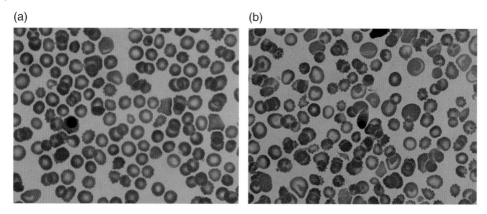

Fig. 1.8 Normal preterm red cells at different gestational ages: (a) baby born at 28 weeks' gestation showing echinocytes, polychromatic macrocytes and one nucleated red blood cell (NRBC); (b) baby born at 25 weeks' gestation showing numerous echinocytes, echinocytic fragments and one NRBC. Note that anisocytosis and poikilocytosis is greater at 25 weeks than at 28 weeks. MGG, ×100.

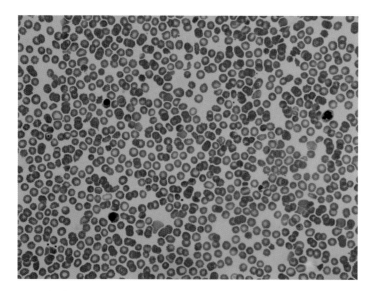

Fig. 1.9 Blood film of a normal preterm baby (born at 28 weeks' gestation) showing a degree of erythroblastosis. MGG, ×40.

Red blood cell metabolism in the fetus and neonate

There are major differences between the metabolism of fetal or neonatal red blood cells and that of adult red blood cells. These differences affect not only the functional properties of the red cells of healthy fetuses and neonates but also the clinical impact of inherited and acquired red cell disorders. Both the glycolytic pathway and the pentose phosphate pathway are affected (see Table 1.1). Overall, glycolysis and glucose consumption are lower in neonatal red blood cells than in adult red blood cells. This occurs despite the increased activity of most glycolytic pathway enzymes, such as glucose-6-phosphate dehydrogenase (G6PD), pyruvate kinase and lactate dehydrogenase (LDH), and is thought to be the result of reduced phosphofructokinase activity. Neonatal red cells also have less ability to generate the reduced form of nicotinamide adenine dinucleotide phosphate (NADPH) via the pentose phosphate pathway and have lower levels of glutathione peroxidase than adult red blood cells. The net result is that neonatal red blood cells are more susceptible than adult cells to oxidant-induced injury.[46]

In addition, neonatal red blood cells have a lower level of methaemoglobin reductase (about 60% of that in adult red blood cells). Methaemoglobin levels are therefore slightly higher in neonates than in adults (mean 4.3 g/l in preterm neonates, 2.2 g/l in term neonates and 1.1 g/l in adults).[35] Neonates are also more likely to develop methaemoglobinaemia because they are susceptible to the toxic effects of chemicals, such as nitric oxide and local anaesthetics, that oxidise haemoglobin-derived iron more rapidly than the maximal possible rate of methaemoglobin reduction (see Chapter 2, Case 2.7).

Iron metabolism in the fetus and neonate

Although stores of iron are adequate at birth in term babies born to well-nourished mothers, this is not always the case in preterm neonates. This is because the majority of fetal total body iron is stored during the third trimester. Estimates have shown that total body iron increases from 35–40 mg at 24 weeks' gestation to 225 mg at term, with the result that preterm neonates, especially those with IUGR, are born with lower iron stores than term neonates.[47,48] These amounts of iron are equivalent to 6 months iron store for a term neonate[49] but only around 2 months for extremely preterm neonates unless they are given supplementary iron. In addition, preterm neonates have an increased requirement for iron both because of their rapid growth rate and because of frequent phlebotomy.[50,51] Therefore, preterm neonates generally develop iron deficiency after 2–4 months if the recommended daily intakes are not maintained.[52] Administration of iron supplements to preterm babies leads to a slightly higher haemoglobin concentration (Hb) and improved iron stores, thereby reducing the risk of subsequent iron deficiency anaemia.[53] The recommended iron intake of preterm infants with a birthweight of 1500–2000 g is 2 mg/kg/ day from 2 to 4 weeks of life using iron-containing human milk fortifier or preterm formula milk and/or iron supplements until at least 6 months of age.[54] For very low birthweight neonates, a higher daily iron intake (2–3 mg/kg/day) is usually recommended, starting at 2 weeks of age.[54]

The regulation of iron status in the neonate, even in those who are born extremely preterm, has recently been shown to depend on the action of hepcidin, erythroferrone (ERFE), ferroportin and EPO, as in adults.[55,56] Thus, hepcidin falls when iron deficiency develops, facilitating increased iron absorption, while hepcidin is upregulated when iron stores are sufficient, triggering degradation of the iron exporter ferroportin, which results in inhibition of iron absorption and mobilisation.[57] Like serum ferritin, hepcidin levels increase with gestational age and in parallel with the increasing iron stores.[58] Hepcidin and prohepcidin levels in term and preterm infants vary in response to inflammation, infection and red blood cell transfusion.[59–61] ERFE, an erythroid hormone, acts as a direct suppressor of hepcidin expression in the liver in response to EPO. Little is known about the role of

ERFE in regulating iron metabolism in neonates but some preliminary data suggest that although the components of the EPO–ERFE–hepcidin–ferroportin axis are present in neonates,[55] ERFE-mediated suppression of hepcidin is impaired, at least in preterm neonates.[62]

Normal values for red blood cell parameters in the fetus and neonate

Haemoglobin concentration and red blood cell indices

Typical normal values for red cell variables in the fetus and neonate are shown in Tables 1.2 and 1.3.[63–68] At birth, the Hb in term infants is high (140–215 g/l), which compensates for the low oxygen concentration in the fetus. The range of normal values for Hb and haematocrit have been updated to reflect the changes in neonatal medicine, including the lower limit of gestation of neonates admitted for neonatal intensive care. Jopling *et al.* published the results of a retrospective study of archived laboratory measurements of Hb and haematocrit from approximately 25 000 neonates analysed on the same equipment in a single group of hospitals between 2002 and 2008.[69] They found an approximately linear increase in both Hb and haematocrit between 22 weeks' and 40 weeks' gestation calculated from

Table 1.2 Impact of gestational age at birth on the principal blood count parameters in healthy neonates*

Gestation at birth	Term (≥37 weeks)	30–36 weeks	26–29 weeks	<26 weeks
Erythropoiesis				
Hb (g/l)	140–215	130–215	115–200	115–185
Hct (l/l)	0.43–0.65	0.40–0.42	0.30–0.58	0.30–0.57
MCV (fl)	98–115	100–117	103–130	104–133
MCH (pg)	32.5–39	33.5–40.5	33.5–43	34.5–44.5
NRBC				
/100 WBC	≤5	≤25	≤25	≤25
×10⁹/l	<1.0	1.0–2.0	2.0–3.0	2.0–3.0
Leucocytes ($\times 10^9$/l)				
Neutrophils				
0–72 hours	3.0–28.0	1.0–25.0	1.0–25.0	1.0–25.0
72–240 hours	2.7–13.0	1.0–12.5	1.3–15.3	1.3–15.3
Monocytes	0.45–3.3	0.20–2.50	0.2–2.20	0.2–2.50
Eosinophils	0.12–1.20	0.06–1.10	0.03–0.90	0.01–0.80
Lymphocytes	3.0–11.0	3.0–11.0	2.5–11.0	3.0–12.0
Blast cells (%)	<5	<8	<8	<8
Platelet count ($\times 10^9$/l)	140–450	140–450	140–450	140–450

* Values for Hb, Hct, MCV and MCH are based on reference ranges in Christensen *et al.*[63] Values for leucocytes and NRBCs are based on reference ranges in references 64–67 and our own hospital laboratory data (unpublished); values for peripheral blood blast cells and platelets are based on Roberts *et al.*[68] Hb, haemoglobin concentration; Hct, haematocrit; MCH, mean cell haemoglobin; MCV, mean cell volume, NRBC, nucleated red blood cell.

Table 1.3 Impact of postnatal age on Hb and Hct values in healthy term and preterm neonates*

	Postnatal age		
	Birth	**2 weeks**	**4 weeks**
Gestation at birth 35–42 weeks			
Hb (g/l)	140–215	110–180	100–170
Hct (l/l)	0.43–0.65	0.32–0.55	0.27–0.48
Gestation at birth 29–34 weeks			
Hb (g/l)	130–215	100–170	80–135
Hct (l/l)	0.40–0.42	0.30–0.48	0.24–0.42

* Values are based on reference ranges in Christensen *et al.* 2009.[63]
Hb, haemoglobin concentration; Hct, haematocrit;

samples collected within 6 hours of birth. In contrast to adults, no differences in Hb or haematocrit were seen between male and female neonates.

In the absence of red cell transfusion, the Hb and haematocrit fall over the first few weeks of life due to the physiological reduction in red blood cell production. In term babies, the average Hb falls from 180 g/l at birth to 140 g/l at the age of 4 weeks,[69] reaching a nadir of around 100 g/l at 2 months of age. Studies of healthy preterm infants carried out almost 50 years ago reported a more rapid fall in Hb than in term babies, reaching a mean of 65–90 g/l at 4–8 weeks postnatal age (reviewed in reference 35). However, these differences are difficult to interpret because of the variable clinical course of preterm infants and the effects of red cell transfusion, particularly in neonates of less than 26 weeks' gestation at birth. More recently, data from non-transfused neonates have confirmed the lower Hb nadir in preterm neonates, with a mean Hb 28 days after birth of approximately 105 g/l in neonates with a gestational age at birth of 29–36 weeks and 130 g/l for term neonates.[69]

The mean cell volume (MCV) of red blood cells in healthy neonates at birth is higher than that in older children and adults and is inversely proportional to gestational age (Table 1.2).[63,68] The average MCV of a term neonate is about 105 fl, while extremely preterm neonates with a gestational age of less than 26 weeks typically have an MCV averaging about 120 fl.[63] Similarly, the mean cell haemoglobin (MCH) at birth is higher in preterm neonates than in term neonates, averaging 40 pg in a preterm neonate of less than 26 weeks' gestation and about 36 pg in a term neonate.[63] The MCV, but not MCH, has been reported to be significantly lower in black preterm compared with white preterm neonates, although this may reflect a higher prevalence of α thalassaemia trait in these neonates as this was not specifically investigated.[70] In contrast to the MCV and MCH, the mean cell haemoglobin concentration (MCHC) does not change significantly during gestation[70] and, unlike in older children, changes in MCHC are not very useful for diagnostic purposes in neonates. In term babies, the MCV and MCH fall slowly over the first few weeks of life, with a lower limit of normal of 77 fl and 26 pg, respectively.[63] The same pattern is seen in preterm neonates although the high frequency of red cell transfusions means that reliable data are not available.

Two newly available automated red cell parameters generated as part of a full blood count, MicroR and HYPO-He, have recently been evaluated in neonates.[71] In adult red blood cells, MicroR provides an automated measure of the percentage of red blood cells with an MCV of <60 fl and HYPO-He measures the percentage of red blood cells with an MCH of <17 pg. Bahr and colleagues created new reference ranges for neonates based on analysis of more than 11 000 blood counts and used them to show that a combination of MicroR and HYPO-He was more sensitive than MCV/MCH in identifying iron deficiency at birth.[71] Further validation of these results in prospective studies and assessment of the impact of gestational age will be needed to determine the value of these new parameters in the diagnosis of neonatal iron deficiency and anaemia.

Reticulocytes and circulating nucleated red blood cells

The reticulocyte count falls rapidly after birth as erythropoiesis declines. In term babies it then starts to increase at 7–8 weeks of age, reaching 35–200×10^9/l (1–1.8%) at 2 months of age; in preterm babies it increases at 6–8 weeks of age.[35] Neonatal reticulocytes, like mature neonatal red blood cells, have a larger volume and lower Hb than adult reticulocytes.[35] Manual reticulocyte counts have now largely been replaced by automated reticulocyte counts based on cell size and ribonucleic acid (RNA) content. Automated reticulocyte counts also provide a measure of the fraction of reticulocytes with the highest RNA content (Immature Reticulocyte Fraction [IRF]), which has been used in neonates to determine whether or not there is increased erythropoietic activity, for example in response to EPO treatment or as a diagnostic aid to haemolysis.[72–74]

Normal ranges for the numbers of circulating nucleated red blood cells (NRBC) in neonates have been compiled by Christensen *et al.*[66] and are generally higher in preterm neonates (2–3×10^9/l) than in term neonates (about 1×10^9/l) (see Table 1.2). Although modern analysers are increasingly able to generate accurate absolute NRBC counts, a useful guide from examination of blood films is that the presence of up to 5 NRBC/100 white blood cells in a term baby and up to 25 NRBC/100 white blood cells in a preterm baby can be considered normal for the first 1–2 days of life. In fact, there seems to be no difference between results obtained when the manual and automated methods are compared.[75] The number of NRBC in the peripheral blood falls rapidly over the first week of life and these cells are no longer seen after the second week of life. By contrast, circulating erythroblasts are increased in a variety of conditions in neonates and their presence can therefore be useful diagnostically because they usually indicate increased erythropoiesis driven either by anaemia or by chronic intrauterine hypoxia, for example due to IUGR (Table 1.4 and Fig. 1.10). It should be noted that NRBC also appear in the peripheral blood as part of a leucoerythroblastic picture, most typically in response to acute perinatal hypoxia (Fig. 1.11).[76,77]

Red blood cell morphology

Even in freshly taken samples, the morphology of neonatal red blood cells is distinctly different to that of adult cells.[35,78] The most typical morphological feature that differs from what is observed at other times of life is the presence of echinocytes (see Fig. 1.8). In healthy neonates, the proportion of echinocytes in blood films made from samples collected during the first week of life is inversely proportional to gestational age at birth.

Table 1.4 Causes of increased numbers of circulating nucleated red blood cells (erythroblasts) in term and preterm neonates

Response to anaemia: haemolytic disorders

Haemolytic disease of the newborn (especially due to anti-D and anti-c)

α thalassaemia major (occasionally, haemoglobin H disease)

Severe congenital dyserythropoietic anaemia (e.g. due to *KLF1* mutations)

Rare severe red cell enzyme deficiencies (e.g. pyruvate kinase deficiency or glucose phosphate isomerase deficiency)

Rare severe red cell membranopathies (e.g. hereditary stomatocytosis or autosomal recessive hereditary spherocytosis)

Response to anaemia: blood loss (mainly acute)

Fetomaternal haemorrhage

Placental abruption

Large cephalohaematoma

Haemorrhage into major organs, e.g. liver

Twin-to-twin transfusion (donor twin)

Response to hypoxia

Chronic *in utero* hypoxia:

    Intrauterine growth restriction

    Maternal hypertension

    Maternal diabetes mellitus

    Down syndrome (mechanism unclear)

Acute perinatal hypoxia:

    Hypoxic ischaemic encephalopathy (leucoerythroblastic)

Neoplasms

Transient abnormal myelopoiesis in Down syndrome*

Congenital leukaemia (non-Down syndrome)

Other

Recovery phase of parvovirus B19 infection

* The increase in circulating erythroblasts is even higher in Down syndrome neonates with transient abnormal myelopoiesis than in Down syndrome neonates in general.

(a)   (b)

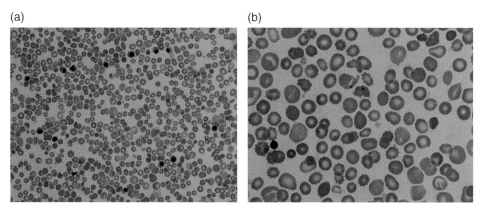

Fig. 1.10 Blood film showing features of hyposplenism resulting from intrauterine growth restriction: (a) low power showing anisocytosis, poikilocytosis, target cells and some fragments (MGG, ×40); (b) high power, two Howell–Jolly bodies are apparent (MGG, ×100).

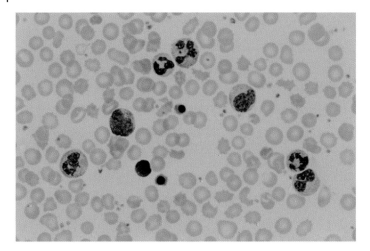

Fig. 1.11 Blood film from a preterm neonate (born at 25 weeks' gestation) on the day of birth showing a leucoerythroblastic picture with NRBC, a myelocyte and promyelocyte as well as toxic granulation of the neutrophils and red cell morphology typical of an extremely preterm neonate. This appearance is typical of perinatal hypoxia. MGG, ×100.

(a)   (b)

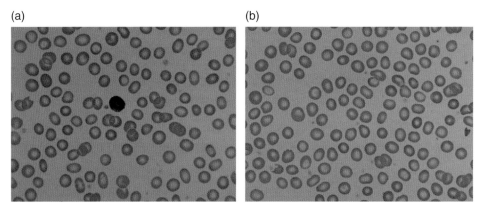

Fig. 1.12 Impact of postnatal age on red cell morphology; blood films from: (a) healthy term baby; (b) neonate at a postnatal age of 4 weeks. MGG, ×100.

Echinocytes gradually disappear from the peripheral blood film over the first few weeks of life so that even very preterm neonates will have few circulating echinocytes by 4 weeks of age (Fig. 1.12). This, together with the universal presence of echinocytes in very preterm neonates, strongly suggests that the changes reflect the unique differences in the cell membrane and metabolism of fetal red blood cells. Indeed, echinocytes are not a useful indicator of red cell pathology in neonates. Instead, other morphological indicators of red cell pathology, such as spherocytes, elliptocytes, target cells and occasionally acanthocytes, are a more reliable diagnostic guide (see Chapter 2).

The presence of a small proportion (typically <5%) of spherocytes and target cells in the first few days of life is normal, particularly in preterm babies, possibly reflecting a degree of functional hyposplenism in the neonate. Consistent with this, these features are more marked in neonates with IUGR, when they are usually accompanied by the presence of Howell–Jolly bodies[34] (see Fig. 1.10). The presence of schistocytes in neonatal blood films may cause confusion. When they are present in large numbers in the first few days of life they may be an indicator of a microangiopathic process, as seen in disseminated intravascular coagulation (DIC), thrombotic thrombocytopenic purpura or Kasabach–Merritt syndrome. On the other hand, the presence of large numbers of schistocytes (10–20%) is very common in well babies for several months after the first few weeks of life (personal observation) and may simply reflect residual damaged fetal erythrocytes yet to be cleared from the circulation (see Fig. 1.12). Care should therefore be taken not to overestimate the significance of schistocytes in well babies with otherwise normal blood counts or mild physiological anaemia.

Blood volume

The normal blood volume at birth varies with gestational age and the timing of clamping of the umbilical cord.[79] In healthy term infants, the average blood volume is 80 ml/kg (range 50–100 ml/kg); however, this can be increased by up to 25% by late clamping of the cord.[79] Estimates of the blood volume in preterm infants show a slightly higher range of 85–106 ml/kg, largely due to an increase in plasma volume.[80–82]

Folic acid and vitamin B$_{12}$

In term and preterm babies of normally nourished mothers, stores of folic acid and vitamin B$_{12}$ are adequate at birth and are maintained after birth in term neonates.[83] However, infants that are breastfed and born to mothers who are vitamin B$_{12}$ deficient, either due to vitamin B$_{12}$ malabsorption or because of a strict vegetarian diet, are at high risk of developing severe vitamin B$_{12}$ deficiency at 4–8 months of life. The prevalence of vitamin B$_{12}$ deficiency at birth varies in different countries from less than 1 in 100 000 in the USA to 1 in 3000–5000 in European countries where neonatal screening studies have been performed.[84–87] Although these infants are asymptomatic in the neonatal period, they develop progressive anaemia and neurological problems over the following months.[88] Although the anaemia is rapidly reversible with intramuscular vitamin B$_{12}$, persistent neurological impairment has been reported,[89] leading some to recommend neonatal screening for presymptomatic identification of vitamin B$_{12}$ deficiency.[90] In preterm infants, folic acid reserves are lower at birth and are depleted more quickly than in term neonates, causing deficiency after 2–4 months if the recommended daily intakes are not maintained. The recommended daily intake for folic acid in preterm neonates is 25–100 µg/kg.[91] As preterm formula milks and breast milk fortifiers provide sufficient folic acid to prevent folate deficiency in preterm infants,[92] further supplementation is not required unless there is chronic haemolysis.

Leucocytes in the fetus and newborn

The leucocytes that form the human blood and immune system in the developing fetus start to appear in the peripheral blood during the first trimester.[93] Monocytes and lymphocytes appear in fetal blood by 8 weeks post-conception, although initially in very low numbers. This is followed by the appearance of neutrophils and eosinophils from around 14–16 weeks post-conception, once haemopoiesis begins to be established in the bone marrow,[9,16] increasing by the end of the third trimester to the lower end of the values reported for leucocyte counts in term neonates. Blast cells are a normal feature in fetal blood, particularly in the second trimester, but are not usually greater than 10%.[94]

Apart from alterations in the numbers of white blood cells in response to infection, leucocyte disorders are not common in neonates. Nevertheless, some diagnostic dilemmas do present in the neonatal period, particularly when there is neutropenia or a rare disorder such as congenital leukaemia is suspected. Careful evaluation of leucocyte morphology can not only help to make an early diagnosis of bacterial infection but can also suggest the type of bacterial infection and provide rapid clues to the presence of congenital viral infection or a rare genetic or metabolic disorder (see Chapter 3). In addition, automated leucocyte differential counts are often inaccurate in neonatal samples, particularly in very preterm neonates, so that validation from a blood film is important.

In contrast to the gestation-related differences in red cell morphology, leucocyte morphology (neutrophils, monocytes, eosinophils, basophils and lymphocytes) is the same in healthy neonates of any gestation as in adults.

Leucocyte production and function in the fetus and neonate

All of the same types of normal leucocyte found in older children can be seen in peripheral blood films of term and preterm neonates (Fig. 1.13), although their frequencies vary from those in older children and also vary both with gestational age and with postnatal age (see Table 1.2). Blast cells are the only cells commonly seen in neonatal blood films that are not usual in blood films from healthy older children or adults (Fig. 1.14).

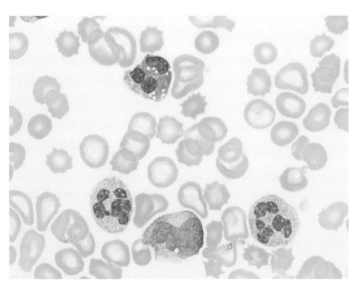

Fig. 1.13 Blood film of a preterm neonate showing normal white cells – two neutrophils, an eosinophil and a monocyte. MGG, ×100.

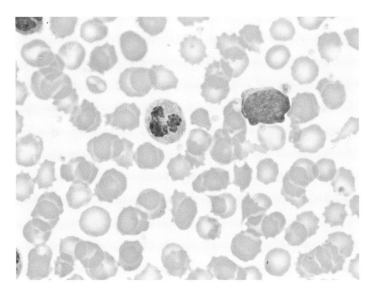

Fig. 1.14   Blood film of a healthy preterm neonate born at 25 weeks' gestation showing a neutrophil and a blast cell. MGG, ×100.

There is increasing recognition that leucocyte function in the fetus and newborn differs from that in adults[95] and that this is almost certain to contribute to the increased susceptibility to infection in neonates, particularly in those that are extremely preterm.[96] As the adaptive immune system only properly develops with antigen exposure after birth, neonates are specifically dependent on the innate immune system as a first line of defence against bacterial and fungal pathogens in particular.[97] Remarkably, all of the cellular components of the innate immune system are established in the human fetus over a small number of weeks late in the first trimester and early second trimester of fetal life.[16]

Neutrophils

At birth, neutrophils are the most plentiful of the circulating leucocytes in healthy neonates, constituting 50–60% of the total circulating white cells, in both term and preterm infants.[64,65,67] The absolute neutrophil count at birth is slightly higher in preterm neonates (averaging about 15×10^9/l) than in term neonates (averaging about 10×10^9/l),[64] and in most preterm neonates (<28 weeks' gestation at birth), the peripheral blood also often contains neutrophil precursors (metamyelocytes, myelocytes and promyelocytes) in small numbers, even when the baby is well (Fig. 1.15).

Neutrophils are produced almost entirely in the bone marrow during fetal life.[16] The numbers of circulating neutrophils in fetal blood samples taken in the first and second trimester are low ($0.1–0.2 \times 10^9$/l),[94] most likely because so much of the bone marrow at this gestation is devoted to expanding B cell production.[8] Thereafter, as granulopoiesis is established in the fetal bone marrow, the numbers of neutrophils gradually rise to reach over 2×10^9/l at the end of the third trimester. Nevertheless, the absolute neutrophil mass per kilogram is less than 25% of adult values in term neonates and slightly lower (20% of adult values) in preterm neonates.[95] This means that reserves of mature neutrophils in the

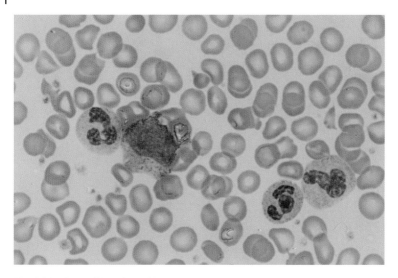

Fig. 1.15 Blood film of a well preterm neonate showing a myelocyte and three normal neutrophils. MGG, ×100.

bone marrow (sometimes referred to as the neutrophil storage pool) are rapidly depleted in neonates. This explains the frequent occurrence of severe neutropenia in preterm neonates as an immediate response to acute bacterial infection or necrotising enterocolitis (NEC) (Fig. 1.16) (see Chapter 3).[98–100] In contrast, adults have large reserves of neutrophils and neutrophil progenitors in the bone marrow, which can be rapidly recruited to boost neutrophil numbers in response to sepsis.

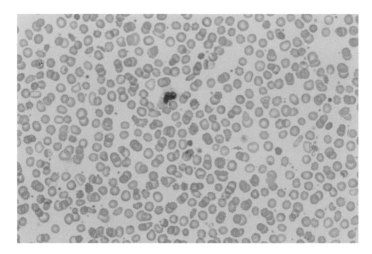

Fig. 1.16 Blood film of a preterm neonate with early clinical signs of necrotising enterocolitis showing severe neutropenia and moderate thrombocytopenia. Note the cytoplasmic vacuolation in the single neutrophil and the presence of large platelets and some schistocytes suggestive of disseminated intravascular coagulation (DIC). MGG, ×40.

Normal ranges for neutrophil counts in neonates were updated by Schmutz *et al.* in 2008.[64] These vary by gestational age at birth (see Table 1.2) and also by postnatal age, particularly over the first 24 hours. In healthy term babies the neutrophil count peaks at around $15.0 \times 10^9/l$ (range $7.5–28.5 \times 10^9/l$) 6–12 hours after birth, with a very similar pattern also seen in healthy preterm babies over 28 weeks' gestation.[64] Normal ranges for very low birthweight neonates less than 28 weeks' gestation are difficult to establish because of the high frequency of medical problems, including infection, in these babies. In practice, the main clinical value of neutrophil normal ranges is to identify neonates with clinically significant neutropenia, especially those with severe congenital neutropenia (SCN), where prompt diagnosis is essential to prevent life-threatening complications. In SCN, the neutrophil count will nearly always be persistently low, although transient and moderate rises sometimes occur in the setting of infection. As a result, serial neutrophil measurements, as well as assessment of a blood film, are essential to rule out acquired disorders associated with neutropenia persisting for more than a week, for example cytomegalovirus (CMV) infection.

Monocytes

There are few monocytes in early second-trimester fetal blood ($<0.06 \times 10^9/l$) but the numbers slowly increase to reach $0.1 \times 10^9/l$ towards the end of the second trimester.[101] Normal ranges for monocyte counts at birth in term and preterm babies are shown in Table 1.2. These show a gradual rise from a mean of $0.75 \times 10^9/l$ in preterm neonates less than 28 weeks' gestation at birth to $1.5 \times 10^9/l$ in term babies.[65] Monocytes play a key role in the innate immune response of neonates to pathogens. Investigations have shown that although the ability of neonatal monocytes to phagocytose microorganisms is not impaired, other aspects of monocyte function in neonates are impaired compared with adult monocytes.[102,103] For example, neonatal monocytes have reduced expression of a number of functionally important cell surface molecules compared with adult monocytes, including HLA-DR, CD80 and L-selectin, which leads to a reduced ability to present antigens efficiently and to migrate to sites of inflammation.[104] In addition, many studies have reported differences in the pattern of pro- and anti-inflammatory cytokine production in neonatal monocytes, which may impair the antimicrobial activity not only of the monocytes themselves, but also of neutrophils,[105–108] although their ability to respond appropriately to bacille Calmette–Guérin (BCG) vaccine appears to be preserved.[109]

Eosinophils

Eosinophils are barely detectable in fetal blood until the middle of the second trimester.[101] Recent data indicate that there is no eosinophil production in fetal liver[9] and that circulating eosinophils are likely to be derived entirely from the bone marrow. The numbers of eosinophils in neonates gradually increase with gestational age from a mean of $0.02 \times 10^9/l$ in preterm infants less than 28 weeks' gestation to $0.06 \times 10^9/l$ in term neonates.[65] Normal ranges for neonatal eosinophil counts are shown in Table 1.2.

Lymphocytes

There are few studies of lymphopoiesis in the human fetus. Although B lymphocytes are found in low numbers in fetal liver and fetal blood by 8 weeks' gestation[110] and gradually increase in number during the second trimester,[111] the bone marrow is the main site of B lymphopoiesis in fetal life.[8] By the second trimester, both fetal liver and fetal bone marrow B cells are polyclonal with equally diversified IgH chain repertoires, although at this stage the main source of IgM natural immunity seems to reside in the fetal liver as the majority of bone marrow B cells are still immature.[112] Two types of fetal B cell have been described in mice (B1 and B2 cells), with B1 cells being specific to fetal life and hypothesised to mainly play a role in innate immunity as they have limited Ig production capacity.[113] Putative B1 B cells have also been described in human fetal liver and bone marrow and in cord blood,[114] but their developmental origin and function are still to be defined.

T cell progenitors are first detected in the thymus at 9 weeks post-conception and mature T cells by 12–13 weeks post-conception followed by T cells appearing in the spleen and lymph nodes by 24 weeks.[115] Regulatory T cells, which are critical for promoting self-tolerance in fetal life, are detected in the thymus at 12 weeks post-conception.[116,117] T lymphocytes are detectable in fetal blood, marrow and thymus during the second trimester[118] and T cell development is largely complete by birth.[119] By term, T lymphocytes form 40–45% of circulating mononuclear cells, with a CD4:CD8 ratio of around 5:1, slightly higher than that in adult blood (3.1:1). The normal ranges for the total lymphocyte count in neonatal blood are the same in term and preterm neonates (see Table 1.2) and remain stable over the first month of life in healthy neonates.[67]

Blast cells

Blast cells, usually resembling myeloblasts, are a normal feature on neonatal blood films (see Fig. 1.14). Their numbers are increased in preterm compared with term babies and in babies with severe infection. A study that evaluated blood films in 123 healthy neonates found an upper limit of 4% for the frequency of circulating blasts in neonatal blood, whereas for sick babies up to 8% blasts were occasionally seen.[68] The causes of increased blast cells in neonates are discussed in Chapter 3 (see Table 3.6).

Leucocyte function in the fetus and neonate

The clinical importance of the immaturity of the innate immune system in neonates is best demonstrated by the fact that the pattern of infections in neonates closely mimics that seen in children with SCN. While neutrophil numbers at birth are similar to those in older children and adults, the lack of neutrophil reserves discussed above is aggravated by the impaired function of neonatal neutrophils.[95] First, recruitment and migration of neonatal neutrophils to sites of infection is impaired compared with adult neutrophils. The processes involved are complex and several aspects are defective in neonatal neutrophils, including chemotaxis, adhesion, rolling and transmigration, which together result in an impaired ability to leave the circulation and enter the tissues.[120–122] Secondly, neonatal neutrophils have an overall reduced ability to generate neutrophil extracellular traps (NETs), which are an important component of the innate immune response that limits the dissemination of a variety of pathogens.[123–125] NETs are extracellular, web-like structures composed of a variety of antimicrobial molecules, such as elastase, myeloperoxidase, lactoferrin and defensins, and are key for protection against infection in neonates, trapping, neutralising and killing bacteria, fungi, viruses and parasites.[126] Thirdly, neonatal neutrophils have lower levels of various antimicrobial granule proteins, such as lactoferrin and bactericidal/

permeability-increasing protein (BPI), particularly in preterm neonates.[95] Recent data suggest that lactoferrin may be particularly important for converting neonatal neutrophils and monocytes to myeloid-derived suppressor cells (MDSC), which are now recognised as being critical in controlling diseases associated with deregulated inflammation in neonates, including NEC.[127,128] Finally, although term neonates are able to phagocytose both Gram-positive and Gram-negative bacteria normally, in preterm neonates phagocytosis of bacteria and of *Candida albicans* is less efficient.[102,129]

Platelets and megakaryocytes in the fetus and neonate

Platelets appear in the circulation at 5–6 weeks' gestation and reach values of $150 \times 10^9/l$ by the end of the first trimester[110,118] and 175–$250 \times 10^9/l$ during the second and third trimesters.[93,130,131] Although some studies have suggested that there is a linear increase in the platelet count with increasing gestational age, a large study of more than 5000 fetal blood samples showed that there was no further significant increase in fetal platelet count through the second and third trimesters.[131] Thus, a platelet count of less than $150 \times 10^9/l$ can be considered abnormal, even in the most preterm neonate.

Developmental megakaryopoiesis and thrombopoiesis

As for most of the other types of blood cell, there are many differences between neonates and adults in the processes that regulate megakaryocyte production (megakaryopoiesis) and platelet production (thrombopoiesis).[132,133] These differences are particularly marked in preterm neonates and likely to contribute to the frequent occurrence of thrombocytopenia in sick neonates; they are important to consider in the investigation and treatment of neonatal thrombocytopenia (see Chapter 4).

   The principal cytokine regulating platelet production in the fetus and newborn, as in adults, is thrombopoietin (TPO).[34] Circulating levels of TPO, which is produced in the liver from early in fetal life,[134,135] are higher in healthy term and preterm neonates than in adults.[136,137] This does not seem to be a compensatory mechanism since TPO-induced signalling is upregulated in cord blood megakaryocytes compared with adult megakaryocytes.[133] Fetal megakaryocytes are also smaller and of lower ploidy than their adult counterparts, which may be the reason that they not infrequently circulate in the peripheral blood in preterm neonates (Fig. 1.17) and that cord blood-derived megakaryocytes produce approximately 50% fewer platelets per cell[138] (reviewed in references 139 and 140). Furthermore, unlike adults, thrombocytopenic neonates can only increase their megakaryocyte number, and not size, in response to consumptive thrombocytopenia.[141] Nevertheless, fetal megakaryocytes appear to be cytoplasmically mature and express increased amounts of messenger RNA for the transcription factor GATA1 and increased surface glycoprotein 1b compared with adult megakaryocytes.[133] These functional differences in fetal and neonatal megakaryocytes are now known to be accompanied by increased expression of genes associated with a number of signalling pathways, including those mediated by transforming growth factor β (TGFβ), insulin-like growth factor (IGF) and Janus kinase 2 (JAK2), in fetal compared with adult megakaryocytes.[142]

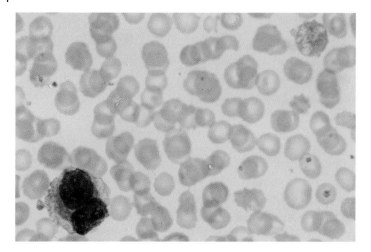

Fig. 1.17 Blood film of a preterm neonate born at 24 weeks' gestation showing a circulating megakaryocyte and giant platelet. MGG, ×100.

There are also developmental differences in megakaryocyte progenitor cells. The numbers of these cells are high early in fetal life and fall towards term and are higher in healthy preterm than term babies.[132,143,144] Additionally, fetal megakaryocyte progenitors have more proliferative potential *in vitro* than those derived from adults, perhaps related to stronger activation of the JAK2 and mTOR pathways in response to TPO stimulation as found in cord blood megakaryocytes.[133] These properties may explain how fetal and neonatal platelet counts are maintained at levels similar to those of adults, at least in the healthy fetus and neonate. The observation of increased numbers of reticulated (young) platelets in fetal compared with adult peripheral blood is consistent with this hypothesis.[145]

Platelet numbers in the neonate and fetus – normal values

Since platelet counts in fetal blood reach normal adult values by the end of the second trimester, it is reasonable to consider that platelet counts of less than 150×10^9/l represent thrombocytopenia in a healthy neonate regardless of gestation at birth. This conclusion has been challenged by a large retrospective analysis of 47 000 neonates, in which a reference range of platelet counts at different gestational ages was determined by excluding the highest and lowest 5th percentile of all observed counts. By this method, the lowest limit of platelet counts was found to be 104×10^9/l for infants of less than 32 weeks' gestation, compared with 123×10^9/l for neonates of greater than 32 weeks' gestation.[146] However, as the study included all neonates, regardless of clinical status, these counts may simply reflect the high frequency of thrombocytopenia in neonatal units, where sepsis and placental insufficiency are common causes for admission, rather than representing a new physiological definition of normal platelet counts in the newborn. Indeed, the mean platelet count was above 200×10^9/l regardless of gestation at birth, consistent with accepted normal ranges for the platelet count in neonates.[143]

Several studies have investigated the clinical relevance of newer automated platelet parameters in neonatal medicine, particularly the immature platelet fraction (IPF). Overall, these studies support the conclusion that in neonates, as in adults, the IPF% provides a measure of the proportion of immature platelets and a surrogate measure of platelet production although the results are variable.[147] MacQueen and colleagues established reference ranges for the IPF% in their hospitals based on more than 20 000 automated results from nearly 9000 neonates.[148] They reported a higher IPF% in the most premature infants (less than 32 weeks' gestation). Consistent with this, they also found that IPF% values were higher in neonates who developed consumptive thrombocytopenia compared with those were considered to have reduced platelet production, suggesting that further clinical studies of the value of the IPF% in neonates might be useful, given the practical difficulties of bone marrow aspiration in the newborn.

Neonatal platelet function

Studies of neonatal platelet function *in vitro* have consistently shown hyporeactivity of neonatal compared with adult platelets to a wide range of platelet agonists, including adenosine diphosphate (ADP), thrombin and thromboxane and especially so to collagen and adrenaline (epinephrine).[132,149] In keeping with this, the number of α-adrenergic receptors on neonatal platelets has been found to be 50% lower than on adult platelets.[150,151] By contrast, expression of the main platelet adhesion receptors appears to be similar in neonatal and adult platelets, with the exception of glycoprotein (Gp) IIb/IIIa, which is expressed at lower levels in neonatal platelets.[152] Importantly, follow-up studies have shown that previously impaired platelet responses in neonates are similar to adult responses within 2 weeks of birth.[152,153] Another point of note is that most studies of neonatal platelet function have been carried out on cord blood platelet-rich plasma. However, more recent studies on whole blood have shown that healthy neonates have robust primary haemostasis overall, despite apparently hypofunctional platelets as assessed using standard techniques in platelet-rich plasma. This may, at least in part, be due to the higher haematocrit and higher levels of von Willebrand factor in neonates. In addition, measures of *in vitro* platelet activation and aggregation in cord blood do not match those obtained when studying peripheral blood.[154] These observations have led some investigators to conclude that the function of neonatal platelets should not be viewed as impaired but, instead, that neonatal platelets function as a component of a generally well-balanced neonatal haemostatic system.[149]

Practical problems in interpreting neonatal blood counts and films

Sample quality/artefacts

One of the commonest practical difficulties in interpreting neonatal blood counts and blood films occurs because of the much higher haematocrit in neonates. First, there is a higher frequency of clotted samples, which most likely reflects the challenge of collecting free-flowing blood samples from neonates, especially those who are very low birthweight and/or preterm. Secondly, the high haematocrit often leads to poor-quality 'thick' or

(a)   (b)

(c)

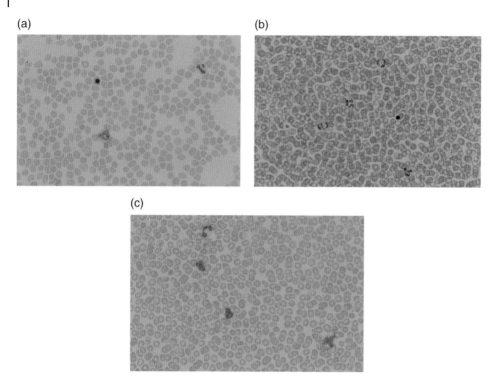

Fig. 1.18   Blood film of a healthy term neonate with a normal blood count and no evidence of haemolysis, showing artefactual changes in red cell morphology apparent on different sections of the blood film. (a) Thin end of the blood film showing apparent 'spherocytes' that are not present on the well-spread section of the film (compare with Fig. 1.18c). A normal neutrophil, monocyte and NRBC can also be seen. (b) Thick end of the same blood film showing overlapping red cells, which make it difficult to interpret the red cell morphology, and apparent target cells and hypochromia that are not present on the well-spread section of the film (compare with Fig. 1.18c). Normal neutrophils and an NRBC are also shown. (c) Good section of the blood film showing normal red cell morphology. Normal white blood cells are also shown. MGG, ×40.

unevenly spread films, which may give the misleading impression of the presence of abnormal red cells, such as spherocytes or target cells, which are not seen when the correctly spread section of the film is reviewed (Fig. 1.18). These effects can often be mitigated by dilution of the sample prior to analysis and preparation of the blood film. Another practical problem is the difficulty of distinguishing the typical changes seen on aged blood samples anticoagulated with ethylene diaminetetra-acetic acid (EDTA) from the normal red cell features typical of preterm babies. It is therefore particularly important to make blood films on neonatal samples as soon as possible.

Site of sampling

The site of sampling also influences blood count analyses in neonates. For example, in the first few hours of life the Hb of venous samples is lower than that of heel-prick samples collected simultaneously,[155] sometimes by up to 20–40 g/l.[35] This difference is greater in preterm neonates and falls with increasing postnatal age, such that by the fifth day of life there is almost no difference in Hb between a well-taken heel-prick sample and a venous sample.[155] Similarly, the haematocrit and red blood cell count at birth are lower in venous blood compared with capillary blood samples collected simultaneously, while there is no difference in the other red cell indices by site of sampling.[155] Neonatal heel-prick samples have also been shown to have white cell, neutrophil and lymphocyte counts about 20% higher than arterial or venous samples; counts are most likely to approximate to those of venous blood if there is a free flow of blood and if early drops, excluding the first, are used for the count.[35] In contrast, the platelet count and mean platelet volume (MPV) are lower in capillary samples than in venous samples.[155,156]

Gestational age and postnatal age

Although the Hb, haematocrit and MCV vary little over the first week of life, there is a gradual loss of other distinctive neonatal red cell features after the first week of life. In particular, the numbers of circulating nucleated red cells fall, as mentioned above, and echinocytes are gradually replaced by red cells with the more typical appearance of adult red cells. Consideration of the postnatal age of a baby is most important when interpreting blood films to help in the identification of infection or the cause of anaemia. For example, maternal chorioamnionitis may cause extremely high neutrophil counts, often with associated toxic granulation, in the newborn infant despite the absence of active infection in the neonate (Fig. 1.19). It seems likely that this is due to maternal cytokines crossing the placenta, although this has not been specifically demonstrated. Importantly, virtually identical changes observed on neonatal blood films after the first week of life are highly likely to reflect active infection in the neonate as any maternal cytokine-driven changes will have resolved by this time.

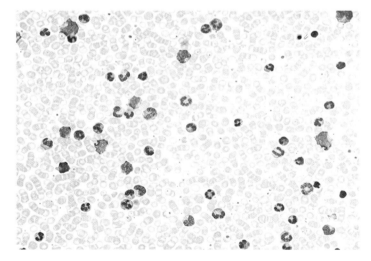

Fig. 1.19 Blood film in maternal chorioamnionitis showing neutrophilia, left shift (myelocytes and promyelocytes) and toxic granulation. MGG, ×40.

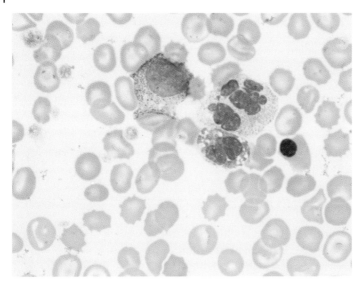

Fig. 1.20 Leucoerythroblastic blood film in a preterm neonate with hypoxic ischaemic encephalopathy showing a myelocyte, an NRBC, an eosinophil and a macropolycyte, likely to be a tetraploid cell. MGG, ×100.

Pregnancy-associated complications and mode of delivery

In addition to being influenced by maternal chorioamnionitis, the white cell count (WBC) at birth is also affected by the mode of delivery, being lower after an elective caesarean section than after either vaginal delivery or caesarean section performed after labour has commenced.[64] Hypoxic ischaemic encephalopathy (HIE) following perinatal hypoxia (e.g. due to the cord being round the neck of the baby) also causes an increased WBC; in this case the blood film is leucoerythroblastic and the neutrophils show varying degrees of toxic granulation, often making it difficult to identify the presence of coexisting infection based on the haematological findings alone (Fig. 1.20).

References

1 Huyhn A, Dommergues M, Izac B, Croisille L, Katz W, Vainchenker W and Coulombel L (1995) Characterization of hematopoietic progenitors from human yolk sacs and embryos. *Blood*, **86**, 4474–4485.

2 Tavian M, Cortes F, Charbord P, Labastie M-C and Péault B (1999) Emergence of the haematopoietic system in the human embryo and foetus. *Haematologica*, **84** (Suppl EHA-4), 1–3.

3 Palis J (2016) Hematopoietic stem cell-independent hematopoiesis: emergence of erythroid, megakaryocytic, and myeloid potential in the mammalian embryo. *FEBS Lett*, **590**, 3965–3974.

4 de Bruijn MF, Speck NA, Peeters MC and Dzierzak E (2000) Definitive hematopoietic stem cells first develop within the major arterial regions of the mouse embryo. *EMBO J*, **19**, 2465–2474.

5 Ivanovs A, Rybtsov S, Welch L, Anderson RA, Turner ML and Medvinsky A (2011) Highly potent human hematopoietic stem cells first emerge in the intraembryonic aorta-gonad-mesonephros region. *J Exp Med*, **208**, 2417–2427.

6 Ivanovs A, Rybtsov S, Anderson RA, Turner ML and Medvinsky A (2014) Identification of the niche and phenotype of the first human hematopoietic stem cells. *Stem Cell Reports*, **2**, 449–456.

7 Marshall CJ and Thrasher AJ (2001) The embryonic origins of human haematopoiesis. *Br J Haematol*, **112**, 838–850.

8 O'Byrne S, Elliott N, Rice S, Buck G, Fordham N, Crump NT *et al.* (2019) Discovery of a CD10 negative B-progenitor in human fetal life identifies unique ontogeny-related developmental programs. *Blood*, **134**, 1059–1071.

9 Popescu D-M, Botting RA, Stephenson E, Green K, Jardine L, Acres M *et al.* (2019) Decoding the development of the blood and immune systems during human fetal liver haematopoiesis. *Nature*, **574**, 365–371.

10 Migliaccio, AG., Migliaccio AR, Petti S, Mavilio F, Russo G, Lazzaro D *et al.* (1986) Human embryonic hemopoiesis. Kinetics of progenitors and precursors underlying the yolk sac–liver transition. *J Clin Invest*, **78**, 51–60.

11 Tavian M, Hallais MF and Peault B (1999) Emergence of intraembryonic hematopoietic precursors in the pre-liver human embryo. *Development*, **126**, 793–803.

12 Charbord P, Tavian M, Humeau L and Peault B (1996) Early ontogeny of the human marrow from long bones: an immunohistochemical study of hematopoiesis and its microenvironment. *Blood*, **87**, 4109–4119.

13 Benz C, Copley MR, Kent DG, Wohrer S, Cortes A, Aghaeepour N *et al.* (2012) Hematopoietic stem cell subtypes expand differentially during development and display distinct lymphopoietic programs. *Cell Stem Cell*, **10**, 273–283.

14 Yuan J, Nguyen CK, Liu X, Kanellopoulou C and Muljo SA (2012) Lin28b reprograms adult bone marrow hematopoietic progenitors to mediate fetal-like lymphopoiesis. *Science*, **335**, 1195–1200.

15 Copley MR, Babovic S, Benz C, Knapp DJHF, Beer PA, Kent DG *et al.* (2013) The Lin28b-let-7-Hmga2 axis determines the higher self-renewal potential of fetal haematopoietic stem cells. *Nat Cell Biol*, **15**, 916–925.

16 Jardine L, Webb S, Goh I, Quiroga Londoño M, Reynolds G, Mather M *et al.* (2021) Intrinsic and extrinsic regulation of human fetal bone marrow haematopoiesis and perturbations in Down syndrome. *Nature*, **598**, 327–331.

17 Roy A, Wang G, Iskander D, O'Byrne S, Elliott N, O'Sullivan J *et al.* (2021) Developmental stage- and site-specific transitions in lineage specification and gene regulatory networks in human hematopoietic stem and progenitor cells. *Cell Rep*, **36**, 109698.

18 Bowie MB, Kent DG, Dykstra B, McKnight KD, McCaffrey L, Hoodless PA and Eaves CJ (2007) Identification of a new intrinsically timed developmental checkpoint that reprograms key hematopoietic stem cell properties. *Proc Natl Acad Sci U S A*, **104**, 5878–5882.

19 Ranzoni AM, Tangherloni A, Berest I, Riva SG, Myers B, Strzelecka PM *et al.* (2021) Integrative single-cell RNA-Seq and ATAC-Seq analysis of human developmental hematopoiesis. *Cell Stem Cell*, **28**, 472–487.e7.

20 Mascarenhas MI, Parker A, Dzierzak E and Ottersbach K (2009) Identification of novel regulators of hematopoietic stem cell development through refinement of stem cell localization and expression profiling. *Blood*, **114**, 4645–4653.

21 Chou S, Flygare J and Lodish HF (2013) Fetal hepatic progenitors support long-term expansion of hematopoietic stem cells. *Exp Hematol*, **41**, 479–490.

22 Hock H, Hamblen MJ, Rooke HM, Schindler JW, Saleque S, Fujiwara Y and Orkin SH (2004) Gfi-1 restricts proliferation and preserves functional integrity of haematopoietic stem cells. *Nature*, **431**, 1002–1007.

23 Hock H, Meade E, Medeiros S, Schindler JW, Valk PJ, Fujiwara Y and Orkin SH (2004) Tel/ Etv6 is an essential and selective regulator of adult hematopoietic stem cell survival. *Genes Dev*, **18**, 2336–2341.

24 Kim I, Saunders TL and Morrison SJ (2007) Sox17 dependence distinguishes the transcriptional regulation of fetal from adult hematopoietic stem cells. *Cell*, **130**, 470–483.

25 Mochizuki-Kashio M, Mishima Y, Miyagi S, Negishi, Saraya A, Konuma T *et al.* (2011) Dependency on the polycomb gene Ezh2 distinguishes fetal from adult hematopoietic stem cells. *Blood*, **118**, 6553–6561.

26 Pietras EM and Passegue E (2013) Linking HSCs to their youth. *Nat Cell Biol*, **15**, 885–887.

27 Rice S, Jackson T, Crump NT, Fordham N, Elliott N, O'Byrne S *et al.* (2021) A human fetal liver-derived infant MLL-AF4 acute lymphoblastic leukemia model reveals a distinct fetal gene expression program. *Nat Commun*, **12**, 6905.

28 Böiers C, Richardson SE, Laycock E, Zriwil A, Turati VA, Brown J *et al.* (2018) A human IPS model implicates embryonic B-myeloid fate restriction as developmental susceptibility to B acute lymphoblastic leukemia-associated ETV6-RUNX1. *Dev Cell*, **44**, 362–377.e7.

29 Jackson TR, Ling R and Roy A (2021) The origin of B-cells: human fetal B cell development and implications for the pathogenesis of childhood acute lymphoblastic leukemia. *Front Immunol*, **12**, 637975.

30 Yan H, Hale J, Jaffray J, Li J, Wang Y, Huang Y *et al.* (2018) Developmental differences between neonatal and adult human erythropoiesis. *Am J Hematol*, **93**, 494–503.

31 Dame C, Fahnenstich H, Freitag P, Hofmann D, Abdul-Nour T, Bartmann P and Fandray J (1998) Erythropoietin mRNA expression in human and neonatal tissue. *Blood*, **92**, 3218–3225.

32 Teramo KA, Klemetti MM and Widness JA (2018) Robust increases in Hb by the hypoxic fetus is a response to protect the brain and other organs. *Pediatr Res*, **84**, 807–812.

33 Tojo Y, Sekine H, Hirano I, Pan X, Souma T, Tsujita T *et al.* (2015) Hypoxia signaling cascade for erythropoietin production in hepatocytes. *Mol Cell Biol*, **35**, 2658–2672.

34 Watts TL and Roberts IAG (1999) Haematological abnormalities in the growth-restricted infant. *Semin Neonatol*, **4**, 41–54.

35 Brugnara C and Platt OS (2009) The neonatal erythrocyte and its disorders. In: Orkin SH, Nathan DG, Ginsburg D, Look AT, Fisher DE and Lux SE (eds), *Nathan and Oski's Hematology of Infancy and Childhood*, 7th edn. WB Saunders, Philadelphia, pp. 21–66.

36 Ohls RK (2002) Erythropoietin in extremely low birthweight infants: blood in versus blood out. *J Pediatr*, **141**, 3–6.

37 Bain BJ (2020) *Haemoglobinopathy Diagnosis*, 3rd edn. Wiley Blackwell, Oxford, pp. 2–4.

38 King AJ and Higgs DR (2018) Potential new approaches to the management of the Hb Bart's hydrops fetalis syndrome: the most severe form of α-thalassemia. *Hematology Am Soc Hematol Educ Program* 2018, **2018**, 353–360.

39 Bard H (1975) The postnatal decline in HbF synthesis in normal full-time infants. *J Clin Invest*, **55**, 395–398.

40 Phillips HM, Holland BM, Jones JG, Abdel-Moiz AL, Turner TL and Wardrop CA (1988) Definitive estimate of rate of hemoglobin switching: measurement of percent hemoglobin F in neonatal reticulocytes. *Pediatr Res*, **23**, 595–597.

41 Vinjamur DS, Bauer DE, Orkin SH (2018) Recent progress in understanding and manipulating haemoglobin switching for the haemoglobinopathies. *Br J Haematol*, **180**, 630–643.

42 Frangoul H, Altshuler D, Cappellini MD, Chen YS, Domm J, Eustace BK *et al.* (2020) CRISPR-Cas9 gene editing for sickle cell disease and β-thalassemia. *N Engl J Med*, **384**, 252–260.

43 Kuruvilla DJ, Widness JA, Nalbant D, Schmidt RL, Mock DM, An G and Veng-Pedersen P (2017) Estimation of adult and neonatal RBC lifespans in anemic neonates using RBCs labeled at several discrete biotin densities. *Pediatr Res*, **81**, 905–910.

44 Böhler T, Leo A, Stadler A and Linderkamp O (1992) Mechanical fragility of erythrocyte membrane in neonates and adults. *Pediatr Res*, **32**, 92–96.

45 Ruef P and Linderkamp O (1999) Deformability and geometry of neonatal erythrocytes with irregular shapes. *Pediatr Res*, **45**, 114–119.

46 Frosali S, Di Simplicio P, Perrone S, Di Guiseppe D, Longini M, Tanganelli D and Buonocore G (2004) Glutathione recycling and antioxidant enzyme activities in erythrocytes of term and preterm newborns at birth. *Biol Neonate*, **85**, 188–194.

47 Siddappa AM, Rao R, Long JD, Widness JA and Georgieff MK (2007) The assessment of newborn iron stores at birth: a review of the literature and standards for ferritin concentrations. *Neonatology*, **92**, 73–82.

48 Lorenz L, Peter A, Poets CF and Franz AR (2013) A review of cord blood concentrations of iron status parameters to define reference ranges for preterm infants. *Neonatology*, **104**, 194–202.

49 Rao R and Georgieff MK (2002) Perinatal aspects of iron metabolism. *Acta Paediatr Suppl*, **91**, 124–129.

50 Niklasson A, Engstrom E, Hard AL, Wikland KA and Hellstrom A (2003) Growth in very preterm children: a longitudinal study. *Pediatr Res*, **54**, 899–905.

51 Widness JA, Madan A, Grindeanu LA, Zimmerman MB, Wong DK and Stevenson DK (2005) Reduction in red blood cell transfusions among preterm infants: results of a randomized trial with an in-line blood gas and chemistry monitor. *Pediatrics*, **115**, 1299–1306.

52 McCarthy EK, Dempsey EM and Kiely ME (2019) Iron supplementation in preterm and low-birth-weight infants: a systematic review of intervention studies. *Nutr Rev*, **77**, 865–877.

53 Mills RJ and Davies MW (2012) Enteral iron supplementation in preterm and low birth weight infants. *Cochrane Database Syst Rev*, CD005095.

54 Domellöf M (2017) Meeting the iron needs of low and very low birth weight infants. *Ann Nutr Metab*, **71** (Suppl 3), 16–23.

55 Bahr TM, Ward DM, Jia X, Ohls RK, German KR, and Christensen RD (2021) Is the erythropoietin-erythroferrone-hepcidin axis intact in human neonates? *Blood Cells Mol Dis*, **88**, 102536.

56 German KR, Comstock BA, Parikh P, Whittington D, Maycock DE, Heagerty PJ *et al.* (2022) Do extremely low gestational age neonates regulate iron absorption via hepcidin? *J Pediatr*, **241**, 62–67.e1.

57 Nemeth E and Ganz T (2021) Hepcidin-ferroportin interaction controls systemic iron homeostasis. *Int J Mol Sci*, **22**, 6493.

58 Lorenz L, Herbst J, Engel C, Peter A, Abele H, Poets CF *et al.* (2014) Gestational age-specific reference ranges of hepcidin in cord blood. *Neonatology*, **106**, 133–139.

59 Yapakci E, Ecevit A, Goekmen Z, Tarcan A and Ozbek N (2009) Erythrocyte transfusions and serum prohepcidin levels in premature newborns with anemia of prematurity. *J Pediatr Hematol Oncol*, **31**, 840–842.

60 Wu TW, Tabangin M, Kusano R, Ma Y, Ridsdale R and Akinbi H (2013) The utility of serum hepcidin as a biomarker for late-onset neonatal sepsis. *J Pediatr*, **162**, 67–71.

61 Lorenz L, Mueller KF, Poets CF, Peter A, Olbina G, Westerman M *et al.* (2015) Short-term effects of blood transfusions on hepcidin in preterm infants. *Neonatology*, **108**, 205–210.

62 Lenhartova N, Ochiai M, Sawano T, Yasuoka K, Fujiyoshi J, Inoue H and Ohga S (2022) Serum erythroferrone levels during the first month of life in premature infants. *J Perinatol*, **42**, 97–102.

63 Christensen R, Henry E, Jopling J and Wiedmeier S (2009) The CBC: reference ranges for neonates. *Semin Perinatol*, **33**, 3–11.

64 Schmutz N, Henry E, Jopling J and Christensen RD (2008) Expected ranges for blood neutrophil concentrations of neonates: the Manroe and Mouzinho charts revisited. *J Perinatol*, **28**, 275–281.

65 Christensen RD, Jensen J, Maheshwari A and Henry E (2010) Reference ranges for blood concentrations of eosinophils and monocytes during the neonatal period defined from over 63 000 records in a multihospital health-care system. *J Perinatol*, **30**, 540–545.

66 Christensen RD, Henry E, Andres RL and Bennett ST (2011) Reference ranges for blood concentrations of nucleated red blood cells in neonates. *Neonatology*, **99**, 289–294.

67 Christensen RD, Baer VL, Gordon PV, Henry E, Whitaker C, Andres RL and Bennett ST (2012) Reference ranges for lymphocyte counts of neonates: associations between abnormal counts and outcomes. *Pediatrics*, **129**, e1165–e1172.

68 Roberts I, Alford K, Hall G, Juban G, Richmond H, Norton A *et al.*; Oxford-Imperial Down Syndrome Cohort Study Group (2013) GATA1-mutant clones are frequent and often unsuspected in babies with Down syndrome: identification of a population at risk of leukemia. *Blood*, **122**, 3908–3917.

69 Jopling J, Henry E, Wiedmeier SE and Christensen RD (2009) Reference ranges for hematocrit and blood hemoglobin concentration during the neonatal period: data from a multihospital health care system. *Pediatrics*, **123**, e333–e337.

70 Alur P, Devapatla SS, Super DM, Danish E, Stern T, Inagandla R and Moore JJ (2000) Impact of race and gestational age on red blood cell indices in very low birth weight infants. *J Pediatr*, **106**, 306–310.

71 Bahr TM, Christensen TR, Henry E, Wilkes J, Ohls RK, Bennett ST *et al.* (2021) Neonatal reference intervals for the complete blood count parameters MicroR and HYPO-He: sensitivity beyond the red cell indices for identifying microcytic and hypochromic disorders. *J Pediatr*, **239**, 95–100.e2.

72 Warwood TL, Ohls RK, Wiedmeier SE, Lambert DK, Jones C, Scoffield SH *et al.* (2005) Single-dose darbepoetin administration to anemic preterm neonates. *J Perinatol*, **25**, 725–730.

73 Christensen RD, Henry E, Bennett ST and Yaish HM (2016) Reference intervals for reticulocyte parameters of infants during their first 90 days after birth. *J Perinatol*, **36**, 61–66.

74 Sottiaux J, Favresse J, Chevalier C, Chatelain B, Hugues J and Mullier F (2020) Evaluation of a hereditary spherocytosis screening algorithm by automated blood count using reticulocytes and erythrocytic parameters on the Sysmex XN-series. *Int J Lab Hematol*, **42**, e88–e91.

75 Rolfo A, Maconi M, Cardaropoli S, Biolcati M, Danise P and Todros T (2007) Nucleated red blood cells in term fetuses: reference values using an automated analyzer. *Neonatology*, **92**, 205–208.

76 Green DW, Hendon B and Mimouni FB (1995) Nucleated erythrocytes and intraventricular hemorrhage in preterm neonates. *Pediatrics*, **96**, 475–478.

77 Buonocore G, Perrone S, Gioia D, Gatti MG, Massafra C, Agosta R and Bracci R (1999) Nucleated red blood cell count at birth as an index of perinatal brain damage. *Am J Obstet Gynecol*, **181**, 1500–1505.

78 Zipursky, A (2003) Transient leukaemia – a benign form of leukaemia in newborn infants with trisomy 21. *Br J Haematol*, **120**, 930–938.

79 Linderkamp O, Nelle M, Kraus M and Zilow EP (1992) The effect of early and late cord clamping on blood viscosity and other hemorheological parameters in full-term infants. *Acta Paediatr*, **81**, 745–750.

80 Kiserud T (2004) The fetal circulation. *Prenat Diagn*, **24**, 1049–1059.

81 Cassady G (1966) Plasma volume studies in low birth weight infants. *Pediatrics*, **38**, 1020–1027.

82 Bauer K, Linderkamp O and Versmold HT (1993) Systolic blood pressure and blood volume in preterm infants. *Arch Dis Child*, **69**, 521–522.

83 Pepper MR and Black MM (2011) B12 in fetal development. *Semin Cell Dev Biol*, **22**, 619–623.

84 Hinton CF, Ojodu JA, Fernhoff PM, Rasmussen SA, Scanlon KS and Hannon WH (2010) Maternal and neonatal vitamin B12 deficiency detected through expanded newborn screening – United States, 2003–2007. *J Pediatr*, **157**, 162–163.

85 Scolamiero E, Villani GR, Ingenito L, Pecce R, Albano L, Caterino M *et al.* (2014) Maternal vitamin B12 deficiency detected in expanded newborn screening. *Clin Biochem*, **47**, 312–317.

86 Reinson K, Kuennapas K, Kriisa A, Vals MA, Muru K and Ounap K (2018) High incidence of low vitamin B12 levels in Estonian newborns. *Mol Genet Metab Rep*, **15**, 1–5.

87 Muetze U, Walter M, Keller M, Gramer G, Garbade SF, Gleich F *et al.* (2021) Health outcomes of infants with vitamin B12 deficiency identified by newborn screening and early treated. *J Pediatr*, **235**, 42–48.

88 Higginbottom MC, Sweetman L and Nyhan WL (1978) A syndrome of methylmalonic aciduria, homocystinuria, megaloblastic anemia and neurologic abnormalities in a vitamin B12-deficient breast-fed infant of a strict vegetarian. *N Engl J Med*, **299**, 317–323.

89 Wighton MC, Manson JI, Robertson E and Chapman E (1979) Brain damage in infancy and dietary vitamin B12 deficiency. *Med J Aust*, **2**, 1–3.

90 Gramer G, Fang-Hoffmann J, Feyh P, Klinke G, Monostori P, Mutze U *et al.* (2020) Newborn screening for vitamin B12-deficiency in Germany–strategies, results, and public health implications. *J Pediatr*, **216**, 165–172.

91 Oliver C, Watson C, Crowley E, Gilroy M, Page D, Weber K *et al.* (2020) Vitamin and Mineral Supplementation Practices in Preterm Infants: A Survey of Australian and New Zealand Neonatal Intensive and Special Care Units. *Nutrients*, **12**, 51.

92 Jyothi S, Misra I, Morris G, Benton A, Griffin D and Allen S (2007) Red cell folate and plasma homocysteine in preterm infants. *Neonatology*, **92**, 264–268.

93 Forestier F, Daffos F and Galacteros F (1986) Haematological values of 163 normal fetuses between 18 and 30 weeks of gestation. *Pediatr Res*, **20**, 342–346.

94 Campagnoli C, Fisk N, Overton T, Bennett P, Watts T and Roberts I (2000). Circulating hematopoietic progenitor cells in first trimester fetal blood. *Blood* **95**, 1967–1972.

95 Lawrence SM, Corriden R and Nizet V (2017) Age-appropriate functions and dysfunctions of the neonatal neutrophil. *Front Pediatr*, **5**, 23.

96 Raymond SL, Stortz JA, Mira JC, Larson SD, Wynn JL and Moldawer LL (2017) Immunological defects in neonatal sepsis and potential therapeutic approaches. *Front Pediatr*, **5**, 14.

97 Levy O (2007) Innate immunity of the newborn: basic mechanisms and clinical correlates. *Nat Rev Immunol*, **7**, 379–390.

98 Koenig JM and Christensen RD (1989) Incidence, neutrophil kinetics, and natural history of neonatal neutropenia associated with maternal hypertension. *N Engl J Med*, **321**, 557–562.

99 Ohls RK, Li Y, Abdel-Mageed A, Buchanan Jr G, Mandell L and Christensen RD (1995) Neutrophil pool sizes and granulocyte colony stimulating factor production in human mid-trimester fetuses. *Pediatr Res*, **37**, 806–811.

100 Christensen RD, Calhoun DA and Rimsza LM (2000) A practical approach to evaluating and treating neutropenia in the neonatal intensive care unit. *Clin Perinatol*, **27**, 577–601.

101 Millar DS, Davis LR, Rodeck CH, Nicolaides KH and Mibashan RS (1985) Normal blood cell values in the early mid-trimester fetus. *Prenat Diagn*, **5**, 367–373.

102 Filias A, Theodorou GL, Mouzopoulou S, Varvarigou AA, Mantagos S and Karakantza M (2011) Phagocytic ability of neutrophils and monocytes in neonates. *BMC Pediatr*, **11**, 29.

103 Tsafaras GT, Ntontsi P and Xanthou G (2020) Advantages and limitations of the neonatal immune system. *Front Pediatr*, **8**, 5.

104 Torok C, Lundahl J, Hed J and Lagercrantz H (1993) Diversity in regulation of adhesion molecules (Mac-1 and L-selectin) in monocytes and neutrophils from neonates and adults. *Arch Dis Child*, **68**, 561–565.

105 Angelone DF, Wessels MR, Coughlin M, Suter EE, Valentini P, Kalish LA *et al.* (2006) Innate immunity of the human newborn is polarized toward a high ratio of IL-6/TNF-α production *in vitro* and *in vivo*. *Pediatr Res*, **60**, 205–209.

106 Tatad AM, Nesin M, Peoples J, Cheung S, Lin H, Sison C *et al.* (2008) Cytokine expression in response to bacterial antigens in preterm and term infant cord blood monocytes. *Neonatology*, **94**, 8–15.

107 Strunk T, Prosser A, Levy O, Philbin V, Simmer K, Doherty D *et al.* (2012) Responsiveness of human monocytes to the commensal bacterium Staphylococcus epidermidis develops late in gestation. *Pediatr Res*, **72**, 10–18.

108 Li YP, Yu SL, Huang ZJ, Huang J, Pan J, Feng X *et al.* (2015) An impaired inflammatory cytokine response to gram-negative LPS in human neonates is associated with the defective TLR-mediated signaling pathway. *J Clin Immunol*, **35**, 218–226.

109 Angelidou A, Diray-Arce J, Conti M-G, Netea MG, Blok BA, Liu M *et al.* (2021) Human newborn monocytes demonstrate distinct BCG-induced primary and trained innate cytokine production and metabolic activation in vitro. *Front Immunol*, **12**, 674334.

110 Hann IM (1991) Development of blood in the fetus. In: Hann IM, Gibson BES and Letsky E (eds), *Fetal and Neonatal Haematology*. Bailliere Tindall, London, pp. 1–28.

111 Roy A, Cowan G, Mead AJ, Filippi S, Bohn G, Chaidos A *et al.* (2012) Perturbation of fetal liver hematopoietic stem and progenitor cell development by trisomy 21. *Proc Natl Acad Sci U S A*, **109**, 17579–17584.

112 Roy A, Bystry V, Bohn G, Goudevenou K, Reigl T, Papaioannou M *et al.* (2017) High resolution IgH repertoire analysis reveals fetal liver as the likely origin of life-long, innate B lymphopoiesis in humans. *Clin Immunol*, **183**, 8–16.

113 Montecino-Rodriguez E and Dorshkind K (2012) B-1 B cell development in the fetus and adult. *Immunity*, **36**, 13–21.

114 Bueno C, Van Roon EHJ, Muñoz-López A, Sanjuan-Pla A, Juan M, Navarro A *et al.* (2016) Immunophenotypic analysis and quantification of B-1 and B-2 B cells during human fetal hematopoietic development. *Leukemia*, **30**, 1603–1606.

115 Haynes BF, Martin ME, Kay HH and Kurtzberg J (1988) Early events in human T cell ontogeny. Phenotypic characterization and immunohistologic localization of T cell precursors in early human fetal tissues. *J Exp Med*, **168**, 1061–1080.

116 Cupedo T, Nagasawa M, Weijer K, Blom B and Spits H (2005) Development and activation of regulatory T cells in the human fetus. *Eur J Immunol*, **35**, 383–390.

117 Michaelsson J, Mold JE, McCune JM and Nixon DF (2006) Regulation of T cell responses in the developing human fetus. *J Immunol*, **176**, 5741–5748.

118 Pahal G, Jauniaux E, Kinnon C, Thrasher AJ and Rodeck CH (2000) Normal development of human fetal hematopoiesis between eight and seventeen weeks' gestation. *Am J Obstet Gynecol*, **183**, 1029–1034.

119 Kumar BV, Connors T and Farber DL (2018) Human T cell development, localization, and function throughout life. *Immunity*, **48**, 202–213.

120 Krause PJ, Herson VC, Boutin-Lebowitz J, Eisenfeld L, Block C, LoBello T *et al.* (1986) Polymorphonuclear leukocyte adherence and chemotaxis in stressed and healthy neonates. *Pediatr Res*, **20**, 296–300.

121 Anderson DC, Rothlein R, Marlin SD, Krater SS AND Smith CW (1990) Impaired transendothelial migration by neonatal neutrophils: abnormalities of Mac-1 (CD11b/CD18)-dependent adherence reactions. *Blood*, **76**, 2613–2621.

122 Nussbaum C, Gloning A, Pruenster M, Frommhold D, Bierschenk S, Genzel-Boroviczény O *et al.* (2013) Neutrophil and endothelial adhesive function during human fetal ontogeny. *J Leukoc Biol*, **93**, 175–184.

123 Yost CC, Cody MJ, Harris ES, Thornton NL, McInturff AM, Martinez ML *et al.* (2009) Impaired neutrophil extracellular trap (NET) formation: a novel innate immune deficiency of human neonates. *Blood*, **113**, 6419–6427.

124 Lipp P, Ruhnau J, Lange A, Vogelgesang A, Dressel A and Heckmann M (2016) Less neutrophil extracellular trap formation in term newborns than in adults. *Neonatology*, **111**, 182–188.

125 Yost CC, Schwertz H, Cody MJ, Wallace JA, Campbell RA, Vieira-de-Abreu A *et al.* (2016) Neonatal NET-inhibitory factor and related peptides inhibit neutrophil extracellular trap formation. *J Clin Invest*, **126**, 3783–3798.

126 Papayannopoulos V (2018) Neutrophil extracellular traps in immunity and disease. *Nat Rev Immunol*, **18**, 134–147.

127 He Y-M, Li X, Perego M, Nefedova Y, Kossenov AV, Jensen EA *et al.* (2018) Transitory presence of myeloid-derived suppressor cells in neonates is critical for control of inflammation. *Nat Med*, **24**, 224–231.

128 Weber R and Umansky V (2019) Fighting infant infections with myeloid-derived suppressor cells. *J Clin Invest*, **129**, 4080–4082.

129 Källman J, Schollin J, Schalèn C, Erlandsson A and Kihlström E (1998) Impaired phagocytosis and opsonisation towards group B streptococci in preterm neonates. *Arch Dis Child Fetal Neonatal Ed*, **78**, F46–F50.

130 Forestier F, Daffos F, Catherine N, Renard M and Andreux JP (1991) Developmental hematopoiesis in normal human fetal blood. *Blood*, **77**, 2360–2363.

131 Hohlfeld P, Forestier F, Kaplan C, Tissot JD and Daffos F (1994) Fetal thrombocytopenia: a retrospective survey of 5,194 fetal blood samplings. *Blood*, **84**, 1851–1856.

132 Ferrer-Marin F, Liu ZJ, Gutti R and Sola-Visner M (2010) Neonatal thrombocytopenia and megakaryocytopoiesis. *Semin Hematol*, **47**, 281–288.

133 Liu ZJ, Italiano J, Ferrer-Marin F, Gutti R, Bailey M, Poterjoy B *et al.* (2011) Developmental differences in megakaryocytopoiesis are associated with up-regulated TPO signalling through mTOR and elevated GATA-1 levels in neonatal megakaryocytes. *Blood*, **117**, 4106–4117.

134 Wolber E-M, Bame C, Fahnenstich H, Hofmann D, Bartmann P, Jelkmann W and Fandrey J (1999) Expression of the thrombopoietin gene in human fetal and neonatal tissues. *Blood*, **94**, 97–105.

135 Walka MM, Sonntag J, Dudenhausen JW and Obladen M (1999) Thrombopoietin concentration in umbilical cord blood of healthy term newborns is higher than in adult controls. *Biol Neonate*, **75**, 54–58.

136 Murray NA, Watts TL, and Roberts IAG (1998) Endogenous thrombopoietin levels and effect of recombinant human thrombopoietin on megakaryocyte precursors in term and preterm babies. *Pediatr Res*, **43**, 148–151.

137 Sola MC, Calhoun DA, Hutson AD and Christensen RD (1999) Plasma thrombopoietin concentrations in thrombocytopenic and non-thrombocytopenic patients in a neonatal intensive care unit. *Br J Haematol*, **104**, 90–92.

138 Hegyi E, Nakazawa M, Debili N, Navarro S, Katz A, Breton-Gorius J and Vainchenker W (1991) Developmental changes in human megakaryocyte ploidy. *Exp Hematol*, **19**, 87–94.

139 Sola-Visner M (2012) Platelets in the neonatal period: developmental differences in platelet production, function, and hemostasis and the potential impacts on therapies. *Hematology Am Soc Hematol Educ Program*, **2012**, 506–511.

140 Roberts IAG and Chakravorty S (2019) Thrombocytopenia in the newborn. In: Michelson A, Cataneo M, Frelinger A and Newman P (eds), *Platelets*, 4th edn. Academic Press, New York, pp. 813–831.

141 Sola-Visner MC, Christensen RD, Hutson AD and Rimsza LM (2007) Megakaryocyte size and concentration in the bone marrow of thrombocytopenic and non-thrombocytopenic neonates. *Pediatr Res*, **61**, 479–484.

142 Davenport P, Liu ZJ and Sola-Visner M (2020) Changes in megakaryopoiesis over ontogeny and their implications in health and disease. *Platelets*, **31**, 692–699.

143 Murray NA and Roberts IAG (1995) Circulating megakaryocytes and their progenitors (BFU-MK and CFU-MK) in term and pre-term neonates. *Br J Haematol*, **89**, 41–46.

144 Saxonhouse MA, Christensen RD, Walker DM, Hutson AD and Sola MC (2004) The concentration of circulating megakaryocyte progenitors in preterm neonates is a function of post-conceptional age. *Early Hum Dev*, **78**, 119–124.

145 Saxonhouse MA, Sola MC, Pastos KM, Ignatz ME, Hutson AD, Christensen RD and Rimsza LM (2004) Reticulated platelet percentages in term and preterm neonates. *J Pediatr Hematol Oncol*, **26**, 797–802.

146 Wiedmeier SE, Henry E, Sola-Visner MC and Christensen RD (2009) Platelet reference ranges for neonates, defined using data from over 47,000 patients in a multi hospital healthcare system. *J Perinatol*, **29**, 130–136.

147 Cremer M, Sallmon H, Kling PJ, Buhrer C and Dame C (2016) Thrombocytopenia and platelet transfusion in the neonate. *Semin Fetal Neonatal Med*, **21**, 10–18.

148 MacQueen BC, Christensen RD, Henry E, Romrell AM, Pysher TJ, Bennett ST and Sola-Visner MC (2017) The immature platelet fraction: creating neonatal reference intervals and using these to categorize neonatal thrombocytopenias. *J Perinatol*, **37**, 834–838.

149 Lorenz V, Ferrer-Marin, Israels SJ and Sola-Visner M (2019) Platelet function in the newborn. In: Michelson A, Cataneo M, Frelinger A and Newman P (eds), *Platelets*, 4th edn. Academic Press, New York, pp. 443–457.

150 Corby DG and O'Barr TP (1981) Decreased alpha-adrenergic receptors in newborn platelets: cause of abnormal response to epinephrine. *Dev Pharmacol Ther*, **2**, 215–225.

151 Caparros-Perez E, Teruel-Montoya R, Lopez-Andreo MJ, Llanos MC, Rivera J, Palma-Barqueros V *et al.* (2017) Comprehensive comparison of neonate and adult human platelet transcriptomes. *PLoS One*, **12**, e0183042.

152 Sitaru AG, Holzhauer S, Speer CP, Singer D, Obergfell A, Walter U, Grossmann R *et al.* (2005) Neonatal platelets from cord blood and peripheral blood. *Platelets*, **16**, 203–210.

153 Bednarek FJ, Bean S, Barnard MR, Frelinger AL and Michelson AD (2009) The platelet hyporeactivity of extremely low birth weight neonates is age-dependent. *Thromb Res*, **124**, 42–45.

154 Grevsen AK, Hviid CVB, Haansen AK and Hvas A-M (2021) Platelet count and function in umbilical cord blood versus peripheral blood in term neonates. *Platelets*, **32**, 626–632.

155 Kayiran SM, Ozbek N, Turan M and Gurankan B (2003) Significant differences between capillary and venous complete blood counts in the neonatal period. *Clin Lab Haematol*, **25**, 9–16.

156 Özbek N, Gürakan B and Kayiran SM (2000) Complete blood cell counts in capillary and venous blood of healthy term newborns. *Acta Haematol*, **103**, 226–228.

2

Red cell disorders: anaemia, jaundice, polycythaemia and cyanosis

Neonatal anaemia

Definition and clinical significance of neonatal anaemia

Anaemia is generally defined as a haemoglobin concentration or haematocrit at least two standard deviations below the mean or below the 5th percentile compared with reference values for age and, if appropriate, gender. For neonates these normal values vary with gestational age at birth (see Table 1.2). For term babies, a haemoglobin concentration (Hb) below 140 g/l is abnormal and could be considered as anaemia, while in preterm babies born before 30 weeks' gestation the lower limit of normal is 115 g/l.

As a first step in assessing the significance and cause of neonatal anaemia, the laboratory result should be considered in light of the clinical findings. Detailed investigations will not be necessary for every neonate with an Hb below the normal range. It is important to consider the possibility of artefactual results, for example due to *in vitro* blood clotting in the sample tube. In addition, haemoglobin measurements on heel-prick samples may be misleading as they can be up to 40 g/l lower than venous samples in the first few hours of life, particularly in term babies.[1] Another major factor determining the Hb at birth is the timing and position of the baby at the time of clamping of the cord (babies held below the placenta receive more blood). In a term baby, the placental vessels typically contain around 100 ml of blood at birth. Since up to 25% of the placental blood is 'transfused' into the baby within the first 15 seconds and 50% by the end of the first minute, even a short delay has the potential to increase the volume of placental blood transfused to the neonate by 50 ml.[2] Indeed, as discussed later in this chapter, a policy of deliberate delay to cord clamping has been investigated in several studies as a strategy for reducing neonatal red cell transfusion requirements.

The clinical significance of neonatal anaemia depends both upon the haemoglobin concentration and on the ability of the haemoglobin to deliver oxygen to the tissues. This, in turn, depends on the characteristics of the haemoglobin–oxygen dissociation curve. In neonates, the two most important parameters that determine the position of the haemoglobin–oxygen dissociation curve are the concentration of haemoglobin F and the level of 2,3-diphosphoglycerate (2,3-DPG) within the red blood cells. At birth, when the

Neonatal Haematology: A Practical Guide, First Edition. Irene Roberts and Barbara J. Bain.
© 2022 John Wiley & Sons Ltd. Published 2022 by John Wiley & Sons Ltd.

Table 2.1 Mechanisms of fetal and neonatal anaemia

- Reduced production (red cell aplasia/dysplasia)
- Increased destruction (haemolysis)
- Blood loss
- Multifactorial (anaemia of prematurity)

predominant haemoglobin is haemoglobin F and the levels of 2,3-DPG are low, the curve shifts to the left, i.e. the affinity of haemoglobin for oxygen is high and so less oxygen is released to the tissues. This can cause particular problems for the most preterm neonates (<28 weeks' gestation) in which haemoglobin F forms more than 90% of the total haemoglobin. As the proportion of haemoglobin F falls, either physiologically or following red cell transfusion, and 2,3-DPG levels rise, the haemoglobin–oxygen dissociation curve gradually shifts to the right and oxygen delivery to the tissues improves.

Anaemia may be caused by reduced red cell production, increased red cell destruction (haemolysis), blood loss or a combination of these factors (Table 2.1). While simple investigations, in particular the full blood count and blood film, remain the cornerstone for identifying the causes of neonatal anaemias, accurate diagnosis of the rarer inherited anaemias has been greatly facilitated by the increasing speed and availability of next generation sequencing.[3,4]

Neonatal anaemia due to reduced red cell production

Reduced red cell production in the neonate may result either from a virtually complete absence of red cells and erythroid progenitors (red cell aplasia) or from qualitatively abnormal red cell production where erythroid progenitors fail to differentiate normally into mature red cells (ineffective erythropoiesis). Red cell aplasia and anaemias due to ineffective erythropoiesis (often also dyserythropoietic) are uncommon in the neonatal period but are important to recognise promptly because they are often severe and, for inherited disorders, are a cause of life-long ill health. The most common causes of red cell aplasia are congenital infections (largely due to parvovirus B19) and the genetic disorder Diamond–Blackfan anaemia (DBA). As both parvovirus B19 and DBA cause highly selective effects on the erythroid lineage, the white cell count and platelet count are usually normal in affected neonates. However, reduced red cell production may also occur as part of a general failure of haemopoiesis. In this situation the neutrophil count, platelet count and Hb are all reduced, for example in congenital leukaemias (see Chapter 3). Apart from parvovirus B19, other infections that can cause anaemia due to reduced red cell production include cytomegalovirus (CMV), toxoplasmosis, congenital syphilis, rubella and herpes simplex, although the anaemia and reticulocytopenia are usually relatively mild.[5,6]

The main diagnostic clues to reduced red cell production in a neonate with anaemia are the combination of a low reticulocyte count ($<20 \times 10^9$/l) with a negative direct antiglobulin test (DAT or Coombs test) (Table 2.2). The principal causes of anaemia due to reduced red cell production in neonates are shown in Table 2.3.

Table 2.2 Diagnostic clues to red cell aplasia in neonates with anaemia

Low reticulocytes)	$<20 \times 10^9/l$
Direct Coombs test	Negative
Bilirubin	Usually normal
Blood film	Red blood cell morphology usually normal

Table 2.3 Causes of failure of red cell production in neonates with anaemia

Red cell aplasia and/or dysplasia	Useful diagnostic tests
Parvovirus B19 infection	Blood film: disproportionate lack of polychromasia and NRBC (in setting of low Hb)
	Maternal parvovirus B19 serology: IgM antibodies during pregnancy indicates *in utero* infection
	Parvovirus B19 DNA (neonate ± mother)
Diamond–Blackfan anaemia	Family history
	Exclude parvovirus B19 infection
	Adenosine deaminase assay (pretransfusion), including parents
	Molecular analysis (ribosomal protein genes*), including parents
	Bone marrow aspirate
Congenital dyserythropoietic anaemia	Family history
	Red cell indices (MCV usually increased)
	Red cell morphology (macrocytosis and poikilocytosis)
	Molecular analysis (known CDA genes)*
	Bone marrow aspirate (characteristic dyserythropoiesis)
	Electron microscopy (bone marrow cells)
Mitochondrial cytopathy: Pearson syndrome	Bone marrow aspirate (vacuolation of erythroid and granulocytic precursors)
	Molecular analysis of leucocytes (mitochondrial genome sequencing)

* If molecular analysis is readily available and clinical suspicion is high, it may be preferable to perform the bone marrow aspirate after molecular analysis as this may allow additional tests (e.g. electron microscopy for suspected CDA) to be performed at the same time.
CDA, congenital dyserythropoietic anaemia; DNA, deoxyribonucleic acid; Hb haemoglobin concentration; Ig, immunoglobulin; MCV, mean cell volume; NRBC, nucleated red blood cells.

Parvovirus B19 and fetal/neonatal anaemia

Population studies indicate that 25–50% of women of reproductive age remain susceptible to parvovirus B19.[7] When the infection occurs in pregnant women who lack immunity, particularly during the first 20 weeks of pregnancy, severe fetal and/or neonatal anaemia due to red cell aplasia develops in up to one-third of affected pregnancies.[7] Although the majority of fetuses are unaffected, it is important to recognise that parvovirus B19 is the cause of 6–7% of cases of non-immune hydrops fetalis and is the commonest infective cause of this condition.[8,9] Typically, the affected fetus or neonate has marked

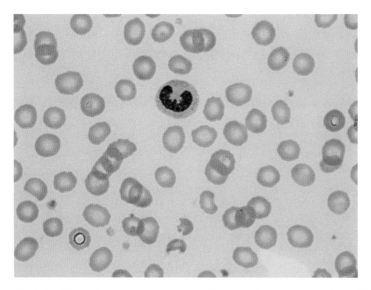

Fig. 2.1 Blood film of a term neonate with anaemia due to parvovirus B19 infection showing normochromic normocytic red cells with occasional schistocytes and an absence of polychromasia. A normal neutrophil is also shown. May–Grünwald–Giemsa (MGG), ×100.

reticulocytopenia (often $<10 \times 10^9$/l) and in severe cases thrombocytopenia can also occur.[5] The red blood cells are morphologically normal and an important diagnostic clue is the absence of polychromasia and circulating nucleated red blood cells (NRBC) despite the presence of severe anaemia (Fig. 2.1). The diagnosis is made by maternal serology and demonstration of B19 DNA in the fetus or neonate by dot-blot hybridisation or polymerase chain reaction (PCR) of peripheral blood (bone marrow aspiration for morphology and parvovirus B19 PCR may be necessary in difficult cases).[9]

Management of fetal parvovirus B19 infection depends on the severity of the anaemia and whether or not the fetus is hydropic. A recent systematic review and meta-analysis showed that the presence of hydrops was the main determinant of mortality and adverse perinatal outcome.[9] The majority of hydropic fetuses were treated by intrauterine transfusion (IUT) whereas this was only used as treatment for approximately 26% of non-hydropic fetuses. The outcome was very good for non-hydropic fetuses, with an *in utero* mortality rate of about 2% and no neonatal deaths. However, almost 25% of fetuses who presented with hydrops due to parvovirus B19 infection died despite IUT, the majority of them prior to delivery, and a further 10% had a poor neurodevelopmental outcome. In addition, a small number of neonates affected by intrauterine parvovirus B19 infection develop chronic red cell aplasia, with or without evidence of persistent B19 DNA by PCR.[5] In such cases, intravenous immunoglobulin (IVIg) has been reported to be effective in treating the anaemia and eradicating persistent viral infection in some,[10] but not all, cases.[11,12]

Genetic red cell aplasia and dysplasia

These two groups of conditions differ in that in red cell aplasia the marrow is hypocellular with reduced progenitor cell numbers, whereas in dysplasia erythropoiesis is active but ineffective and dysplastic. Apart from DBA, the genetic causes of congenital red cell aplasia and dysplasia are extremely rare. They include congenital dyserythropoietic anaemia (CDA) and Pearson syndrome. The other inherited bone marrow failure syndromes, such as Fanconi anaemia, are rarely manifest at birth. Similarly, congenital atransferrinaemia nearly always presents later in childhood or in adulthood, although rare cases presenting as early as 2 months have been described.[13] These genetic causes of congenital red cell aplasia/dysplasia can normally be distinguished from each other through a combination of their distinctive bone marrow morphology, family history and the presence, or not, of additional congenital anomalies. However, precise diagnosis increasingly relies on targeted or whole genome sequencing gene panels on neonatal and parental blood samples.[14,15]

Diamond–Blackfan anaemia

The incidence of DBA is estimated at 5–7 cases per million live births.[16] DBA has a clear family history in 20% of cases (autosomal dominant or recessive) and appears to be sporadic in the remaining 80%.[16] It usually presents as increasing anaemia over the first few weeks or months of life but approximately 25% of cases present with anaemia at birth[16,17] and the most severe cases manifest as second-trimester anaemia or hydrops fetalis.[18,19] Around 40% of neonates with DBA have associated congenital anomalies, particularly craniofacial dysmorphism, neck anomalies, congenital heart disease, urogenital anomalies and thumb malformations, such as a triphalangeal thumb, while around 25% have intrauterine growth restriction (IUGR).[17] Several of these anomalies are also seen in Fanconi anaemia. However, the diagnosis is usually clear as Fanconi anaemia very rarely presents in the fetus or the newborn and the blood count usually shows pancytopenia rather than anaemia.

Recent studies indicate that about 75% of cases of DBA are due to defects in the synthesis and function of structural ribosomal proteins (RP). To date, heterozygous mutations in 19 different genes with good evidence of pathogenicity have been reported in DBA patients.[14] The majority of cases are associated with pathogenic variants in RP genes that encode either the small RP subunit (*RPS7, RPS10, RPS17, RPS19, RPS24, RPS26, RPS27, RPS28* and *RPS29*) or the large RP subunit (*RPL5, RPL11, RPL15, RPL18, RPL26, RPL27, RPL35* and *RPL35a*). *RPS19* mutations are the commonest (25% of all DBA). Recently, mutations in two X-linked genes (*GATA1* and *TSR2*) have also been shown to cause DBA in a small proportion of patients.[20,21] In up to 50% of patients, the molecular basis for the disease has proved elusive, even after using a targeted panel to screen all 80 RP genes for mutations[11] or using whole exome sequencing.[22]

The blood film in neonates with DBA typically shows normochromic red cells with an absence of polychromasia and nucleated red cells despite severe anaemia (Case 2.1, see page 88). Reticulocytopenia is usually severe but reticulocyte counts of 20–30×10^9/l are sometimes seen. These findings are not specific for DBA but if investigations exclude parvovirus B19 infection and/or if there are typical DBA-associated congenital anomalies or a relevant family history, neonates with persistent anaemia and a low reticulocyte count should have specific investigations for DBA. These include molecular testing for RP gene mutations (many laboratories now offer next generation sequencing for DBA diagnosis) and/or a bone marrow examination, which will demonstrate the lack of erythroid precursors characteristic of this disease. In case of doubt, or where molecular testing is not available, measurement of red cell adenosine deaminase (ADA) levels, which are elevated in most affected patients, may be useful.[14,23]

In the neonatal period, the only treatment of DBA is red cell transfusion, although corticosteroids are used in older infants and children.[23] DBA is almost always a life-long condition although rare spontaneous remissions later in childhood or in adulthood have been reported. Bone marrow transplantation is the only long-term curative option but carries a significant mortality and this must be balanced against the morbidity of life-long red cell transfusion or corticosteroids.[23]

Pearson syndrome

This rare condition nearly always presents within a few days or weeks of birth. It is caused by mutations or deletions in mitochondrial DNA and presents with anaemia, neutropenia, thrombocytopenia and failure to thrive.[24] Most affected neonates have low birthweight with metabolic acidosis and exocrine pancreatic deficiency; abnormal liver and renal function are common. The bone marrow is typically hypercellular with erythroid and megakaryocyte dysplasia (Fig. 2.2), including micromegakaryocytes, and basophilic stippling in erythroblasts (Fig. 2.3). The most useful haematological clue to the diagnosis is the highly characteristic vacuolation of early erythroid and granulocytic cells in the marrow aspirate (Figs 2.2 and 2.4). Vacuolated dysplastic normoblasts and neutrophils can also be seen occasionally in peripheral blood films (Figs 2.5 and 2.6). Confirmation of the diagnosis requires mitochondrial genome sequencing, which can be performed very rapidly in specialised centres. It is important to note that whole exome sequencing may miss mitochondrial gene deletions.[25] Interestingly, some reports have identified large mitochondrial gene deletions in a small sub-group of patients considered to have DBA. When these cases were re-evaluated they were found to be cases of Pearson syndrome which had been misdiagnosed as DBA.[26] Unfortunately, the prognosis for children with this condition is very poor, with few surviving beyond the second year of life.

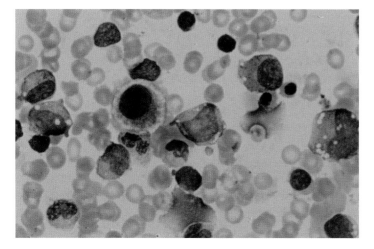

Fig. 2.2 Bone marrow film of a neonate with Pearson syndrome showing vacuolation of erythroid and myeloid cells and a dysplastic megakaryocyte. MGG, ×100.

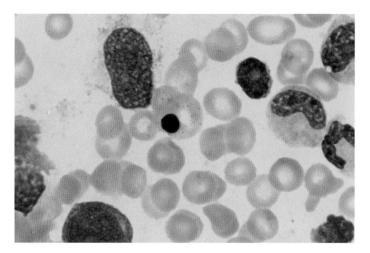

Fig. 2.3 Basophilic stippling in a bone marrow erythroblast (centre field) from a neonate with Pearson syndrome. MGG, ×100.

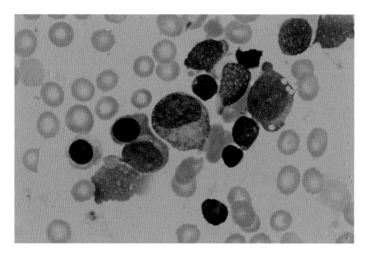

Fig. 2.4 Dyserythropoietic erythroblasts in the bone marrow of a neonate with Pearson syndrome showing prominent vacuolation of a proerythroblast. MGG, ×100.

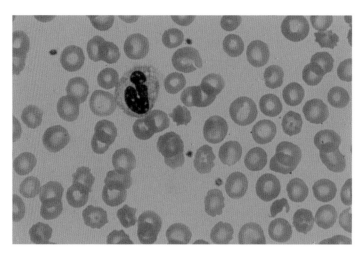

Fig. 2.5 Peripheral blood film of a neonate with Pearson syndrome showing vacuolation in a dysplastic neutrophil. MGG, ×100.

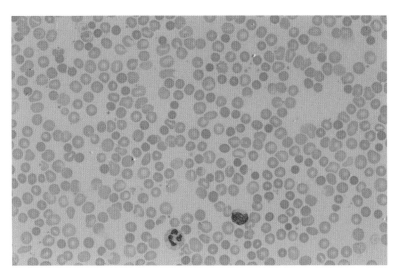

Fig. 2.6 Peripheral blood film of a neonate with Pearson syndrome showing a dysplastic neutrophil with vacuolation. MGG, ×40

Congenital dyserythropoietic anaemias

Congenital dyserythropoietic anaemias are now conventionally classified into three main types (I, II and III) with additional variant types of CDA that do not conform to the criteria for types I–III being recognised (reviewed in reference 27). While most cases of CDA present during childhood, type I, II and some variant CDA can all present with neonatal anaemia and/or hydrops fetalis in association with fetal anaemia.[28–31] Although in older children the anaemia is typically macrocytic, the blood film in neonates with CDA usually shows normocytic red cells with variable anisopoikilocytosis (Fig. 2.7; Case 2.2, see page 90). The peripheral blood findings are non-specific and often the most notable feature is the relative

(a)   (b)

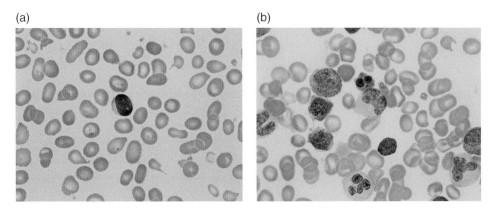

Fig. 2.7 Congenital dyserythropoietic anaemia (CDA): (a) blood film of a term neonate with CDA showing normochromic red cells with anisopoikilocytosis (note the absence of polychromasia); (b) bone marrow film of the same child at age 3 months showing cytoplasmic bridging between two basophilic normoblasts and a normoblast with a dumbbell-shaped nucleus. MGG, ×100.

absence of polychromasia despite moderate or even severe anaemia. The bone marrow aspirate shows increased erythropoiesis with varying degrees – depending on the type of CDA – of dyserythropoiesis, including megaloblastic changes, binucleate or multinucleate erythroblasts, internuclear chromatin bridges, nuclear irregularity and pale staining chromatin. Diagnosis on the basis of morphology alone is unreliable except in very experienced hands and molecular analysis, with or without electron microscopy, is essential for genetic counselling and planning treatment.[3] Next generation sequencing is increasingly used to make a definitive diagnosis.[32]

Most cases of CDA type I are autosomal recessive and caused by bi-allelic mutations of either the *CDAN1* gene or the *CDIN1* (*C15orf41*) gene, although the genetic basis for occasional cases remains unknown.[32] CDA type I is not usually diagnosed in the neonatal period. However, as retrospective series suggest that anaemia and jaundice are common in neonates subsequently diagnosed with the condition, CDA type I should be considered in the differential diagnosis of unexplained, persistent neonatal anaemia.[33] CDA type I also occasionally presents with severe anaemia *in utero* and should be considered in the differential diagnosis of unexplained hydrops fetalis.[34–36] Some patients have nail or skeletal abnormalities, particularly syndactyly of the fingers or toes which may provide a useful clue to the diagnosis.[37] The characteristic haematological features of CDA type I are macrocytic anaemia together with the presence of binucleate macrocytic erythroblasts and internuclear bridging in the bone marrow.[32] Despite the severity of the anaemia in the neonatal period, the majority of infants become transfusion-independent by the age of 4 months.[33]

CDA type II is an autosomal recessive anaemia caused by bi-allelic mutations in the *SEC23B* gene. The anaemia is typically normocytic with a hypercellular bone marrow containing bi- and multinucleated erythroblasts.[38] Approximately 60% of patients have anaemia and jaundice in the neonatal period, although the diagnosis is often unclear until later in childhood, and almost half of affected individuals have a history of neonatal red cell transfusion.[38] Occasional cases of severe fetal anaemia and hydrops have been reported.[28,39] The severity of CDA type II varies from life-long transfusion dependence (in about 20% of cases) to asymptomatic disease.[38]

CDA type III, which is very rare, is characterised by moderate to severe macrocytic anaemia and marked erythroblast multinuclearity on bone marrow examination. This type of CDA has not been reported to present in neonates. CDA type III is caused by bi-allelic mutations in the *KIF23* gene.[27]

Several variant forms of CDA have also been described, some of which present in fetal or neonatal life. These include an X-linked syndrome of severe anaemia and thrombocytopenia due to somatic mutations in the *GATA1* transcription factor gene[40] and a severe anaemia presenting in fetal or neonatal life due to bi-allelic mutations in the *KLF1* gene.[31,41] Although the majority of affected individuals with bi-allelic *KLF1* mutations present with severe normocytic anaemia and jaundice at or before birth, occasional patients with milder disease do not present until adulthood.[31] Despite the severity of the fetal/neonatal anaemia, only occasional neonates with bi-allelic *KLF1* mutations remain transfusion-dependent.[31,42] Variant forms of CDA may also present with neonatal anaemia in conjunction with other syndromic features, including mutations in *MVK*, the mevalonate kinase gene,[43] mutations in *COX4I2*, encoding a component of the cytochrome c oxidase complex,[44] and mutations in the *VPS4A* gene which predominantly cause severe neurodevelopmental delay.[45]

Neonatal anaemia due to increased red cell destruction

Haemolysis is the commonest cause of anaemia in term babies and second only to anaemia of prematurity in preterm babies. The presence of haemolysis is an important sign because, even if mild or transient, this may be the first evidence of a more serious disorder that would otherwise be manifest later in infancy or childhood (e.g. red cell enzymopathies). In addition, there may be implications for future siblings (e.g. haemolytic disease of the fetus and newborn [HDFN]). Initial investigations of suspected haemolysis in a neonate should include a full blood count, a blood film, a reticulocyte count and a Coombs test.

The main diagnostic clues suggesting a haemolytic anaemia are increased numbers of reticulocytes and/or circulating nucleated red cells, unconjugated hyperbilirubinaemia and a positive Coombs test (since this is only positive in cases of immune haemolytic anaemia) (Table 2.4). In most cases there are also characteristic changes in the morphology of the red cells in a blood film (e.g. spherocytes in hereditary spherocytosis; see Fig. 2.13). The main cause of immune haemolytic anaemia is HDFN (Table 2.5). Maternal autoimmune haemolytic anaemia (AIHA) may also cause a positive Coombs test in the neonate but clinical evidence of haemolysis or anaemia in the baby is unusual in this situation. The main causes of non-immune neonatal haemolysis are red cell membrane disorders and red cell enzymopathies (see Table 2.5). Occasionally, neonatal anaemia occurs in haemoglobinopathies, and haemolysis is one of the causative factors (see below). A number of congenital and nosocomial infections can also cause neonatal haemolytic anaemia including CMV, toxoplasmosis, congenital syphilis, rubella, herpes simplex and malaria. Although simple investigations are often sufficient to identify the cause of haemolysis in a neonate, rarer disorders require specialist investigations, including next generation sequencing.

Immune haemolysis, including haemolytic disease of the fetus and newborn

Haemolytic disease of the fetus and newborn results from maternal alloantibodies against paternally derived fetal red cell antigens crossing the placenta and binding to the fetal red cells, causing haemolysis and anaemia. Overall, recent estimates indicate that up to 1 in 600 pregnancies is affected by maternal red cell alloimmunisation.[46] The principal alloantibodies causing HDFN are those against ABO blood group antigens (anti-A, anti-B), Rh antigens (anti-D, anti-c or anti-E), Kell antigens (mainly anti-K), Kidd antigens (anti-Jk^a or anti-Jk^b), Duffy antigens (anti-Fy^a) and antigens of the MNS blood group system (including anti-U). ABO HDFN due to anti-A or anti-B antibodies is the most common type of immune haemolytic disease in the perinatal period but is usually a fairly mild disease.[47]

Table 2.4 Diagnostic clues to haemolysis in neonates with anaemia and/or jaundice

Increased reticulocyte count	Usually $>150 \times 10^9$/l
Direct Coombs test	Positive if immune
Jaundice	Unconjugated hyperbilirubinaemia
Blood film	Red blood cell morphology usually abnormal and provides helpful guide to likely diagnosis
Family history and ethnic origin	Often useful, including history of jaundice, anaemia, splenectomy, transfusions or gallstones

Table 2.5 Causes of neonatal haemolytic anaemias

Causes of haemolysis in neonates with anaemia	Useful diagnostic tests
Immune – haemolytic disease of the newborn	Coombs test Blood group of mother and baby Neonatal blood film (spherocytes, polychromasia) Maternal red cell antibody screen Maternal immune (IgG) anti-A/anti-B (if ABO haemolytic disease suspected) Eluate of antibody from neonatal red cells
Red cell membrane disorders	Neonatal blood film Parental FBC, reticulocyte count and blood films EMA dye-binding test (largely replaced osmotic fragility testing) Molecular analysis for pathogenic variants in genes known to cause primary red cell membrane disorders (e.g. *SPTA1*, *SPTB*, *EPB41*)
Red cell enzymopathies	Neonatal blood film Parental FBC, reticulocyte count and blood films G6PD enzyme activity assay PK enzyme activity assay (helpful to assay levels in parental samples at the same time) Molecular analysis for pathogenic variants in genes known to cause red cell enzymopathies (e.g. *PKLR*, *GPI*)
Haemoglobinopathies	Neonatal blood film HPLC Family studies if results difficult to interpret Consider mass spectrometry or molecular analysis of globin genes if haemoglobinopathy strongly suspected but no diagnosis on HPLC (e.g. unstable haemoglobin)
Other inherited disorders, e.g. congenital thrombotic thrombocytopenic purpura, congenital haemolytic uraemic syndrome	Neonatal blood film Plasma ADAMTS13 activity assay Molecular analysis for pathogenic variants in genes known to cause congenital TTP (ADAMTS13) or HUS (cobalamin C)
Infections associated with neonatal haemolysis	Blood film Microbiological tests for neonatal bacterial infection or congenital bacterial, viral or parasitic infection Cytomegalovirus Disseminated herpesvirus Adenovirus Rubella* Syphilis Malaria Toxoplasmosis
Microangiopathic, e.g. Kaposiform haemangioendothelioma with or without Kasabach–Merritt phenomenon; vascular anomalies (renal artery stenosis, coarctation of the aorta)	Blood count and coagulation screen to look for consumptive coagulopathy Blood film Imaging

* Equivocal evidence to support haemolysis as a cause of anaemia.
EMA, eosin-5-maleimide; FBC, full blood count; G6PD, glucose-6-phosphate; HPLC, high performance liquid chromatography; HUS, haemolytic uraemic syndrome; Ig, immunoglobulin: PK, pyruvate kinase; TTP, thrombotic thrombocytopenic purpura.

In contrast, anti-D is the most frequent alloantibody that causes severe haemolytic anaemia, affecting 1 in 1000 pregnancies even in countries where routine antenatal and postnatal anti-D prophylaxis has been widely implemented.[48] Anti-K antibodies are less common but can cause severe fetal and neonatal anaemia because they inhibit erythropoiesis as well as causing haemolysis.[49]

ABO haemolytic disease of the fetus and newborn This condition is almost always confined to offspring of women of blood group O or A_2 who are group A or group B. In recent years, several cases of unanticipated ABO HDFN have arisen in neonates born to surrogate mothers, for example in a baby of blood group AB who was born to a group O surrogate mother and whose biological mother was group B.[50] ABO alloimmunisation of the fetus is confined to the 1% of group O women who have high-titre immunoglobulin G (IgG) antibodies. In contrast to HDFN due to other red cell antibodies, ABO HDFN frequently occurs during a first pregnancy and the recurrence rate in subsequent pregnancies is very high (almost 90%).[51] In infants of European ancestry, haemolysis due to anti-A is more common (1 in 150 births) than that due to anti-B, which is more common in infants of African ancestry.[52] In contrast to cases due to Rh antibodies, where anaemia usually accompanies jaundice, ABO haemolysis is usually characterised by hyperbilirubinaemia without significant anaemia. Several case reports, as well as personal experience, suggest that haemolysis due to anti-B tends to be more severe than that due to anti-A and may even cause hydrops fetalis[53,54] (Case 2.3, see page 93). The blood film in ABO haemolytic disease characteristically shows very large numbers of spherocytes with little or no increase in NRBC (Figs 2.8 and 2.9) (Table 2.6).

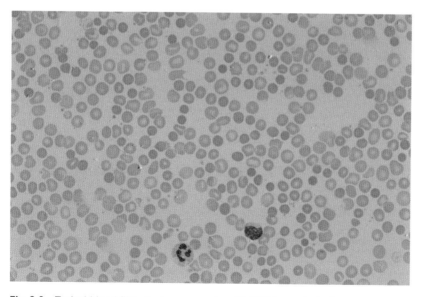

Fig. 2.8 Typical blood film of a term neonate with ABO haemolytic disease of the fetus and newborn (HDFN) showing large numbers of spherocytes. Note that no nucleated red blood cells (NRBC) are visible in this image and very few were seen on other fields. MGG, ×40.

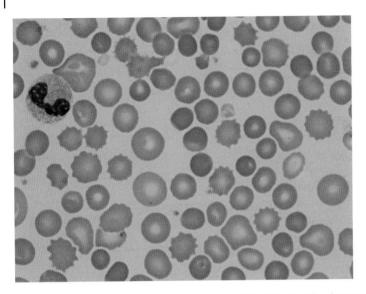

Fig. 2.9 Blood film of a preterm neonate with ABO HDFN showing large numbers of spherocytes as well as some macrocytes, echinocytes and polychromasia (note the absence of NRBC). MGG, ×100.

Table 2.6 Laboratory features of ABO and Rh haemolytic disease of the fetus and newborn

	ABO	Rh
Haemoglobin concentration	Usually normal	Usually reduced and falls rapidly in first few hours or days
Coombs test	Occasionally negative	Always positive
Reticulocytes	Usually increased	Usually increased
Erythroblastosis	Uncommon	Nearly always
Spherocytes	Easily seen on blood films in very large numbers	Often inconspicuous
Causative antibodies	Anti-A (usually mild) Anti-B (sometimes severe)	Anti-D (often severe) Anti-c (often severe) Anti-C Anti-E

Rh haemolytic disease of the fetus and newborn Rh haemolytic disease of the fetus and newborn remains the most common cause of severe disease.[55] In neonates, Rh HDFN presents with early-onset, rapidly worsening jaundice together with progressive anaemia. In severe cases there is hepatosplenomegaly. Occasionally, affected neonates develop widespread skin deposits due to extramedullary haemopoiesis, giving an appearance described as 'blueberry muffin' baby,[56] although this finding is not specific to Rh HDFN as it is also seen in other conditions with extramedullary haemopoiesis, such as congenital

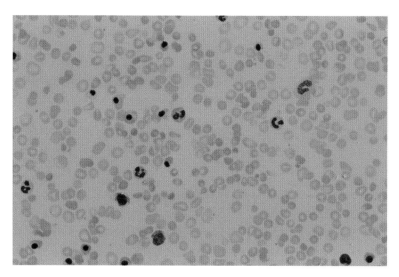

Fig. 2.10 Blood film of a term neonate with severe Rh HDFN showing large numbers of NRBC, including two early normoblasts, polychromasia and some spherocytes (compare with Fig. 2.8). MGG, ×40.

leukaemia (see Figs 3.26 and 3.28). In contrast to ABO HDFN, the blood film in Rh HDFN typically shows marked polychromasia due to reticulocytosis, large numbers of circulating erythroblasts, which are often dyserythropoietic, and variable numbers of spherocytes (Figs 2.10–2.12) (see Table 2.6). In the most severe cases, Rh HDFN, presents *in utero* with rapidly progressive anaemia and hydrops fetalis.[52]

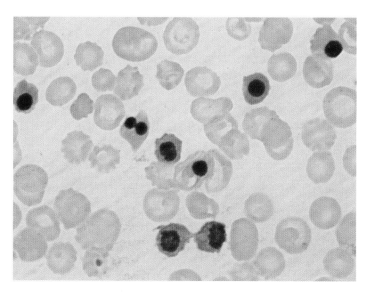

Fig. 2.11 Blood film of a preterm neonate with Rh HDFN showing large numbers of erythroblasts, including several dyserythropoietic cells, and marked polychromasia (note the lower frequency of spherocytes compared with ABO HDFN). MGG, ×100.

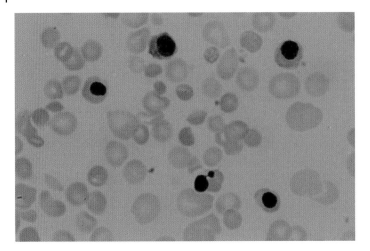

Fig. 2.12 Blood film of a term baby with severe Rh HDFN showing dyserythropoietic NRBC. MGG, ×100.

Management of haemolytic disease of the fetus and newborn Effective management of pregnancies affected by red cell alloimmunisation relies on close cooperation between obstetric, neonatal and haematology teams and many countries have developed national guidelines to ensure best practice for management of the fetus and the neonate.[57–59] For fetuses at risk, monitoring to assess the degree of anaemia using cerebral middle cerebral artery (MCA) Doppler velocity measurements is typically performed every 1–2 weeks. Once anaemia is suspected, based on increasing MCA velocity, invasive testing via cordocentesis is performed to obtain an accurate measure of the fetal Hb/haematocrit, and IUT and/or delivery is planned, depending on the gestation, previous history and fetal wellbeing.[52,59]

All neonates at risk should have cord blood taken for measurement of Hb and bilirubin and a Coombs test, and should remain in hospital or under close outpatient supervision until hyperbilirubinaemia and/or anaemia have been properly managed.[57–59] Neonates with haemolysis due to Rh HDFN should receive phototherapy from birth, because the bilirubin can rise steeply; this avoids the need for exchange transfusion in some infants. In haemolytic disease due to anti-K, anaemia is usually more prominent than jaundice and only minimal phototherapy may be necessary despite severe anaemia.[60] ABO HDFN usually just requires phototherapy, as significant anaemia is uncommon.

The indications for exchange transfusion in HDFN are:

- severe anaemia (Hb <100 g/l at birth); and/or
- severe or rapidly increasing hyperbilirubinaemia.[61]

Irradiated blood must be used for infants who have previously received IUT, to prevent the risk of transfusion-associated graft-versus-host disease (TA-GvHD). IVIg has been used to reduce the need for exchange transfusion but the value of this approach remains to be proven in clinical trials.[62] Neonates with haemolytic disease due to anti-Rh antibodies may develop 'late' anaemia at a few weeks of age, requiring 'top-up' transfusion. Late anaemia occurs particularly in neonates who have received one or more IUTs.[63] This is seen both in HDFN due to anti-D and that due to anti-K and is attributable, at least in part, to suppression by transfusion of the anaemia-induced compensatory increase in erythropoiesis[64] and possibly also by red cell alloantibodies present in maternal breast milk.[65] Although recombinant EPO has been reported to reduce the need for top-up transfusion for late anaemia, it is not effective when haemolysis is brisk and there are no data from randomised trials to support the routine use of EPO in this situation.[66] Folic acid (500 μg/kg daily) should be given to all babies with haemolysis at least until they reach 3 months of age,[60] but iron supplementation is unnecessary as the vast majority of neonates with red cell alloimmunisation have iron overload at birth.[67]

Neonatal haemolytic anaemia due to red cell membrane disorders

A number of genetic red cell membrane disorders can present in the neonatal period with haemolytic anaemia (Table 2.7). In neonates, haemolysis due to a red cell membrane disorder usually presents with jaundice, with or without anaemia, and the blood film shows abnormal red cell morphology. The changes in red cell morphology are often very characteristic and allow a provisional diagnosis to be made simply by reviewing the blood film. As for other genetic red cell disorders, the family history is usually extremely useful. In the majority of cases, it is possible to elicit a history of neonatal jaundice or anaemia in several generations of close family members or sometimes of splenectomy or cholecystectomy during childhood or early adulthood. A summary of the main features of red cell membrane disorders presenting with anaemia and/or jaundice is shown in Table 2.7. It is important to note that occasional cases of coinheritance of a red cell membrane disorder with a genetic defect in bilirubin metabolism, such as Gilbert syndrome, may have very severe hyperbilirubinaemia in the neonatal period.[68]

The main clues to the type of red cell membrane disorder are the family history and the characteristic shape of the red cells in a blood film. Many of the classical biochemical and functional tests used for the diagnosis of red cell membrane disorders, such as red cell membrane electrophoresis and osmotic fragility, have largely been replaced by molecular analysis using next generation sequencing, which is generally much more precise. However, newer functional tests, such as flow cytometric analysis of eosin-5-maleimide (EMA) dye binding or osmotic gradient ektacytometry, still play an important role, especially in cases where the pathogenicity of newly identified molecular variants in red cell membrane genes is uncertain.[3,69–71]

Hereditary spherocytosis   Hereditary spherocytosis is the most common of the red cell membrane disorders causing symptomatic anaemia, affecting 1 in 2000 to 1 in 5000 live births to parents of northern European extraction.[72] The disorder is caused by mutations in one or more of five genes that encode red cell cytoskeleton and transmembrane proteins: α spectrin (*SPTA1*), β spectrin (*SPTB*), ankyrin-1 (*ANK1*), band 3 anion transport protein (*SLC4A1*) and erythrocyte membrane protein band 4.2 (*EPB42*) (reviewed in reference 70). In 75% of families, hereditary spherocytosis is inherited in an autosomal dominant fashion. In the remaining cases, inheritance is non-dominant and there is usually no family history, either because of autosomal recessive inheritance or because of the presence of a *de novo* autosomal dominant mutation. Autosomal recessive hereditary spherocytosis can be

Table 2.7 Red cell membrane disorders presenting with anaemia and/or jaundice in the neonatal period

Condition	Diagnostic clues and useful tests
Hereditary spherocytosis	
Autosomal dominant hereditary spherocytosis	Spherocytosis with negative Coombs test and/or maternal blood Group A, B or AB
	Usually a strong family history – of HS, gallstones and/or neonatal jaundice or anaemia
	Relatively common (1 in 2000–5000 in White Europeans)
Autosomal recessive hereditary spherocytosis	Presents with severe neonatal anaemia and/or hydrops fetalis
	Usually no family history of anaemia or jaundice
	Some patients with bi-allelic *SLC4A1* mutations have renal tubular acidosis
Hereditary elliptocytosis	
Hereditary pyropoikilocytosis	Anaemia usually marked in neonatal period
	Due to microspherocytes and other schistocytes, the MCV is typically very low (<70 fl) and platelet counts may be artefactually high
	Homozygous/compound heterozygous for α spectrin variants
	Often no family history but one or both parents usually have blood film typical of HE
Hereditary elliptocytosis with infantile poikilocytosis	Elliptocytosis with marked poikilocytosis and anaemia (Hb is normal in typical common HE)
	Heterozygous for an HE α spectrin variant common in Black Africans
	Often no family history but one parent usually has blood films typical of HE
Southeast Asian ovalocytosis	
Southeast Asian ovalocytosis	Blood film shows stomatocytosis with a population of macro-ovalocytes
	Caused by heterozygous mutations in *SLC4A1*
	Jaundice common
	Mild (or no) anaemia; often have increased MCH
	Family history, including origin from areas where the disease is prevalent (e.g. Thailand)
Hereditary stomatocytosis	
Overhydrated hereditary stomatocytosis	May present with hydrops fetalis
	MCHC may be decreased or normal
	Blood film shows stomatocytes
	Pseudohyperkalaemia (when sample stored at 4°C overnight)

Hb, haemoglobin concentration; HE, hereditary elliptocytosis; HS, hereditary spherocytosis; MCH, mean cell haemoglobin; MCHC, mean cell haemoglobin concentration; MCV, mean cell volume.

Table 2.8 Genes mutated in autosomal recessive and autosomal dominant or sporadic hereditary spherocytosis (HS)

Gene mutated in HS	Proportion of cases of HS*	Autosomal recessive HS	Autosomal dominant or sporadic HS
Alpha spectrin (*SPTA1*)	<5%	Yes	No
Beta spectrin (*SPTB*)	15–30%	Yes	Yes
Ankyrin-1 (*ANK1*)	30–60%	Yes	Yes
Band 3 (*SLC4A1*)	20–30%	Yes	Yes
Band 4.2 (*EPB42*)	<5%	Yes	No

* Proportion of cases in Europe and the USA; these frequencies are very different in the Japanese population, where 45–50% of HS cases are due to mutations in *EPB42*.
Data summarised from reference 73.
HS, hereditary spherocytosis.

caused by bi-allelic mutations in any of the five membrane genes, whereas autosomal dominant disease is seen only for mutations in *SPTB*, *ANK1* and *SLC4A1* (Table 2.8).[73] The autosomal recessive forms of hereditary spherocytosis are typically very severe, presenting as hydrops fetalis or severe neonatal haemolytic anaemia (see Table 2.7).[74–76]

Most neonates with hereditary spherocytosis will have jaundice, although this is not usually severe and is easily controlled with phototherapy. However, neonates with hereditary spherocytosis who coinherit the trait for Gilbert syndrome, a common polymorphism in the promoter region of the uridine diphosphate–glucuronosyltransferase gene (*UGT1A1*), often develop severe jaundice and may need exchange transfusion to prevent the development of kernicterus.[77,78] The Hb in hereditary spherocytosis is usually normal at birth but around one-third of neonates will develop significant anaemia in the neonatal period.[79] The anaemia is usually moderate (70–100 g/l).

The diagnosis of hereditary spherocytosis may be made from the neonatal blood film alone where the family history is known, the film is good quality and other causes of spherocytosis have been excluded. Typically, the blood film in neonates with hereditary spherocytosis shows spherocytes with little or no polychromasia (Figs 2.13 and 2.14). Only one-third of neonates with hereditary spherocytosis will have a reticulocyte count of >10% and circulating NRBC are not usually increased unless there is moderate or severe anaemia.[80] The diagnosis of hereditary spherocytosis is sometimes difficult in neonates, especially in milder cases, because low numbers of spherocytes may be seen in healthy babies for the first few weeks of life. In addition, the blood film typically has an appearance identical to that of ABO HDFN (see Fig. 2.14b). Although the Coombs test is nearly always positive in ABO HDFN, occasional neonates will have both hereditary spherocytosis and ABO incompatibility. For these reasons, it is advisable to confirm suspected cases of hereditary spherocytosis. The most reliable and widely used method, which has been extensively validated in neonatal samples, is the EMA binding test. This is a rapid, flow cytometry-based test that measures the uptake of the fluorescent EMA by band 3 in the red cell membrane. Reduced EMA dye binding is a very sensitive and specific screening test for certain red cell membrane defects, which is positive in about 90% of cases of hereditary

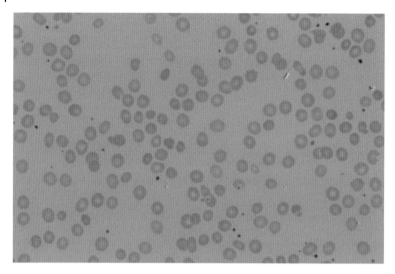

Fig. 2.13 Blood film of a neonate with hereditary spherocytosis showing spherocytes and one button-mushroom poikilocyte. MGG, ×50.

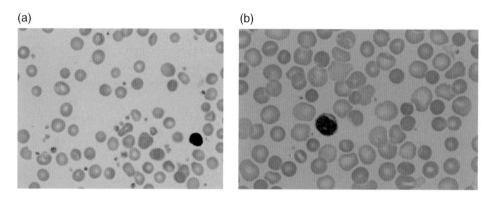

Fig. 2.14 (a) Blood film of a neonate with hereditary spherocytosis showing moderate numbers of spherocytes (note the absence of polychromasia and NRBC in this case where the haemolysis was very mild). MGG, ×100. (b) Blood film of a neonate with ABO HDFN showing almost identical appearance with moderate numbers of spherocytes. MGG, ×100.

spherocytosis, including neonates.[81,82] In most cases no other diagnostic tests will be required. However, in difficult cases, for example where the clinical features are atypical and/or the family history is either unavailable or does not fit the clinical picture, further investigations should be considered, including next generation sequencing.[70]

The management of hereditary spherocytosis depends on the severity of the anaemia and the jaundice. For those neonates that do develop anaemia, up to 75% will require one or two transfusions during the neonatal period before a transfusion-free plateau Hb of 80–100 g/l is achieved after several months.[79] Jaundice is normally readily controlled by phototherapy and exchange transfusion is rarely required. Folic acid supplementation (500 μg/kg daily) is recommended for all affected infants with evidence of chronic haemolysis. The majority of children and adults with hereditary spherocytosis are not transfusion-dependent. However, chronic haemolysis, even when mild, predisposes these patients to a number of long-term complications including gallstones, splenomegaly, leg ulcers, parvovirus-associated red cell aplastic crisis and episodic acute anaemia due to haemolytic crises, usually provoked by infection (reviewed in detail in reference 73).

Hereditary elliptocytosis and hereditary pyropoikilocytosis These disorders are caused by autosomal dominant mutations in the genes encoding α or β spectrin (*SPTA1, SPTB*) or erythrocyte membrane protein band 4.1 (*EPB41*).[70] The prevalence of hereditary elliptocytosis has been estimated at 1 in 2000 to 1 in 4000 of the population but this varies considerably in different parts of the world.[73] For example, hereditary elliptocytosis is more common in areas of endemic malaria, particularly in people of African and Mediterranean origin.[83]

The clinical manifestations of hereditary elliptocytosis and related syndromes are complex in that at least three different types of disease manifestation are recognised; any of these may present in the neonatal period. The most frequent presentation, particularly in neonates of African descent, is common hereditary elliptocytosis, an autosomal dominant condition which rarely has any clinical manifestations apart from the presence of elliptocytes in the blood film. The diagnosis in the neonatal period is therefore made as an incidental finding when a blood film is reviewed for another reason, such as screening for the presence of infection. No further investigations or haematological follow-up are necessary and folate supplementation is not indicated.

The more severe forms of hereditary elliptocytosis are summarised in Table 2.7. Neonates who are homozygous or compound heterozygous for hereditary elliptocytosis mutations have severe, transfusion-dependent haemolytic anaemia that presents in fetal life or within a few days of birth. Almost all of these neonates have hereditary pyropoikilocytosis (HPP), which is typically caused by bi-allelic (homozygous or compound heterozygous) variants, especially in *SPTA1*, that disrupt spectrin self-association.[84,85] Rare cases of HPP caused by bi-allelic *SPTB* mutations[86] or digenic inheritance of *SPTA1* and *SPTB* mutations have been reported.[85,87,88]

Hereditary pyropoikilocytosis is the most common form of severe hereditary elliptocytosis. It presents in the neonatal period with marked, persistent transfusion-dependent haemolytic anaemia. The diagnosis is usually easily made from the low mean cell volume (MCV), which may be as low as 25 fl, and the blood film, which show extreme poikilocytosis with large numbers of bizarre, fragmented red cells, microspherocytes and elliptocytes (Fig. 2.15a). Examination of the parental blood films is very helpful since one or both parents typically has common hereditary elliptocytosis (Figs 2.15b,c).[89] It is important to note that HPP can also occur when both parental blood films appear to be normal, for example as a result of a *de novo* mutation in combination with a silent spectrin mutation, such as the α^{LELY} variant (Case 2.4, see page 95). The treatment of neonates with HPP is red cell transfusion. Transfusions should continue on a regular basis until the child is old enough to undergo splenectomy, to which there is an excellent response with all patients rendered transfusion-independent.[85]

Hereditary elliptocytosis with infantile poikilocytosis is the second most severe form of hereditary elliptocytosis in the neonatal period. It occurs in a very small proportion of

(a)

(b)

(c)

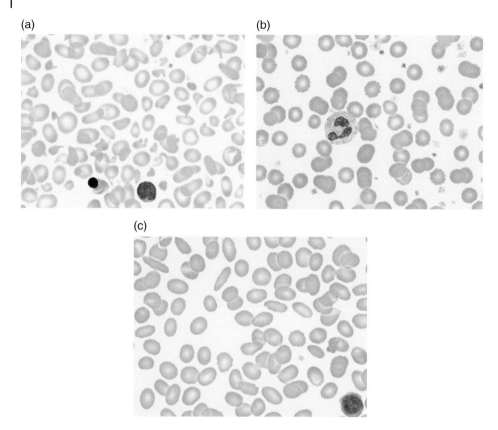

Fig. 2.15 Blood films of a neonate with hereditary pyropoikilocytosis and her parents. The baby was noted to be jaundiced at 36 hours of age and on day 5 had a haemoglobin concentration (Hb) of 133 g/l, a low mean cell volume (MCV) of 85 fl and a reticulocyte count of 125–175 × 10⁹/l. (a) Blood film of the neonate showing marked anisopoikilocytosis with ovalocytes, elliptocytes and schistocytes; a single NRBC and occasional spherocytes can also be seen. (b) Blood film of the mother who was haematologically normal but was heterozygous for the low expression allele *SPTA1* c.[5572C>G:6531-12C>T]; p. (Leu1858Val), known as α spectrin^LELY (low expression Lyon allele). (c) Blood film of the father who had hereditary elliptocytosis and was heterozygous for *SPTA1* c.460_462dup; p. (Leu155dup). The neonate showed compound heterozygosity for these two *SPTA1* mutations. MGG, ×100.

neonates with common hereditary elliptocytosis due to mono-allelic α spectrin variants. Typically, affected neonates have moderately severe haemolytic anaemia with marked poikilocytosis as well as elliptocytes. Occasionally the jaundice is severe enough to require exchange transfusion. Most neonates require red cell transfusion for anaemia but become transfusion-independent as the poikilocytosis and anaemia resolve over the first 3–6 months of life; apart from elliptocytes in the blood film the blood results are completely normal by the age of 12 months. The diagnosis is suggested when one, but not both, parents have typical common hereditary elliptocytosis with elliptocytes in the blood film and no anaemia or jaundice. However, diagnosis is often finalised only when the natural history confirms that this is not a case of HPP and/or molecular diagnosis is performed.

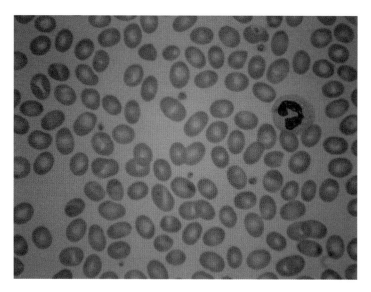

Fig. 2.16 Blood film of an older patient with Southeast Asian ovalocytosis showing ovalocytes, macro-ovalocytes and distinctive stomatocytes. MGG, ×100.

Southeast Asian ovalocytosis This condition is characterised by striking morphological abnormalities in the blood of children and adults with ovalocytes, macro-ovalocytes and distinctive stomatocytes (Fig. 2.16). It results from homozygosity for a mutation in *SLC4A1*, which causes haematological abnormalities but without clinical consequences beyond the neonatal period. However, about half of heterozygous neonates have haemolytic anaemia and hyperbilirubinaemia.[90] Homozygosity causes hydrops fetalis and usually intrauterine death.[91]

Neonatal haemolysis due to red cell enzymopathies

There are many aspects of the clinical and haematological presentation of the inherited red cell enzymopathies that are unique to the neonatal period. These differences are important for tailoring our diagnostic approach in this age group and also for our understanding of their clinical and haematological impact. First, from a diagnostic point of view, the initial presentation of these disorders in neonates is usually with jaundice. Anaemia, if it occurs, is not usually present at birth and many neonates never develop anaemia even when the jaundice is severe. Secondly, in contrast to red cell membrane disorders, there are usually no diagnostic changes on the neonatal blood film. Thirdly, with the exception of glucose-6-phosphate dehydrogenase (G6PD) deficiency, inherited red cell enzyme disorders are rare. G6PD deficiency, on the other hand, is common, with millions of affected individuals worldwide. Importantly, the G6PD gene is on the X chromosome and therefore the vast majority of neonates with G6PD deficiency are male. Furthermore, the geographical distribution of G6PD deficiency maps to the prevalence of malaria and therefore most, but not all, affected neonates are of African, Mediterranean, Asian or Arabic descent.

Although G6PD deficiency is by far the most common of the inherited red cell enzymo-pathies that present in the neonatal period, awareness of the rarer disorders is extremely important as they are often difficult to diagnose and yet can be associated with very severe disease (Table 2.9).[92]

Table 2.9   Red cell enzymopathies presenting with neonatal anaemia and/or jaundice

Red cell enzymopathies	Diagnostic clues and useful tests
Glucose-6-phosphate dehydrogenase deficiency (*G6PD* gene)	Neonatal jaundice, often severe, despite normal blood film and Hb, presenting in the first 5 days of life in a male infant
	Mother typically of African, Caribbean, Mediterranean, Arabic or Indian subcontinent origin
	May also present in neonates a few weeks of age with sudden and profound drop in Hb due to acute oxidative haemolysis, often in association with infection (or drugs/chemicals)
	Family history of anaemia usually absent but there may be a history of neonatal jaundice
Pyruvate kinase deficiency (*PK* gene)	Family history of anaemia, often severe and sometimes transfusion-dependent
	May present with neonatal hepatic failure and severe cholestasis
	Males and females equally affected
	No ethnic predisposition
Infantile pyknocytosis	Sudden onset of severe anaemia at 2–4 weeks of age, typically with Hb drop of 40–50 g/l over a few days; transfusion often required (usually only 1–2 transfusions)
	More common in preterm babies
	May occur in twins/siblings but otherwise no family history
	Self-limiting and confined to the neonatal period
	Blood film shows features of oxidative haemolysis but G6PD and PK activity are normal
	No genetic cause identified; glutathione peroxidase levels are often reduced
Rare enzyme deficiencies (gene mutated): Glucose phosphate isomerase (*GPI*) Hexokinase (*HK*) Pyrimidine-5′-nucleotidase (*NT5C3A*) Phosphofructokinase (*PFK*) Phosphoglycerate kinase (*PGK*) Triosephosphate isomerase (*TPI*)	Chronic non-spherocytic haemolytic anaemia Family history of severe, often transfusion-dependent haemolytic anaemia and/or consanguinity Associated features, e.g. neurological problems

G6PD, glucose-6-phosphate dehydrogenase; Hb, haemoglobin concentration; PK, pyruvate kinase.

Glucose-6-phosphate dehydrogenase deficiency The prevalence of G6PD deficiency is particularly high in individuals from Central Africa (20% of males) and the Mediterranean (10% of males) but is also seen in the Indian subcontinent, the Far East and the Middle East (reviewed in reference 93). In neonates, G6PD deficiency typically presents with jaundice during the first few days of life, with a peak incidence on day 2 or 3.[94] Neonatal jaundice due to G6PD deficiency is often severe, despite an Hb that is normal or only slightly reduced and severe anaemia is rare.[95,96] Although the majority of affected neonates are boys, female carriers are sometimes identified through neonatal jaundice screens because these babies also occasionally develop severe neonatal jaundice.[97] The blood film is usually completely normal with no irregularly contracted cells, reticulocytosis or erythroblastosis. However, in the small proportion of neonates who develop anaemia due to G6PD deficiency, the blood film shows typical changes of oxidative haemolysis (Fig. 2.17).

It is not clear why some, but not all, G6PD-deficient neonates develop neonatal jaundice as this does not appear to correlate with the level of G6PD enzyme activity in the red cells, although this is controversial.[97] The pathogenesis of the jaundice is also unclear as most babies with G6PD deficiency have no evidence of haemolysis. Current views are that the jaundice is likely to be of hepatic origin and to reflect inefficient bilirubin conjugation rather than haemolysis.[98]

The diagnosis of G6PD deficiency is made by assaying G6PD on a peripheral blood sample, the result being interpreted in the light of any elevation of the reticulocyte count above normal neonatal levels and the higher normal range in neonates. It is essential to perform the G6PD assay before any red cell transfusions are given (or once any transfused cells have been cleared from the circulation, which may take up to 8 weeks). Mutation analysis of the *G6PD* gene should be considered for atypical cases – for

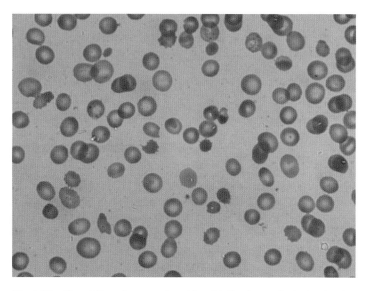

Fig. 2.17 Blood film of a neonate with oxidative haemolysis due to glucose-6-phosphate dehydrogenase (G6PD) deficiency showing irregularly contracted cells and a bite cell. MGG, ×40.

example those presenting with severe anaemia where there is no evidence of either HDFN or red cell membranopathy. Some mutations are associated with chronic non-spherocytic hemolytic anaemia and mutation analysis is especially useful for establishing the diagnosis in these cases.

Management of neonatal G6PD deficiency requires close monitoring of the bilirubin to prevent kernicterus, particularly when interactions with other risk factors for neonatal hyperbilirubinaemia, such as Gilbert syndrome, HDFN or hereditary spherocytosis are present. If exchange transfusion is required for severe hyperbilirubinaemia, conventional guidelines for exchange transfusion can be followed.[61] It is important to provide information to the parents/carers of affected neonates as to which specific medicines, chemicals and foods may precipitate haemolysis (these are listed in Table 2.10). In countries where malaria is endemic, G6PD deficiency should be excluded before giving primaquine for malaria eradication due to the high risk of drug-induced haemolysis in affected G6PD-deficient individuals. It is also useful to be aware that acute haemolysis due to exposure of neonates to naphthalene-containing mothballs has been reported[99] and that consumption of fava beans or quinine-containing drinks by breastfeeding mothers may cause haemolysis in G6PD-deficient neonates.[100,101] Folate supplementation is not routinely indicated in G6PD-deficient neonates because, in the vast majority of cases, G6PD deficiency does not cause chronic haemolysis. However, for those infants with one of the uncommon variants of G6PD deficiency associated with chronic non-spherocytic haemolytic anaemia, such as G6PD Volendam,[102] folic acid supplements should be given as described above for the red cell membrane disorders.

Table 2.10 Drugs and chemicals that may precipitate haemolysis in neonates and infants with G6PD deficiency

Chemicals	Methylene blue
	Naphthalene (mothballs)
	Fava beans (mother)*
Antibiotics	Nitrofurantoin*
	Some sulfonamides, e.g. sulfasalazine*
	Quinolones (ciprofloxacin*, nalidixic acid*)
	Chloramphenicol[†]
	Trimethoprim*[†]
	Isoniazid
Antimalarials	Primaquine*
	Chloroquine[†]
	Quinine[†]
Other medication	Rasburicase
	Dapsone*
	Aspirin*[†]

* Avoid in breastfeeding mothers.
[†] Not absolutely contraindicated but use with caution.

Pyruvate kinase deficiency In contrast to G6PD deficiency, pyruvate kinase (PK) deficiency is fairly rare, with an estimated incidence of 1 in 20 000 in Caucasians.[92] As a result, even large neonatal centres are only likely to identify one case of PK deficiency every 5 years. PK deficiency is transmitted in an autosomal recessive fashion and is due to bi-allelic mutations in the *PKLR* gene that encodes the PK enzyme.[103] More than 120 different *PKLR* variants have been described and the frequency of novel pathogenic variants that have not previously been reported is high (approximately 20%).[104] PK deficiency is clinically heterogeneous, varying from anaemia severe enough to cause hydrops fetalis to a mild unconjugated hyperbilirubinaemia (Case 2.5, see page 98). However, the *PKLR* genotype does not seem to correlate with the frequency of complications *in utero* or in the newborn period.[104] A recent study of the natural history of PK deficiency in over 250 patients found that perinatal complications were common in PK deficiency, including anaemia that required transfusion and hyperbilirubinemia as well as hydrops fetalis and prematurity.[103] This study clearly shows that jaundice is a common finding in neonates with PK deficiency as the majority of neonates (93%) were treated with phototherapy and almost half (46%) required exchange transfusion.[103] In severe cases, extramedullary haemopoiesis, presenting as a typical violaceous, papular facial rash, has been reported.[105]

The diagnosis of PK deficiency is made by measuring pretransfusion red cell PK activity. In mild cases enzyme activity may be only modestly reduced and in such cases it can be useful to assay PK levels in the parents. However, mutation analysis of the *PKLR* gene is increasingly used as the definitive diagnostic tool either by directly sequencing the gene or as part of a targeted next generation sequencing gene panel.[3,104] The blood film is sometimes distinctive, with small numbers of markedly echinocytic cells (Fig. 2.18), but more often shows non-specific changes of non-spherocytic haemolysis. Occasional cases of

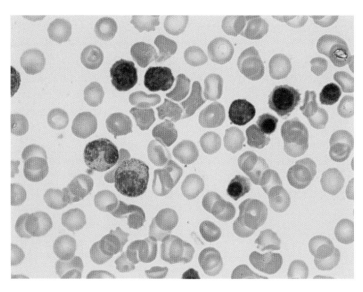

Fig. 2.18 Blood film of a neonate with pyruvate kinase (PK) deficiency showing marked erythroblastosis and polychromasia and occasional echinocytes. There is also left shift. MGG, ×100.

PK deficiency present with extreme and persistent neonatal hyperbilirubinemia and hepatic failure with or without evidence of haemolysis,[106] making the diagnosis extremely difficult.[103]

Management of PK deficiency in the neonatal period depends on the severity of the jaundice and anaemia. As mentioned above, the majority of affected neonates will require phototherapy for jaundice and almost half will require exchange transfusion. Just over 50% of children remain transfusion-dependent.[107] For those that are transfusion-independent, folic acid supplements should be given to prevent deficiency due to chronic haemolysis.[103] Splenectomy later in childhood reduces the transfusion requirement in 90% of cases. However, management of PK deficiency in children is likely to change in the near future with the promising results of a new small molecule allosteric activator of the PK enzyme (mitapivat), which has been shown to increase red cell enzyme activity and Hb in PK-deficient adults.[108]

Infantile pyknocytosis   This poorly understood condition causes acute haemolysis confined to the neonatal period and accounts for about 10% of cases due to red cell enzyme deficiencies.[109] In the original report of this disorder, infantile pyknocytosis was defined as the presence of 'distorted, irregular, densely stained erythrocytes, presenting with several to many spiny projections' in a neonate with self-limiting acute haemolytic anaemia.[110] These morphological features, and the natural history, strongly point to a red cell enzyme defect. However, the genetic basis of infantile pyknocytosis remains unknown. Recent targeted next generation sequencing has excluded mutations in most of the red cell enzyme genes associated with neonatal haemolytic anaemia, including *PKLR*, *G6PD*, hexokinase (*HK1*), phosphoglycerate kinase (*PGK1*), phosphofructokinase (*PFKL*), glucose phosphate isomerase (*GPI*), triosephosphate isomerase (*TPI1*) and *NT5C3A*, the gene encoding pyrimidine-5′-nucleotidase.[111] In many cases affected neonates are found to have reduced levels of glutathione peroxidase (reference 112 and unpublished data) but no mutations in the *GPX1* gene encoding the enzyme have been reported, even when specifically tested.[111] Infantile pyknocytosis is more common in preterm neonates and when it occurs in twins, both are usually affected. The anaemia associated with infantile pyknocytosis is often moderately severe and may require one or two red cell transfusions; it then gradually resolves by the age of 2–3 months. The blood film typically shows changes of oxidative haemolysis during the neonatal period but returns to normal as the haemolysis resolves (Case 2.6, see page 100). Measurement of glutathione peroxidase levels in affected neonates may be useful (parental levels are normal) but the diagnosis is usually easily made from the blood film and natural history. There are no reports of recurrence of haemolysis beyond the neonatal period in babies with infantile pyknocytosis and care should be taken to exclude other causes of haemolytic anaemia in any cases where the haemolysis does not resolve, or recurs, after the age of 3 months.

Other red cell enzymopathies   The other red cell enzymopathies reported to present in the neonatal period are all rare and are shown in Table 2.9. Several of these disorders cause very severe fetal and/or neonatal haemolytic anaemia. Glucose phosphate isomerase (GPI) and hexokinase (HK) deficiencies, which are autosomal recessive conditions, have both been reported to present with severe neonatal haemolytic anaemia including hydrops fetalis.[113–116] Deficiency of pyrimidine-5′-nucleotidase due to mutations in the *NT5C3A* gene usually causes mild chronic haemolytic anaemia and does not present until adolescence; however, about 15% of cases have neonatal jaundice and this diagnosis should be considered in unexplained neonatal haemolysis where the blood film shows prominent basophilic stippling.[117] As phosphofructokinase (PFK) deficiency can involve red cells, muscle or both, depending on the PFK subunit affected, the disease may manifest as haemolytic anaemia and/or myopathy. In severe cases the myopathy causes death during infancy as a result of respiratory insufficiency and other complications.[118] Phosphoglycerate kinase (PGK) deficiency is a sex-linked disorder that largely affects males and occasionally presents in the neonatal period with jaundice and non-spherocytic haemolytic anaemia. More often PGK deficiency presents in older children and clinically has a variable combination of chronic haemolytic anaemia, developmental delay and myopathy.[119] Triosephosphate isomerase (TPI) deficiency causes neonatal haemolytic anaemia in around one-third of patients. This is important to recognise because the haemolytic anaemia often presents many months before the devastating neurological features of this disorder become apparent.[120]

Other causes of neonatal haemolytic anaemia

Other causes of neonatal haemolytic anaemia are shown in Table 2.5. These include infections, rare extrinsic causes of haemolysis, such as thrombotic thrombocytopenic purpura (TTP) and cavernous haemangiomas (Kasabach–Merritt syndrome). Exposure to oxidant drugs and chemicals can cause haemolysis even in babies without G6PD deficiency. It has been reported, for example, in a neonate exposed to higher than recommended levels of methylene blue during creation of a gastrointestinal anastomosis (Case 2.7, see page 103).[121]

Neonatal haemolytic anaemia due to infection   As well as perinatally acquired bacterial infection, a number of congenital infections have been reported to cause neonatal anaemia via a haemolytic mechanism, including CMV, herpes simplex and rubella viruses, syphilis, malaria and toxoplasmosis (see Table 2.5). While there is good evidence for significant neonatal haemolytic anaemia due to syphilis, malaria and toxoplasmosis, solid evidence of haemolysis due to CMV infection is scanty.

Perinatally acquired syphilis remains a significant clinical problem in many countries, affecting an estimated 713 600–1 575 000 pregnancies worldwide (reviewed in reference 122). Just over half of all neonates born with congenital syphilis will have Coombs-negative haemolytic anaemia, which may persist for weeks after treatment.[122] Although fatal cases are uncommon, severe cases may present with hydrops fetalis.[123] Congenital toxoplasma infection may also present with severe neonatal haemolytic anaemia and/or hydrops fetalis.[124,125] Despite the prevalence of malaria in pregnant women, congenital malaria is surprisingly rare, even in countries where malaria is endemic, and it is exceptionally rare in non-endemic countries,[126,127] perhaps because of protective IgG antibodies in the mother.[128] Congenital malaria presents with anaemia, jaundice, hepatosplenomegaly and non-specific signs such as poor feeding, lethargy and fever.[126,127,129] Typically, the first signs of malaria arise at 10–28 days of age, although presentation within the first few hours or as late as 8 weeks of age has been reported.[130]

CMV has been shown to cause haemolytic anaemia in infants[131] but this seems to be very rare in neonates. In most case series in neonates where anaemia and/or an increased transfusion requirement is reported, there is insufficient evidence to indicate the mechanism of the anaemia and other causes, such as the side effects of anti-viral drugs, may be responsible.[132] In one well-documented case, concomitant CMV infection increased the extent of haemolysis in a neonate with immune haemolytic anaemia secondary to maternal lupus.[133] Similarly, although acute haemolysis has been reported in children with herpes simplex infection[134] and a small proportion of neonates with congenital herpes simplex have anaemia, there is no definite evidence that this is caused by haemolysis.[135] This is also the case for congenital rubella. Neonates with congenital rubella syndrome may have hepatosplenomegaly and jaundice but anaemia is not usually a feature,[136] although older children may develop autoimmune haemolytic anaemia in response to acute rubella infection.[137]

Neonatal anaemia due to extrinsic causes of red cell destruction Neonates may also develop microangiopathic haemolytic anaemia (MAHA) secondary to extrinsic damage to neonatal red cells. The three major types of disorder associated with MAHA in neonates are congenital TTP, atypical haemolytic uraemic syndrome (aHUS) and congenital haemangiomas.

Hereditary TTP typically presents in the neonatal period with severe haemolysis and hyperbilirubinaemia although, as in many very rare disorders, the diagnosis is often delayed by several years (reviewed in reference 138). Hereditary TTP is caused by bi-allelic mutations in the *ADAMTS13* gene.[139] In neonates, severe haemolytic anaemia is the most common presentation together with severe thrombocytopenia and red cell fragmentation seen in the blood film. Over one-third of the cases reported in a recent series required exchange transfusion in the neonatal period due to severe haemolysis in the first 2 days of life.[140] In most of these cases there was a single acute episode of haemolysis and thrombocytopenia; in at least one case the apparent trigger was the altered pattern of blood flow (high sheer stress) through a persistent patent ductus arteriosus, although the trigger for the other cases could not be identified. The diagnosis of inherited TTP should therefore be considered in any neonate with unexplained Coombs-negative severe hyperbilirubinaemia and thrombocytopenia. Infusions of fresh frozen plasma (FFP) are the mainstay of treatment of recurrent episodes of haemolysis and thrombocytopenia in childhood and beyond.[138]

Atypical haemolytic uraemic syndrome is another rare disorder that may present in the neonatal period with MAHA and thrombocytopenia but with the additional problem of acute kidney injury. Most forms of aHUS are associated with dysregulation of the alternative complement pathway and about two-thirds of patients have mutations or likely-pathogenic variants in genes encoding complement pathway proteins, including complement factor H (*CFH*), complement factor I (*CFI*), membrane cofactor protein (encoded by *CD46*), complement factor B (*CFB*) or complement factor 3 (*C3*).[141] As for TTP, the blood film shows red cell fragmentation together with severe thrombocytopenia with no evidence of disseminated intravascular coagulation (DIC) on the coagulation screen. Early diagnosis is important because affected neonates respond well to treatment with the C5 inhibitor ecluzimab.[141–143] A recent report suggests that measurement of the Fragmented Red Cell (FRC) count now available on some blood count analysers may be useful to alert clinicians to a potential diagnosis of aHUS in neonates.[144]

Microangiopathic haemolytic anaemia may also be part of the presentation of a group of disorders known as kaposiform haemangioendotheliomas (KHE) and tufted angiomas, which are rare vascular tumours derived from capillary and lymphatic endothelium.[145] The majority of such tumours affect the extremities or the torso.[146] In 50% of cases these tumours present in the neonatal period and around two-thirds of these will have associated consumptive coagulopathy and thrombocytopenia (known as the Kasabach–Merritt phenomenon [KMP]).[146,147] Although the coagulopathy and thrombocytopenia are the main haematological findings in KMP, some affected neonates do have a microangiopathic anaemia.[148] It is now clear that KMP is confined to cases of KHE and tufted angiomas and is not seen in the more common benign infantile haemangiomas.[147] KHE with KMP rarely, if ever, regresses spontaneously and treatment in the neonatal period is usually with a combination of prednisolone and vincristine.[147] Platelet transfusion should be avoided unless there is active bleeding or a surgical procedure is required.[147]

Neonatal anaemia due to haemoglobinopathies and other microcytic anaemias

Clinically significant haemoglobinopathies that present with anaemia or jaundice in the newborn are summarised in Table 2.11. These are predominantly α thalassemia syndromes and structural defects of the α globin chain or γ thalassaemias and γ globin structural variants. The mechanism of anaemia varies between different haemoglobinopathies and is often multifactorial. The most clinically severe haemoglobinopathies that present in the fetal or neonatal period are α thalassaemia major, in which all four α globin genes are deleted and, uncommonly, haemoglobin H disease, in which three α globin genes are deleted or mutated.[149] Alpha thalassaemia trait, where two α globin genes are deleted, and which is much more common, is often easy to suspect in the neonatal period since the MCV is reduced below the lower limit of normal and other causes of microcytosis in neonates (see Table 2.12) are very rare. Non-thalassaemic structural α and γ globin gene mutations, which are clinically silent in adults and children, can cause transient neonatal haemolytic anaemia because the variant haemoglobin is unstable, whereas the β globin haemoglobinopathies (sickle cell disease and β thalassaemia major) do not cause haemolysis or anaemia in neonates and rarely manifest clinically until after 6–8 weeks of age. Methaemoglobinaemia due to rare inherited mutations in an α or a γ globin gene causing the production of haemoglobin M (see also Table 2.16) can also present in the neonatal period and is discussed at the end of this chapter.

Alpha thalassaemia major (haemoglobin Bart's hydrops fetalis)

Alpha thalassaemia is one of the most common inherited disorders, with a worldwide carrier rate of approximately 5%.[150] The most significant form predominantly affects families of Southeast Asian origin, where the carrier rate approaches 40%, although it is also common in parts of India and the Mediterranean (Greece, Turkey, Cyprus and Sardinia).[151] Alpha thalassemia is most commonly caused by one of more than 50 deletions affecting either one (referred to as α⁺ thalassaemia) or both (referred to as α⁰ thalassaemia) of the α globin genes on one copy of chromosome 16.[152] The severity of α thalassaemia depends on the number of affected α globin genes. Where both parents are carriers of α⁰

Table 2.11 Haemoglobinopathies presenting with anaemia and/or jaundice in the neonatal period*

Condition	Genetic defect *Useful diagnostic tests*
Alpha globin disorders	
Alpha thalassaemia major	Deletion of four α globin genes
	Red cell indices
	Red cell morphology
	HPLC
	Investigation of parents
Haemoglobin H disease* including that associated with the α globin variants, haemoglobin Constant Spring and haemoglobin Paksé	Deletion and/or mutation of three α globin genes
	Red cell indices
	Red cell morphology
	HPLC (further investigation indicated if haemoglobin Bart's is >10%)
	investigation of parents
Unstable α chain variants	Hb Hasharon (α_2Asp14→Hisβ_2)
	Red cell morphology
	HPLC and/or mass spectrometry
Gamma globin disorders	
Unstable γ chain variants	Mutation of the $^G\gamma$ or $^A\gamma$globin gene
	HPLC
Gamma beta delta thalassaemia	Deletion of the β globin gene cluster
	Red cell indices
	Red cell morphology
	HPLC (no abnormality)
	Investigation of parents

* Beta globin disorders can be identified by screening in the neonatal period but almost never have clinical features at this age; presentation of haemoglobin H disease in the neonatal period is not common.
HPLC, high performance liquid chromatography.

thalassaemia, their offspring may be homozygous for α^0 and inherit no normal α globin genes; deletion of all four α globin genes results in α thalassaemia major, which has the most severe presentation and nearly always manifests *in utero* when it typically presents with severe second-trimester fetal anaemia and hydrops fetalis with an average Hb of 64 g/l.[153] As the principal haemoglobin produced by affected fetuses is haemoglobin Bart's (tetramers of fetal γ globin chains, γ_4), this condition is often known as haemoglobin Bart's hydrops fetalis syndrome (BHFS) to distinguish it from other causes of hydrops fetalis with severe anaemia.[154] The main clinical features of this syndrome are severe pallor with jaundice, cardiac failure, pleural and pericardial effusions, ascites, hepatosplenomegaly and respiratory distress.[154]

The cause of the severe anaemia in BHFS is multifactorial and includes reduced haemoglobin synthesis, reduced haemoglobin stability (haemoglobin Bart's), dyserythropoiesis

Table 2.12 Causes of neonatal microcytic anaemia

Red cell disorder	Diagnostic clues and useful tests
Inherited sideroblastic anaemias	Family history
	High serum iron, transferrin saturation and ferritin
	Low hepcidin
	Molecular analysis for mutations in the following genes:
	ALAS2 (X-linked)
	SLC25A38 (autosomal recessive)
	TRNT1 (autosomal recessive)
Haemoglobinopathies – α thalassaemias (see Table 2.11)	Mother typically of Far Eastern, African, Mediterranean, Arab, Caribbean or Indian subcontinent origin
	Neonatal anaemia (and hydrops) only if α thalassaemia major or haemoglobin H disease
Red cell membrane disorders – hereditary pyropoikilocytosis (see Table 2.7)	Anaemia usually marked
	MCV is typically very low (<70 fl)
	Homozygous/compound heterozygous for α spectrin variants
	Often no family history but parents may have blood films typical of hereditary elliptocytosis
Chronic *in utero* blood loss (see Table 2.13)	Twin-to-twin transfusion (donor twin)
	Chronic fetomaternal haemorrhage

MCV, mean cell volume.

due to precipitation of γ and β chains within the erythroid cells and hypersplenism, which together cause a dramatic anaemia that is partly haemolytic.[149] Furthermore, oxygen delivery to the tissues is severely reduced, not only by the low Hb, but also by the high oxygen affinity of haemoglobin Bart's.[155] Infants with BHFS almost always die either *in utero* (23–38 weeks) or shortly after birth[154] (Case 2.8, see page 105). This condition also carries a serious risk to the mother of the affected fetus, including mortality, with up to 50% developing severe pre-eclampsia, at least in part because of placentomegaly.[156]

Affected fetuses are usually identified on routine ultrasound scanning at 20–21 weeks' gestation by the clinical findings of fetal ascites, pleural effusion, pericardial effusion or hydrops fetalis.[154] These findings in a pregnancy at risk of α thalassaemia should at once prompt fetal blood sampling to determine the Hb and findings on high performance liquid chromatography (HPLC). The diagnosis of α thalassaemia major is confirmed when HPLC shows predominantly haemoglobin Bart's and haemoglobins F and A are absent. Depending on the extent of the α globin cluster deletion, some affected fetuses (e.g. with the homozygous Southeast Asian variant, which is the commonest cause of BHFS) will also have up to 20% embryonic haemoglobin Portland ($\zeta_2\gamma_2$), which is the only functional oxygen-carrying haemoglobin in these fetuses,[155] and sometimes haemoglobin H. The blood film shows hypochromic, often microcytic red cells with vast numbers of circulating NRBC (Fig. 2.19). The mean cell haemoglobin (MCH) and mean cell haemoglobin concentration (MCHC) are reduced but the MCV is not always reduced. Checking the blood counts of the parents will immediately identify whether they are at risk of having a child with α thalassaemia

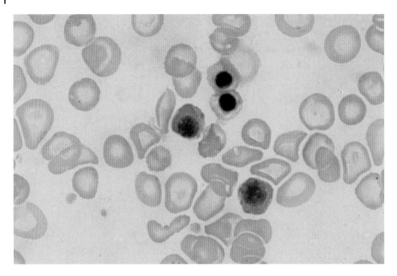

Fig. 2.19 Blood film of a preterm neonate with haemoglobin Bart's hydrops fetalis on day 1 of life showing markedly hypochromic red cells, many of which are microcytic, as well as polychromasia and four NRBC. Two of the NRBC show clearly defective haemoglobinisation. MGG, ×100.

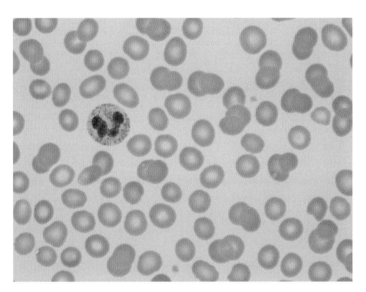

Fig. 2.20 Blood film of the mother of the neonate whose film is shown in Fig. 2.19, showing microcytosis and mild hypochromia. The mother had deletion of two of four α genes on one chromosome 16 (αα/--^{SEA}). MGG, ×100.

major; both parents will have microcytosis, with the MCV usually below 74 fl and MCH usually less than 24 pg (Fig. 2.20).

The only long-term survivors of α thalassaemia major are those who have received IUT followed by regular postnatal transfusions and/or a bone marrow transplant.[154] Affected children also have a high incidence of hypospadias, limb defects and atrial septal defects and others have severe neurological problems. If IUT is delayed until anaemia is severe, neonatal pulmonary hypoplasia is a cause of early mortality.[154] The diagnosis of α thalassaemia major should be suspected in any case of severe fetal anaemia that presents in the second trimester, and any case of hydrops fetalis with severe anaemia in which the parents come from high-prevalence areas, particularly Southeast Asia. In addition to the typical presentation, some neonates have had severe anaemia without hydrops fetalis. Antenatal screening of pregnant women and, when relevant, their partners should lead to prediction of the possibility of haemoglobin Bart's hydrops fetalis, with termination of pregnancy usually being offered when the diagnosis is confirmed.

Increasing awareness of BHFS, and the increase in cases in countries such as the USA where this condition used to be extremely rare, has led to major changes in the treatment options available and to the development of consensus guidelines for the perinatal management of patients with BHFS.[157] These note that lack of awareness of the improving outcome has meant that parents of affected fetuses may not be offered IUT. A recent international conference (https://conference.globalcastmd.com/ucsf-alpha-thalassemia-major/archive) reviewed existing knowledge regarding the prenatal screening, perinatal care, and maternal and childhood outcomes of patients with α thalassaemia major, and summarised their recommendations for management of the condition.[157] These include recommendations for preconceptual (or early antenatal) screening of couples at risk and the offer of fetal blood sampling in all cases of hydrops fetalis in pregnancies at risk in order to make a rapid diagnosis on the basis of blood count and HPLC, with IUT at the same time if the family wishes to pursue intervention in order to boost oxygen delivery to the tissues and minimise complications. These guidelines also suggested that couples at risk should be counselled about the options for a future pregnancy, including the possibility of preimplantation genetic diagnosis.[157]

Haemoglobin H disease in the newborn

This disorder is usually caused by deletion and/or mutation of three α globin genes. In most cases affected individuals are compound heterozygotes for two different mutations rather than homozygotes for a moderately severe molecular defect. Haemoglobin H disease varies considerably in severity. In general, the phenotype correlates very well with the degree of α globin chain deficiency and non-deletional types of haemoglobin H disease are more severe than the more common deletional types.[158,159] The most severe cases present with severe neonatal haemolytic anaemia and, occasionally, with hydrops fetalis.[160–163] This includes haemoglobin H/Constant Spring ($--/\alpha^{CS}\alpha$); haemoglobin Constant Spring is the most common non-deletion α-thalassaemia in Southeast Asia and Southern China and this compound heterozygous state is an important cause of hydrops fetalis.[164] A diagnosis of haemoglobin H disease in the newborn period is suggested by the presence of hypochromic, microcytic anaemia together with jaundice and the presence of large amounts of haemoglobin Bart's (γ_4) and as well as some haemoglobin H (β_4). The heterogeneity of haemoglobin H disease makes genetic counselling particularly difficult. Most cases resulting from simple deletion of the α globin genes are mildly affected and prenatal diagnosis may not be appropriate; virtually all severe cases have at least one non-deletional allele.[161–163] Awareness of the potential severity of coinheritance of α^0 thalassaemia alongside non-deletional α thalassaemia alleles, such as in haemoglobin

H/Constant Spring, in at-risk populations should lead to careful *in utero* monitoring of affected pregnancies for signs of hydrops fetalis as prompt IUT has been shown to prevent fetal morbidity and mortality.[164]

Neonatal haemolysis due to unstable α chain variants

While most α chain mutations do not cause clinically significant disorders either in the newborn or in older children, occasional variants do cause problems specifically in the newborn. In particular, they are a rare cause of unexplained neonatal jaundice and anaemia.[165] The best known example is haemoglobin Hasharon (p.Asp>HisHBA2:c.142G>C), which is mildly unstable (due to a higher propensity for dissociation into subunits) and is found mainly in Ashkenazi Jewish families. The interaction between Hasharon α chains and γ chains in the fetal form of haemoglobin Hasharon results in an unstable haemoglobin that manifests as neonatal haemolytic anaemia.[166] The haemolysis is transient, resolving with the transition from the fetal to the adult form of haemoglobin Hasharon trait at several months of age. The haemolysis is usually mild and, in practice, most infants with α chain mutations are detected only as part of routine neonatal screening. However, the diagnosis may be difficult to establish because of the instability of the abnormal haemoglobin produced; mass spectrometry or molecular analysis is usually more reliable than HPLC.

Neonatal haemolysis due to unstable γ chain variants

At least 130 different γ chain variants have been described, many of which either cause transient neonatal haemolytic anaemia or are picked up as a result of neonatal haemoglobinopathy screening programmes.[167] The most well-known unstable γ chain variants are haemoglobin F Poole[168] and haemoglobin F Bonheiden,[169] which both cause haemolytic anaemia with Heinz bodies (red cell inclusions composed of denatured haemoglobin) confined to the first few weeks of life. The anaemia completely resolves as γ chains are replaced by the production of normal β chains. Hydrops fetalis has also been reported in a unique family where triplets, who were homozygous for haemoglobin Taybe, were born at 27 weeks' gestation with microcytic anaemia (Hb 71–95 g/l), generalised oedema and ascites.[170]

Heterozygosity for εγβδ thalassaemia

Although rare, the diagnosis of heterozygous εγβδ thalassaemia (often referred to as γδβ thalassaemia) should be considered in neonates with unexplained haemolytic anaemia associated with microcytic hypochromic red cells and erythroblastosis.[171,172] Sometimes there is hepatosplenomegaly and the blood film may show basophilic stippling. These conditions result either from large deletions that remove the entire β globin gene cluster[172] or from deletions in which the structural genes are left intact but important regulatory elements are removed.[173] Homozygosity has not been reported and would be incompatible with life. Heterozygous neonates often require red cell transfusion but generally become transfusion-independent after the first few months of life.[171] IUT has also occasionally been required.[174]

Beta globin disorders in the neonatal period

Beta globin disorders usually present in the neonatal period as a result of neonatal haemoglobinopathy screening results rather than with clinical problems, which usually do not develop until after the first few months of life.

Beta thalassaemias Beta thalassemia major, even when caused by homozygous β^0 mutations, typically has no overt clinical or haematological abnormalities at birth. As the Hb falls over the second and third months of life, infants feed more slowly and the rate of weight gain slows. Increasing anaemia is accompanied by noticeable pallor and the development of splenomegaly together with the appearance of polychromasia and circulating erythroblasts. Although there are no consistent or reliable abnormalities in the red cell indices or blood film in neonates with this condition, an interesting report published more than 60 years ago does suggest that subtle features, including very mild anaemia, may be present in some affected neonates,[175] although possibly because of concomitant causes of anaemia in those cases. A diagnosis of β thalassaemia major is strongly suggested by the absence of haemoglobin A on HPLC, especially in a term neonate, and where both parents have been shown to have β thalassaemia heterozygosity. Neonates with β thalassaemia trait have no abnormal haematological findings either in the red cell indices or in the blood film; microcytosis and hypochromia normally become evident by 6 months of age. Antenatal (or preconceptual) screening should be offered to all couples at risk of having a child affected by β thalassaemia major.

Sickle cell disease Babies with sickle cell disease (sickle cell anaemia and compound heterozygous states causing a sickling disorder) are generally not anaemic at birth and have no consistent abnormalities of red cell morphology in blood films examined in the first few weeks of life. Target cells are occasionally present in neonates with sickle cell disease, particularly those with haemoglobin S/haemoglobin C compound heterozygosity. HPLC in neonates with sickle cell anaemia ($\beta^S \beta^S$) typically shows 15–20% haemoglobin S and the absence of haemoglobin A (Fig. 2.21), in contrast to neonates with sickle cell trait ($\beta \beta^S$) where there is approximately 10% haemoglobin A together with a similar amount of haemoglobin S (Fig. 2.22). In cases where clinically evident sickle cell disease has been diagnosed during the neonatal period, the most frequent findings are jaundice, fever, pallor, respiratory distress and abdominal distention.[176]

Neonatal microcytic anaemia

The differential diagnosis of neonatal microcytosis and microcytic anaemias is shown in Table 2.12). This includes specific red cell membrane disorders, such as HPP, discussed earlier, most of the haemoglobinopathies that present in the neonatal period, and chronic *in utero* blood loss as discussed later. A small number of rare sideroblastic anaemias present with hypochromic microcytic anaemia in the neonatal period.

Sideroblastic anaemias presenting in the neonatal period Congenital sideroblastic anaemia is a rare disease caused by mutations of genes involved in haem and iron–sulphur cluster formation, and mitochondrial protein biosynthesis. While the majority of these disorders present later in childhood or in adulthood, a number present in the neonatal period with microcytic anaemia with or without syndromic features.[177] A recent European survey of congenital sideroblastic anaemia identified neonatal presentations in some cases of X-linked sideroblastic anaemia (XLSA) due to mutations in the *ALAS2* gene, in some cases with autosomal recessive sideroblastic anaemia caused by bi-allelic mutations in

Peak Name	Calibrated Area %	Area %	Retention Time (min)	Peak Area
Unknown	---	0.8	0.88	15638
F	84.7*	---	1.20	1615500
Unknown	---	0.1	2.18	2154
Unknown	---	0.3	2.33	6307
Ao	---	0.6	2.53	11641
A2	0.5*	---	3.60	11097
S-window	---	17.9	4.35	363461

Total Area: 2,025,798

F Concentration = 84.7* %
A2 Concentration = 0.5* %

*Values outside of expected ranges

Analysis comments:

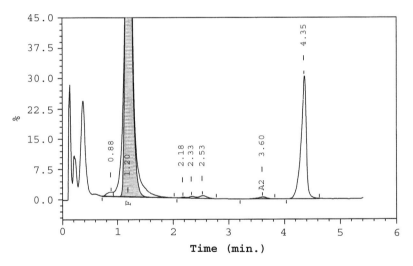

Fig. 2.21 High performance liquid chromatography (HPLC) on a BioRad Variant II instrument of a neonate with sickle cell anaemia (SS) showing 84.7% haemoglobin F, no haemoglobin A and an estimated 17.9% in the haemoglobin S window. The complex peaks to the left are post-translationally modified haemoglobin F. Note the very low percentage of haemoglobin A_2, which is expected in a neonate.

the *SLC25A38* gene and in cases with mutation of the *TRNT1* gene.[177] The same report noted that a molecular defect could not be identified in almost one-third of patients with congenital sideroblastic anaemia, including several that presented in the neonatal period. Of note, several series have demonstrated that congenital sideroblastic anaemia caused by *SLC25A38* mutations is nearly always associated with severe microcytic anaemia in

Peak Name	Calibrated Area %	Area %	Retention Time (min)	Peak Area
Unknown	---	0.1	0.59	4048
Unknown	---	0.6	0.88	20528
F	75.3*	---	1.20	2429277
P3	---	0.7	1.75	22043
Unknown	---	0.1	2.16	2822
Ao	---	15.3	2.57	512392
A2	0.5*	---	3.65	19061
S-window	---	9.9	4.37	329424

Total Area: 3,339,595*

F Concentration = 75.3* %
A2 Concentration = 0.5* %

*Values outside of expected ranges

Analysis comments:

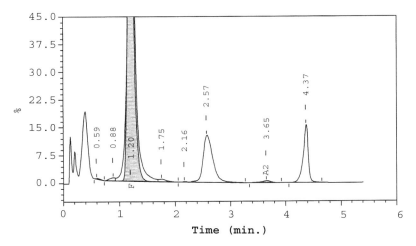

Fig. 2.22 HPLC on a BioRad Variant II instrument of a neonate with sickle cell trait (AS) showing 75.3% haemoglobin F, 15.3% haemoglobin A and 9.9% in the haemoglobin S window. Note that in sickle cell trait the S percentage is lower than the A percentage.

the neonatal period.[177–179] Infants with anaemia due to *SLC25A38* mutations usually require red cell transfusion during the neonatal period and remain transfusion-dependent thereafter. Congenital sideroblastic anaemia due to *TRNT1* mutations is also associated with severe neonatal microcytic anaemia in virtually all reported cases. This syndromic disorder, first termed SIFD syndrome, is characterised by a tetrad of congenital sideroblastic anaemia, B cell immunodeficiency, periodic fevers and developmental delay.[180] Severe cases of SIFD due to mutations in *TRNT1* may present with hydrops

Table 2.13 Useful diagnostic tests in neonatal anaemia due to blood loss

Neonatal anaemia due to blood loss	Diagnostic clues and useful tests
Fetomaternal haemorrhage: acute or chronic	Maternal Kleihauer test or measurement of haemoglobin F-containing cells in the maternal circulation by flow cytometry
	Neonatal blood film (erythroblastosis; dimorphic if acute on chronic blood loss)
Fetofeto haemorrhage (twin-to-twin transfusion)	Blood count on both twins
	Blood film on both twins – donor twin will have erythroblastosis and, if chronic blood loss, may have hypochromic red cells
Fetal/neonatal haemorrhage: cephalohaematoma, intra-abdominal bleeding, pulmonary haemorrhage	Blood film: erythroblastosis if large recent haemorrhage
	Imaging to identify the site of bleeding

fetalis due to progressive fetal anaemia.[181] Affected infants remain transfusion-dependent and haemopoietic stem cell transplantation is usually recommended as a curative approach for both the anaemia and immunodeficiency.[181]

Neonatal anaemia due to blood loss

Blood loss as a cause of neonatal anaemia may be very obvious (for example, a cephalohaematoma or rupture of the umbilical cord) but more often the blood loss is concealed and easy to miss unless specifically sought (for example a fetomaternal bleed). Usually, the most serious blood loss occurs prior to delivery and important causes of this are twin-to-twin transfusion and fetomaternal haemorrhage. Acute perinatal blood loss as a cause of unexpected severe neonatal anaemia and severe hypovolaemic shock is often missed initially, leading to a delay in treatment and a significant risk of neonatal death or severe anoxic brain damage leading to neurological damage.[182,183] Recent data suggest that up to 40% of cases of severe fetomaternal haemorrhage are missed[184] and awareness of this complication amongst obstetricians is often low.[185] Although much less dramatic, chronic neonatal blood loss secondary to iatrogenic blood letting is also important to consider as this is by far the most common cause of anaemia in hospitalised neonates and strategies are now available to minimise this.[186]

The main causes of neonatal anaemia due to blood loss are shown in Table 2.13.

Twin-to-twin transfusion

This occurs in monochorionic twins with monochorial placentas where there are two amniotic sacs (diamniotic).[187] In this situation, the twins share a placenta within which there are multiple vascular anastomoses that allow blood to flow between the twins either in fetal life or during delivery.[188] Although blood flow between the twins is balanced in most cases, in up to 20% of cases net blood flow is towards one of the twins. When this occurs before birth this is known as twin-to-twin transfusion syndrome (TTTS) or twin anaemia–polycythaemia sequence (TAPS), depending upon the size of the vascular anastomoses and the associated clinical sequelae; when bleeding between the twins occurs during delivery, it is known as peripartum TTTS (reviewed in reference 189).

Twin-to-twin transfusion affects around 10% of monochorionic twin pregnancies.[190] Bleeding in TTTS usually occurs during the second trimester and carries a very high mortality rate if left untreated.[191] The diagnosis is based on the ultrasound findings, which predominantly show oligohydramnios in the donor twin and reciprocal polyhydramnios in the recipient twin. The presence of haematological problems in neonates affected by TTTS depends on the type of antenatal treatment. While twins treated with laser coagulation surgery generally have no significant difference in Hb levels, for TTTS twins treated conservatively (expectant management or serial amnioreduction), donor twins typically have a significantly lower Hb at birth than recipient twins; a recent study reported a median inter-twin difference of 36 (16–60) g/l.[192] In conservatively managed cases, around one-third of donor twins will require red cell transfusion for anaemia soon after delivery, while recipient twins may develop severe hyperviscosity–polycythaemia, leading to ischaemic limb necrosis.[193] A recent retrospective study showed that even after fetal laser coagulation surgery, residual patent anastomoses mean that around 50% of donor twins will require red cell transfusion at birth, and one-third of recipient twins will have severe hyperviscosity/polycythaemia and require exchange transfusion.[193] Nevertheless, recent data show that treatment with fetoscopic laser coagulation has significantly improved the outcome from a mortality rate of up to 80% to 30–40%, although about 10% of survivors will have impaired neurodevelopmental outcome, including cerebral palsy.[193]

Twin anaemia–polycythaemia sequence is a newly described form of chronic inter-twin blood transfusion.[194,195] This also leads to anaemia in the donor twin and polycythaemia in the recipient but without signs of oligo- or polyhydramnios, respectively. In contrast to TTTS, TAPS is caused by bleeding through very small placental vascular anastomoses (diameter <1 mm), allowing slow transfusion of blood from one twin to the other, without the major haemodynamic imbalance seen in TTTS. In some cases TAPS can occur with, or following treatment of, TTTS, when it typically manifests during the second and third trimesters of pregnancy. The diagnosis may be made antenatally by identifying differences in the MCA peak systolic velocity, with increased velocity predicting anaemia in the donor twin while reduced velocity in the recipient is associated with polycythaemia.[196] The diagnosis of TAPS after birth is based on the extent of differences in Hb at birth in monochorionic twins. Generally accepted postnatal criteria are an inter-twin Hb difference >80 g/l and either a donor/recipient reticulocyte count ratio of >1.7 and/or the presence of minuscule placental anastomoses (diameter <1 mm).[197] In this situation, the donor twin is smaller, pale and lethargic and may have overt cardiac failure. By contrast, the recipient twin is often plethoric, with polycythaemia, hyperviscosity, hyperbilirubinaemia and, in the most severe cases, DIC.[193] The majority of donor twins will require short-term red cell transfusion by the end of the first day of life but, unlike TTTS, emergency transfusion at birth is not usually needed as the anaemia is chronic. Recipient twins, on the other hand, will frequently require exchange transfusion for severe polycythaemia to reduce the risk of limb ischaemia, skin necrosis and brain injury.[198–201]

Bleeding may also occur acutely during labour with signs similar to those of fetomaternal haemorrhage. However, acute peripartum TTTS is very uncommon, affecting around 1.5–2.5% of monochorionic twins and little is known about the pathogenesis.[202]

Fetomaternal haemorrhage

Most significant fetomaternal bleeds occur during the third trimester, either spontaneously or secondary to trauma, and involve very small quantities of blood (0.5 ml or less).[185] The risk of fetomaternal haemorrhage is increased by invasive procedures, including caesarean section, fetal blood sampling, amniocentesis and chorionic villus sampling, as well as by obstetric complications such as placental abruption, placenta praevia, vasa praevia, choriocarcinoma and chorioangioma.[203,204] Fetomaternal haemorrhage may also follow falls or major trauma, such as road traffic accidents, where haemorrhage can be massive and rapid leading to a high rate of fetal loss.[205] Massive fetomaternal haemorrhage, usually defined as the loss of more than 20% of the blood volume or >30 ml fetal blood transfused into the maternal circulation (Case 2.9, see page 107), may cause intrauterine death or the baby may be born with hydrops fetalis or circulatory shock.[206,207] In some cases the baby appears well, but pale, at birth and collapses a few hours later. Careful questioning of the mother may elicit a history of reduced or absent fetal movements, bleeding or trauma.

As fetomaternal haemorrhage can have a devastating outcome, both in the acute setting and secondary to long-term neurological damage, prompt diagnosis is crucial. The diagnosis should be considered in any neonate with unexpected severe neonatal anaemia with or without signs of hypovolaemic shock. In fact, the presence of moderate or severe anaemia at birth in an otherwise well baby with no or minimal jaundice is a key diagnostic clue. The most useful diagnostic tests are a Coombs test to exclude immune haemolysis, a reticulocyte count to exclude red cell aplasia, a Kleihauer test or flow cytometry on maternal blood to quantify the number of haemoglobin F-containing fetal red cells in the maternal circulation, and a blood film,[207] which shows large numbers of NRBC, particularly where there has been a large acute bleed (Fig. 2.23a,b). The Kleihauer (or Kleihauer–Betke) test has been the mainstay of laboratory methods for estimating the volume of fetal haemorrhage for more than 50 years. This test relies on the principle that adult (maternal) red blood cells normally contain almost entirely haemoglobin A, which is

(a) (b)

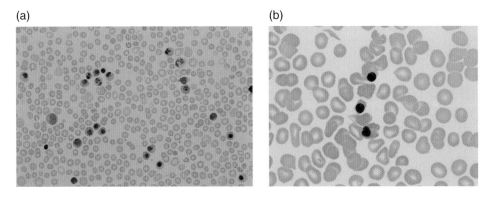

Fig. 2.23 Blood film of two term neonates with anaemia secondary to fetomaternal haemorrhage showing (a) a very marked increase in erythroblasts and marked polychromasia on the first day of life and (b) three erythroblasts as well as an occasional spherocyte and mild polychromasia on day 3 of life. Note that the dyserythropoiesis shown by several erythroblasts is a feature of 'stress erythropoiesis'. MGG, (a) ×40; (b) ×100.

(a)   (b)

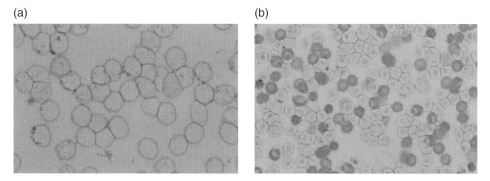

Fig. 2.24 Kleihauer–Betke test. (a) This image shows maternal red blood cells containing almost entirely haemoglobin A after acid elution *in vitro* causes the appearance of colourless 'ghost' cells. (b) This image shows the positive control in which fetal red blood cells have been added prior to acid elution and, as these contain largely haemoglobin F which is resistant to acid elution, these are shown here stained deep pink. ×100.

sensitive to acid elution *in vitro*, giving rise to colourless 'ghost' cells (Fig. 2.24a); by contrast, fetal red cells contain mostly haemoglobin F, which is resistant to acid elution and stains a deep pink colour (Fig. 2.24b). The Kleihauer test remains very widely used as it is rapid and inexpensive and can be performed without expensive equipment.[208] However, careful attention to detail and controls are essential as systematic evaluation has shown both over- and under-estimation of fetomaternal haemorrhage.[209] In addition, the results are difficult to interpret where the mother herself has increased haemoglobin F-containing cells ('F-cells'), for example due to maternal hereditary persistence of fetal haemoglobin (HPFH) or HPFH/sickle trait.[210,211] Newer, more accurate methods, such as anti-haemoglobin F flow cytometry are a promising alternative, although their use is limited by equipment and staffing costs.[212]

Where chronic fetal blood loss has occurred, the baby is often well at birth but may present with cardiac failure. In this situation, the blood film shows hypochromic, microcytic red cells as well as circulating erythroblasts (Fig. 2.25) and the Kleihauer result may be difficult to interpret. In some cases, however, chronic fetomaternal blood loss is followed by an acute bleed, with resultant severe anaemia (Hb <50 g/l) and a high risk of long-term brain injury.[213] Another potential confounding factor is when there is ABO incompatibility between the mother and baby and the baby is disproportionately anaemic.[214,215] In such cases, the fetal cells may be rapidly destroyed within the maternal circulation and a high index of suspicion of fetomaternal haemorrhage as a cause of neonatal anaemia is needed, in order to perform the Kleihauer test as soon as possible.

Choriocarcinoma is a very rare cause of massive fetomaternal haemorrhage, which it is important to consider in all cases as the presence of unexplained severe neonatal anaemia may provide the first clue to the diagnosis.[216] It may also present as fetal hydrops, IUGR or intrauterine fetal death.[217] The presence of choriocarcinoma is often not recognised at delivery because the tumour is not visible macroscopically.[218] Despite the risk to the fetus and newborn, recent data show a cure rate in affected women of almost 100% even in the presence of metastases.[219]

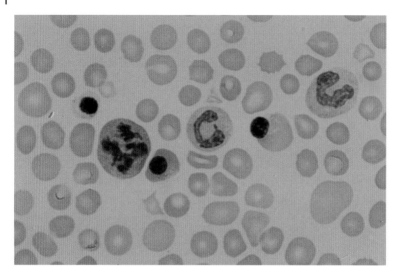

Fig. 2.25 Blood film of a term neonate born with severe anaemia (Hb 50 g/l) showing three normoblasts, an erythroblast containing a mitotic figure, polychromasia and a mixture of normochromic and hypochromic red cells as well as some spherocytes. The Kleihauer–Betke test estimated the fetal blood loss at less than 30 ml and a diagnosis of acute fetomaternal haemorrhage on a background of chronic fetomaternal haemorrhage was suspected. MGG, ×100.

Neonatal anaemia due to blood loss at or after delivery

Anaemia due to blood loss around the time of delivery is usually due to obstetric complications, including placenta praevia, placental abruption or incision of the placenta during caesarean section or, alternatively, is due to bleeding from the umbilical cord caused by trauma or inadequate cord clamping. In these circumstances, the babies are often extremely ill, with circulatory shock, anaemia worsening rapidly after birth, large numbers of circulating NRBC and DIC. One of the most serious causes of acute fetal blood loss is vasa praevia, an anomaly of placentation which results in aberrant fetal blood vessels running across the internal os of the cervix. These vessels are at risk of rupture during labour when the supporting membranes rupture because they are unsupported by the umbilical cord or placental tissue.[220] The classic presentation is with painless vaginal bleeding in the mother, but the diagnosis can easily be missed because the volume of blood is relatively small and it is impossible to distinguish fetal from maternal blood by appearance. The incidence of vasa praevia is estimated to be around 1 in 2500 pregnancies and the condition carries a fetal mortality of almost 50%.[220] The presence of vasa praevia can be detected antenatally using vaginal ultrasound, although this is not routine practice. Nevertheless, recent studies have shown that prenatal diagnosis in centres with prenatal diagnosis expertise can be associated with 100% neonatal survival by performing early caesarean section.[221]

Acute neonatal anaemia may also be due to internal haemorrhage in the baby, usually in association with a traumatic delivery. This may be immediately evident, for example cephalohaematoma, or less obvious, for example pulmonary or intra-abdominal haemorrhage. In such babies, particularly if there is no history of trauma, it is important to consider whether there an underlying bleeding diathesis, such as haemophilia or vitamin K deficiency. Inherited and acquired coagulation disorders that may present with bleeding at birth or during the neonatal period are discussed in Chapter 4.

Anaemia of prematurity

Anaemia of prematurity refers to the normal physiological fall in Hb over the first 4–8 weeks of life in a preterm neonate. The pathogenesis is multifactorial and includes the shorter lifespan of fetal red blood cells, the relatively low EPO concentrations in the first few weeks of life and the rapid growth of the baby during this period as well as iatrogenic anaemia due to phlebotomy for diagnostic investigations.[1,186] Phlebotomy losses are typically highest in very low birthweight neonates (<1500 g at birth) who have been estimated to lose 11–22 ml/kg per week during the first 6 weeks of life, equivalent to 15–30% of their circulating blood volume.[222] Nutritional deficiency no longer plays a significant role, at least in well-resourced countries, due to routine prophylactic supplementation with iron and folic acid.[223] The clinical impact of anaemia of prematurity has been the subject of a large number of studies which, together, suggest a significant association between the extent of anaemia and brain injury, necrotising enterocolitis (NEC) and retinopathy of prematurity.[224–227] The relationship between the degree of anaemia and tissue hypoxia-related damage, as well as the impact of different red cell transfusion strategies and the timing and dose of EPO administration, is described in detail in recent reviews.[228–230]

The diagnosis of anaemia of prematurity is usually straightforward. Typically, a well preterm baby has a slowly falling Hb with an unremarkable blood film showing normochromic, normocytic red blood cells, a slightly low reticulocyte count (e.g. 20×10^9/l) and no NRBC. However, where top-up red cell transfusion is being considered, it is important to first exclude other potential causes of anaemia using clinical features and a diagnostic algorithm such as shown in Fig. 2.26.

Management of anaemia of prematurity

Strategies for the management of this neonatal anaemia vary in different countries, different centres and also between clinicians. Of the three main approaches, there is increased use of the most conservative approach (watchful waiting) as the complications and costs of the other two approaches are increasingly recognised – top-up red cell transfusion and administration of erythropoiesis-stimulating agents, such as EPO and darbepoetin.[230] Whatever option is chosen, it should be combined with appropriate measures to minimise the severity and duration of anaemia, including limiting iatrogenic blood loss by using blood logs, strict criteria for routine blood tests and miniaturised assays.[231–233] There is also increasing interest in delayed clamping of the umbilical cord at delivery to increase the Hb/haematocrit at birth. In addition, all preterm neonates should be given iron supplementation (3 mg/kg/day from 4–6 weeks of age or iron-fortified formula with 0.5–0.9 mg/dl iron) and folate supplementation (50 µg daily or 500 µg once weekly).[234]

Delayed clamping of the cord to minimise neonatal anaemia   A recent systematic review of delayed (30 seconds or more) versus early clamping of the cord at delivery in preterm infants included 18 randomised studies.[235] Although shown to be a safe option, the effects of this approach on the haematocrit at birth was very small (an increase of 2.7%) while the proportion

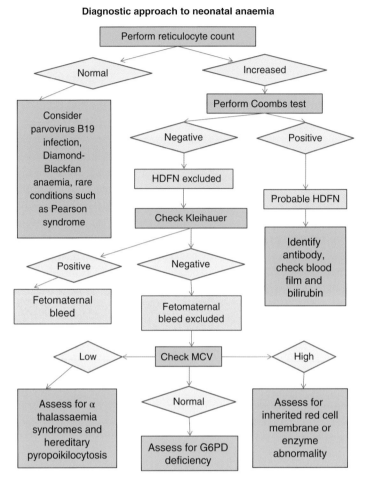

Fig. 2.26 Diagram showing a suggested approach to the diagnosis of neonatal anaemia. G6PD, glucose-6-phosphate dehydrogenase; HDFN, haemolytic disease of the fetus and newborn; MCV, mean cell volume.

of neonates who were transfused fell by 10%. Nevertheless, this review also showed that in-hospital mortality was significantly reduced (risk ratio 0.68).[235] Importantly, the outcome of two of the randomised studies suggests that neurodevelopmental outcome is improved, and some countries, including the UK (https://www.resus.org.uk/library/2021-resuscitation-guidelines/newborn-resuscitation-and-support-transition-infants-birth) and the USA, now recommend delaying cord clamping for at least 30–60 seconds for uncompromised preterm and term neonates (https://www.acog.org/clinical/clinical-guidance/committee-opinion/articles/2020/12/delayed-umbilical-cord-clamping-after-birth). The safety and efficacy of delayed cord clamping and cord 'milking' in preterm infants less than 29 weeks' gestation at birth is not yet clear,[236] awaiting the outcome of several ongoing trials.[237]

Top-up red cell transfusion This remains the mainstay of treatment for anaemia of prematurity. However, increasing recognition of the importance of limiting transfusion to the neonates most likely to benefit from this treatment is leading to more widespread adoption of restrictive transfusion policies. The indications, principles and hazards of neonatal transfusion are briefly summarised below.

Erythropoiesis-stimulating agents to treat and prevent neonatal anaemia   The two erythropoiesis-stimulating agents currently available for use in neonates are recombinant human EPO and darbepoetin, a re-engineered form of EPO with a longer half-life. There have been many controlled trials of erythropoiesis-stimulating agents for prevention of early and late neonatal anaemia, which have recently been the subject of Cochrane systematic reviews.[228,229] There is no doubt that recombinant EPO is biologically effective in that it stimulates erythropoiesis in virtually all preterm infants and there is no evidence that preterm or term neonates are physiologically insensitive to EPO. EPO is also able to reduce red cell transfusion requirements in preterm infants.[228] The recent Cochrane reviews also found that the effects of EPO administration varied depending upon when treatment was started. In particular, early EPO treatment, before the age of 8 days, reduced the number of red blood cell transfusions as well as the total transfusion volume and donor exposure.[228] Early administration of EPO also reduced the risk of intraventricular haemorrhage (IVH), periventricular leucomalacia and NEC without a significant increase in the rate of retinopathy of prematurity. However, early administration of EPO is not currently recommended for routine use, largely because it is not clear that the modest reduction in transfusions is clinically meaningful. In addition, a large randomised study (PENUT; NCT01378273) recently reported that there was no neurodevelopmental benefit for high dose EPO administered within the first 24 hours of life until 32 weeks corrected gestational age.[238] The results of late administration are also modest and the benefits remain unproven.[229] Specifically, EPO started between 8 days and 28 days of life causes a small reduction in the number of red blood cell transfusions but has no significant effect on donor exposure. Given that EPO does have some impact on reducing transfusion requirements, it is possible that future changes in transfusion practice in response to safety concerns or parental acceptance may lead to a more defined role for erythropoiesis-stimulating agents in neonatal medicine.

At present, the main indications for EPO in neonates are to prevent anaemia in those who have received IUT for alloantibody-mediated anaemia[14] and in a non-emergency situation where red cell transfusions are against the parents' wishes but are not essential (e.g. preterm babies of Jehovah's witnesses).[239] The recommended dose is 300 µg/kg as a single subcutaneous injection three times per week starting in the first week of life as the Hb does not start to rise until 10–14 days of treatment. Iron supplements (3 mg/kg/day) should be started as soon as possible to prevent the rapid development of iron deficiency in EPO-treated infants (the dose may need to be increased up to a maximum of 9 mg/kg/day if iron deficiency develops on the standard dose).[240]

A simple diagnostic approach to neonatal anaemia

As discussed earlier, red cell disorders associated with neonatal or fetal anaemia present in three main ways: with an isolated low Hb, with jaundice due to haemolysis or with hydrops fetalis. A diagnostic algorithm to help identify which of these causes is most likely, which can be excluded and what further investigations are most appropriate is shown in Figure 2.26. A list of the haematological causes of hydrops fetalis and the most helpful diagnostic clues is shown in Table 2.14.

Table 2.14 Haematological causes of hydrops fetalis

Condition	Diagnostic clues and useful tests
Failure of normal red cell production	
Parvovirus B19	Inappropriately low reticulocyte count
Diamond–Blackfan anaemia	Blood film: characteristic red cell morphology
Congenital dyserythropoietic anaemia, e.g. CDA type II, CDA type IV (*KLF1* mutations)	(CDA and Southeast Asian ovalocytosis)
Rare genetic syndromes, e.g. Southeast Asian ovalocytosis; *IKZF1* mutation/deletion	Congenital anomalies (DBA) Pancytopenia, immune defects (*IKZF1* mutation)
Haemolytic disease of the newborn	
Rh (mainly anti-D and anti-c)	Known maternal alloantibodies
ABO (rare cause of hydrops and mainly due to anti-B)	Positive Coombs test
Other blood groups: anti-Kell	Previously affected sibling
Red cell membrane disorders	
Hereditary stomatocytosis	Family history
Hereditary spherocytosis (rarely)	Blood film: characteristic red cell morphology
Hereditary xerocytosis (rarely)[241]	Negative Coombs test
Red cell enzymopathies*	
Pyruvate kinase deficiency	PK deficiency may present with unexplained
Glucose phosphate isomerase deficiency	neonatal hepatic failure; often difficult to establish the diagnosis from initial enzyme activity assays
Haemoglobinopathies	
Alpha thalassaemia major (haemoglobin Bart's hydrops fetalis)	Typical red cell indices and blood film abnormalities
Haemoglobin H disease, including related to haemoglobin Constant Spring	Family history and ethnic origin
Chronic fetal blood loss	
Twin-to-twin transfusion	Monochorionic twins
	Discrepant Hb between the twins
Storage disorders	Hepatosplenomegaly
	Metabolic problems
	Family history
	Blood film (lymphocyte vacuolation)
Malignancies	
Transient abnormal myelopoiesis in Down syndrome	TAM: hepatosplenomegaly, ascites, pleural/pericardial effusions and/or skin rash in severe cases; leucocytosis and increased blast cells are the most reliable haematological feature; anaemia is uncommon
Congenital acute myeloid or acute lymphoblastic leukaemia	Acute leukaemia: hepatosplenomegaly, skin nodules, leucocytosis, increased blast cells, rapidly progressing anaemia and thrombocytopenia
Haemophagocytic lymphohistiocytosis	HLH: hepatosplenomegaly, fever, multiorgan failure, disseminated intravascular coagulation

* G6PD deficiency in neonates most often presents with jaundice with few or no red cell morphological abnormalities and a normal Hb.
CDA, congenital dyserythropoietic anaemia; DBA, Diamond–Blackfan anaemia; G6PD, glucose-6-phosphate dehydrogenase; Hb, haemoglobin concentration; HLH, haemophagocytic lymphohistiocytosis; PK, pyruvate kinase; TAM, transient abnormal myelopoiesis.

Table 2.15 Causes of neonatal polycythaemia

Condition	Diagnostic clues and useful tests
Chronic intrauterine hypoxia	
Intrauterine growth restriction	Clinical evidence of intrauterine growth restriction: low birthweight, reduced end-diastolic blood flow
Maternal hypertension	Maternal history
Maternal diabetes	Marked erythroblastosis despite high Hb
	Associated mild/moderate thrombocytopenia resolving within 7–10 days ± mild, self-limiting neutropenia
	Howell–Jolly bodies
Chromosomal disorders	
Trisomy 21	Typical facies and associated congenital anomalies
Trisomy 18	Other typical neonatal haematological abnormalities, e.g.
Trisomy 13	thrombocytopenia, dysplastic white cells and increased blast cells
Twin-to-twin transfusion	Discrepant Hb concentrations in monochorionic twins (>30 g/l) – one twin plethoric and the other pale in severe cases
Endocrine disorders	
Thyrotoxicosis	Thyrotoxicosis: IUGR, goitre, exophthalmos, stare, craniosynostosis,
Congenital adrenal hyperplasia	flushing, heart failure, tachycardia, arrhythmias, hypertension, hypoglycaemia
	CAH: arrythmias, vomiting, hyponatraemia, hypoglycaemia; ambiguous genitalia (females)
Delayed clamping of the cord	Relevant history of delayed clamping and no evidence of alternative causes

CAH, congenital adrenal hyperplasia; Hb, haemoglobin concentration; IUGR, intrauterine growth restriction.

Neonatal polycythaemia

For practical purposes, in both term and preterm infants, polycythaemia can be defined as a central venous haematocrit of greater than 0.65, because there is an exponential rise in blood viscosity above this level.[242] However, even at haematocrits greater than 0.70, only a minority of neonates have clinical signs of hyperviscosity, such as lethargy, hypotonia, hyperbilirubinaemia and hypoglycaemia.[243] In severe cases, skin necrosis has been reported and polycythaemia is also likely to be a contributory factor in the pathogenesis of NEC and in thrombotic disorders such as neonatal seizures, stroke and renal vein thrombosis.[244]

Causes of polycythaemia are shown in Table 2.15. The most common cause is chronic fetal hypoxia secondary to IUGR, maternal hypertension/pre-eclampsia or maternal diabetes. Neonates with Down syndrome are also frequently polycythaemic and this is secondary to the effects of trisomy 21 on fetal erythropoiesis rather than congenital heart disease.[245] Another important cause of severe polycythaemia is TAPS (see earlier) where there has been chronic inter-twin transfusion throughout the second and third trimesters of pregnancy.[189]

Treatment is controversial and is not necessary in infants with very minor signs (for example borderline hypoglycaemia or poor peripheral perfusion). Infants with neurological signs and a haematocrit greater than 0.65 should have a partial exchange transfusion (using a crystalloid solution such as normal saline) to reduce the haematocrit to 0.55. There is no evidence to support the use of FFP or albumin for this procedure.[61]

Haematological causes of cyanosis

Although cyanosis in neonates is nearly always due to underlying cardiac or respiratory compromise, there are several rare and well-recognised haematological causes of cyanosis (Table 2.16), which may cause diagnostic confusion. Cyanosis (or pseudocyanosis) is present at birth with α and γ chain methaemoglobins.[246] The skin colour, brownish/slate, differs slightly from cyanosis due to an increased percentage of deoxyhaemoglobin. In the case of the γ chain variants haemoglobin F-M-Osaka, haemoglobin F-M-Fort Ripley and F-M-Circleville, the cyanosis disappears as β chain synthesis takes over from γ chain synthesis. With α chain variants the cyanosis persists. Haemoglobin M-Iwate and haemoglobin M-Boston are not only methaemoglobins but also have a low oxygen affinity so that there is both pseudocyanosis and true cyanosis. In addition, there are two γ chain variants – haemoglobin F-M-Fort Ripley and haemoglobin F-M-Osaka – that are methaemoglobins and also unstable. Neonatal methaemoglobinaemia can be acquired rather than inherited. Neonates are more susceptible to oxidation of haemoglobin than older infants and adults, both because haemoglobin F is more susceptible to oxidation than haemoglobin A and because methaemoglobin reductase activity is relatively low.

Principles of red cell transfusion in neonates

The decision to transfuse a neonate with anaemia depends on the cause and natural history of the anaemia as well as the severity, the rate of fall in Hb, the postnatal and gestational age of the neonate and the clinical signs. The majority of red cell transfusions

Table 2.16 Haematological causes of cyanosis

Low-affinity haemoglobin
   α chain variants, e.g. haemoglobin Titusville
   γ chain variants, e.g. haemoglobin Toms River, haemoglobin F-Sarajevo

Methaemoglobinaemia
Variant haemoglobin (Haemoglobin M)
   α chain variants, e.g. haemoglobin M-Iwate
   γ chain variants, e.g. haemoglobin F-M-Osaka, haemoglobin F-M-Fort Ripley
Cytochrome b5 reductase (methaemoglobin reductase) deficiency
Oxidant exposure (high-dose methylene blue, local anaesthetic)

Table 2.17 Indications for red cell transfusion in the neonatal period*

Postnatal age	Haemoglobin threshold for transfusion
0–7 days	100–120 g/l (if oxygen-dependent)
	<100 g/l (if oxygen-independent)
8–14 days	95–100 g/l (if oxygen-dependent)
	<75–85 g/l (if oxygen-independent)
15 days onwards	85 g/l

* Based on the recommendations of the British Committee for Standards in Haematology.[61]

administered to neonates are small 'top-ups' for anaemia of prematurity and/or to compensate for phlebotomy losses. Increasing recognition of the hazards of transfusion in neonates has led to re-evaluation of transfusion thresholds (see recent reviews).[247–249] Many countries have developed expert-based consensus guidelines for neonatal transfusion which incorporate available evidence, much of which does not yet come from controlled trials. Two large randomised controlled trials of liberal versus restrictive transfusion policies in preterm neonates have recently been designed. The first, the Effect of Transfusion Thresholds on Neurocognitive Outcome of ELBW infants trial (ETTNO trial; NCT01393496), which was completed in October 2018, showed that using a liberal rather than restrictive red cell policy did not reduce the likelihood of death or disability at the age of 24 months.[250] The Transfusion of Prematures trial (TOPs trial; NCT01702805) is due to complete in August 2023. In the meantime, the indications for top-up transfusion and exchange transfusion recommended by the British Committee for Standards in Haematology are summarised in Table 2.17.

The main risks of transfusion in neonates include: metabolic complications, such as hyperkalaemia and hypocalcaemia; transfusion-transmitted infections, such as CMV infection if CMV-unscreened blood products are used; and immunological complications, such as TA-GvHD which, though rare in neonates, has a high mortality.[230] Many of these risks can be reduced by the use of 'paedipacks' of up to six small-volume red cell transfusion bags prepared from a single donor unit. The use of paedipacks reduces transfusion exposure for multiply transfused preterm neonates; although it may mean using older red blood cells, this has not been shown to adversely affect neonatal outcome.[61] In the UK, transfusion of CMV-seronegative blood products is also recommended for all transfusions in neonates up to 44 weeks corrected gestational age. The optimal transfusion volume for neonatal top-up transfusions has not been established but most guidelines recommend 10–20 ml/kg because higher volumes may cause clinical problems due to volume overload. IUTs require irradiated blood and, when IUT has been necessary, except in a dire emergency, transfusion of the neonate should continue to be with irradiated components to prevent TA-GvHD. The frequency of the most serious hazards of transfusion, such as transfusion-related acute lung injury (TRALI) and transfusion-associated circulatory overload (TACO), that are well recognised in older patients, is unknown in neonates.

Illustrative cases

(For abbreviations used in the text of the illustrative cases, see page 110.)

Case 2.1   Diamond–Blackfan anaemia

Case history

A 5-week-old girl presented with vomiting, failure to thrive and anaemia. She had been born at term after an uneventful pregnancy and was the first child of unrelated Caucasian parents. There was no family history of anaemia, jaundice or other haematological disorder. The blood group of the mother was group A, Rh D-negative. Routine antenatal screening did not detect any red cell alloantibodies in maternal serum during the pregnancy and prophylactic anti-D was given at 28 weeks' gestation following standard recommendations. On examination, the infant was pale but not jaundiced. Her weight was 2.65 kg at birth (<9th centile) and had dropped to the 2nd centile at the time of presentation. She had no hepatosplenomegaly but was noted to have microphthalmia and a hypoplastic left thumb.

Preliminary investigations

FBC: WBC 4.5 × 10^9/l, Hb 76 g/l, RBC 2.49 × 10^{12}/l, MCV 98.6 fl, MCH 30.4 pg, reticulocytes 28 × 10^9/l, neutrophils 1.1 × 10^9/l, platelets 136 × 10^9/l. The blood film showed normochromic, normocytic red cells (Case 2.1, Fig. 1). There was no polychromasia despite the low Hb and no NRBC were seen on the film. The Coombs test was negative. White blood cell and platelet morphology were normal.

Together, the findings suggested a differential diagnosis of red cell aplasia due to:

- Parvovirus B19 infection
- Diamond–Blackfan anaemia
- Fanconi anaemia.

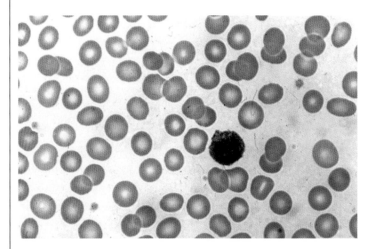

Case 2.1, Fig. 1   Blood film. MGG, ×100 objective.

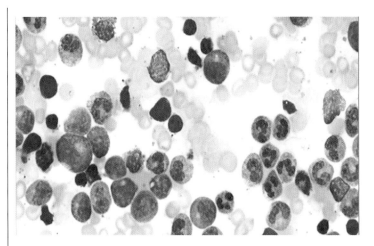

Case 2.1, Fig. 2   Bone marrow aspirate. MGG, ×60.

A peripheral blood sample showed no evidence of B19 DNA in the infant, making a diagnosis of parvovirus-induced anaemia unlikely and a bone marrow aspirate was performed (Case 2.1, Fig. 2).

Further investigations

Investigation	Result	Normal values/comments
Haemoglobin F (age 8 weeks)	30%	5–10%
Adenosine deaminase	140 nmol/h/mg haemoglobin	40–100 nmol/h/mg haemoglobin
Chromosomal breakage studies (DEB)	Normal	NA
Bone marrow aspirate	Normocellular, severe erythroid hypoplasia	NA
Molecular analysis of ribosomal protein genes	Mutation in *RPL26*	While molecular analysis is not essential for diagnosis, it is useful for family counselling, e.g. identification of *de novo* vs inherited disease and for donor selection if HSCT is planned

DEB, diepoxybutane; HSCT, haemopoietic stem cell transplantation; NA, not applicable.

Management

The presence of a heterozygous pathogenic mutation in *RPL26* together with the haematological findings were diagnostic of Diamond–Blackfan anaemia. Both parental blood counts were normal and neither had the same *RPL26* mutation indicating that this was a *de novo* mutation. Regular red cell transfusions were started to maintain her Hb between 80 and 110 g/l, resulting in improved wellbeing and weight gain. By the age of 15 months her weight was maintained between the 10th and 25th centiles and she achieved all her normal developmental milestones. After receiving routine vaccination with the MMR vaccine, she was started on prednisolone 2 mg/kg daily, to which she had a good response, and her red cell transfusions were discontinued. Although she remained transfusion-free, with an Hb of 95–105 g/l on a maintenance dose of prednisolone of 0.5 mg/kg on alternate days, she became steroid refractory at the age of 4 years and resumed regular red cell transfusions. She subsequently had a successful haemopoietic stem cell transplantation from her HLA-identical younger brother after *RPL* gene mutational analysis confirmed that he was unaffected.

For further information see references 15 and 251–253.

Case 2.2 A congenital dyserythropoietic anaemia

Case history

A newborn girl was admitted to the local special care baby unit after being noted to have tachypnoea a few hours after birth. She was a term baby and both the pregnancy and delivery had been uneventful. She was the second child of non-consanguineous, Caucasian parents. Her older brother was healthy and there was no family history of note. On examination, she looked generally well and was not jaundiced or obviously anaemic. She had no hepatosplenomegaly and no congenital anomalies were noted. Routine investigations excluded an acute infection but revealed a mild anaemia.

FBC: WBC 10.5 × 10^9/l, Hb 125 g/l, RBC 3.49 × 10^{12}/l, MCV 105.6 fl, MCH 34.5 pg, reticulocytes 84 × 10^9/l, neutrophils 3.1 × 10^9/l, platelets 336 × 10^9/l.

As the reticulocyte count was normal and the Coombs test was negative, she was discharged home and the anaemia was not investigated further. A blood film was not made.

At the age of 18 months she was referred to the paediatric clinic because a routine blood count taken during a recent viral infection had again shown moderate anaemia (Hb 89 g/l). She had been a healthy child who was gaining weight and developing normally with no history of intercurrent illnesses. She now had two brothers (aged 6 years and 2 months) who were both healthy. On examination, her height and weight were on the 50th centile and she had no dysmorphic features. She had no abnormal physical signs apart from slight pallor. In particular, she was not jaundiced and had no hepatosplenomegaly.

Preliminary investigations

FBC: WBC 8.4 × 10^9/l, Hb 89 g/l, MCV 89 fl, MCH 28 pg, reticulocytes 28 × 10^9/l, neutrophils 3.1 × 10^9/l, platelets 412 × 10^9/l. The serum bilirubin was normal (16 µmol/l) as were her urea and electrolytes. The blood film was normochromic with anisopoikilocytosis; there were no spherocytes and no polychromasia or circulating nucleated red cells were seen (Case 2.2, Fig. 1). White blood cell and platelet morphology were normal.

A differential diagnosis of red cell aplasia or dysplasia was made:

- Transient erythroblastopenia of childhood
- Diamond–Blackfan anaemia
- Congenital dyserythropoietic anaemia.

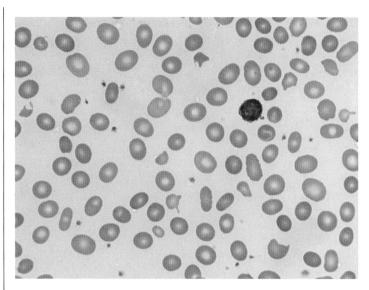

Case 2.2, Fig. 1   Blood film. MGG, ×100.

Transient erythroblastopenia of childhood is an uncommon cause of self-limiting red cell aplasia in children under the age of 4 years. The median age at presentation is 19 months and cases in infants under the age of 6 months are rare.[254] Anaemia in TEC is typically severe (30–40 g/l) and reticulocytes are typically absent at the time of presentation.[254] The majority of children have a history suggestive of a viral infection within the previous 2 weeks.[254] In most cases a specific causative virus is not identified. Parvovirus B19 has been implicated in a few cases[255] but normally only causes anaemia due to red cell aplasia in patients with congenital haemolytic anaemia. It is important to note that TEC due to HHV-6 may cause erythroblast morphological changes resembling CDA,[256] although the natural history will clarify the diagnosis as spontaneous recovery from TEC normally occurs within 1–2 months.[254]

A diagnosis of parvovirus-induced red cell aplasia was considered very unlikely in the absence of an underlying congenital haemolytic anaemia but parvovirus serology was performed to confirm this and no parvovirus B19 IgM or IgG antibodies were detected. A repeat full blood count 3 weeks after presentation showed no change and a presumptive diagnosis of DBA was made on the basis of persistent moderate anaemia and reticulocytopenia. At that point a bone marrow aspirate was performed and showed markedly increased erythropoiesis and dyserythropoiesis including binucleated forms, ruling out DBA and suggesting a diagnosis of CDA (Case 2.2, Fig. 2). Granulopoiesis was normal and megakaryocyte numbers and morphology were normal, consistent with this. HHV6 serology was negative.

Further investigations

Since the bone marrow aspirate suggested a diagnosis of CDA, bone marrow electron microscopy was performed. This showed abnormal erythroblast morphology consistent with CDA but was not considered typical of type I, II or III CDA. Samples from the

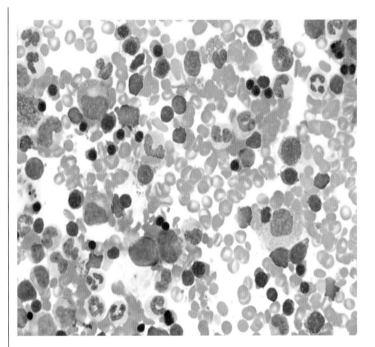

Case 2.2, Fig. 2   Bone marrow aspirate. MGG, ×40.

patient and her parents were then sent for next generation sequencing using a targeted panel of red cell genes.[3] No pathogenic variants in any of the genes known to cause CDA (*CDAN1*, *SEC23B*, *KIF23*, *CDIN1* (*c15orf41*), *KLF1* and *GATA1*) were found. Subsequently, her older brother was found to have moderate asymptomatic anaemia (Hb 91 g/l) with identical peripheral blood and bone marrow findings. Since both parents had normal blood counts and blood films, this suggests an autosomal recessive pattern of inheritance and samples are currently being analysed by whole genome sequencing to try to identify the molecular basis for this anaemia.

Diagnostic notes

- The diagnosis of CDA is often difficult because the blood film changes are not diagnostic.
- Molecular analysis, usually involving red cell targeted next generation sequencing panel, is increasingly used to establish or confirm a diagnosis of CDA and is essential for family studies, prenatal diagnosis and guiding management.
- Bone marrow morphology and electron microscopy remains useful for evaluating newly described variants in known CDA genes or new genes.

For further information see references 3 and 257–261.

Case 2.3   Haemolytic disease of the fetus and newborn due to anti-B

Case history

A term baby born after an uneventful pregnancy was noted to be pale at birth and developed increasing jaundice over the first 24 hours of life. Both of his parents originated from Ghana. He had two older siblings who were both well and there was no family history of anaemia or other haematological abnormality. On questioning, his mother remembered that her first child, a boy, had also developed severe jaundice at birth that has been treated by phototherapy. On examination, there were no clinical findings apart from pallor and moderately severe jaundice. In particular, there was no evidence of hydrops; he was not shocked; his birthweight was normal (3.4 kg), there was no evidence of hepatosplenomegaly, no skin rash and no dysmorphic features.

A provisional diagnosis of neonatal haemolytic anaemia was made on the basis of the severe jaundice and pallor in the absence of clinical signs suggestive of acute blood loss. The diagnoses considered initially were:

- Immune haemolysis
- Inherited red cell enzyme deficiency
- Inherited red cell membrane disorder (HPP or hereditary elliptocytosis with infantile poikilocytosis).

Preliminary investigations

FBC: WBC 45×10^9/l, Hb 55 g/l, MCV 128 fl, MCH 39.5 pg, reticulocytes 280×10^9/l, neutrophils 8.1×10^9/l, platelets 168×10^9/l.

Biochemistry: bilirubin 390 μmol/l.

The blood film showed large numbers of spherocytes, polychromasia and increased numbers of circulating erythroblasts (Case 2.3, Fig. 1). The true WBC count (corrected for circulating erythroblasts) was 18.4×10^9/l and white blood cell and platelet morphology were normal. The blood film appearances and raised MCV excluded a diagnosis of HPP.

Further investigations

Investigation	Result	Normal values/comment
Coombs test	Positive	Positive result indicates immune haemolysis; the Coombs test is occasionally negative in HDFN due to anti-A or anti-B antibodies[257]
Maternal blood group	O Rh D-positive	NA
Baby's blood group	B Rh D-positive	NA
Maternal serology	High-titre IgG anti-A and anti-B	~1% of group O pregnant women have high-titre IgG antibodies[258]

HDFN, haemolytic disease of the fetus and newborn; Ig, immunoglobulin; NA, not applicable.

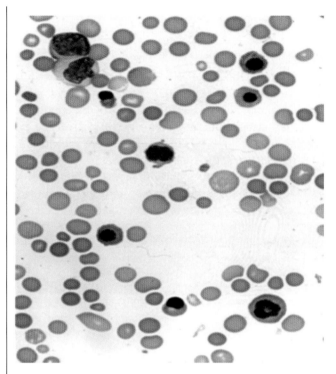

Case 2.3, Fig. 1 Blood film. MGG, ×40.

A final diagnosis of HDFN due to anti-B was made in view of the positive Coombs test in conjunction with the blood film appearances, maternal/baby blood groups and the maternal serology. Where haemolysis is very severe and/or the diagnosis is in doubt, a diagnosis of HDFN due to anti-B can be confirmed by performing a red cell eluate on the neonatal red cells to demonstrate the antibody specificity. However in this case, exchange transfusion was performed without awaiting this result in view of the severity of the anaemia and hyperbilirubinaemia. G6PD enzyme activity was assayed on a pretransfusion blood sample to exclude concomitant G6PD deficiency as this is known to increase the severity of the hyperbilirubinaemia but the level was 10.3 U/g Hb (normal range 7.0–10.4 U/g Hb).

Diagnostic notes

- Fetomaternal haemorrhage is not normally accompanied by marked hyperbilirubinaemia.
- Severe haemolytic anaemia at birth is unusual in G6PD deficiency.
- The principal haemoglobinopathies causing severe anaemia in neonates are α globin disorders (α thalassaemia major/haemoglobin Bart's hydrops fetalis or, much less often, haemoglobin H disease) which would not be compatible with the clinical picture of severe haemolytic anaemia in a relatively well term baby.

For further information see references 53 and 262–264.

Case 2.4   Hereditary pyropoikilocytosis (α spectrin^{LELY})

Case history

A 4-week-old girl was referred to the paediatric clinic because of failure to thrive. She had been born at term after an uneventful pregnancy. Her mother was blood group A Rh D-positive. She was well at birth and was discharged home on day 2 of life with resolving mild jaundice. She was the second child of unrelated Caucasian parents (first child, age 9 years, was well) and there was no family history of note. On examination, she was sleepy and pale but not clinically jaundiced; she had mild splenomegaly (spleen palpable 1.5 cm below left costal margin). She had no dysmorphic features.

Preliminary investigations

FBC: WBC 8.7×10^9/l, Hb 50 g/l, MCV 65.6 fl, MCH 26 pg, reticulocytes 210×10^9/l, platelets 761×10^9/l. The blood film showed marked anisopoikilocytosis, polychromasia, microspherocytes and fragmented red cells (Case 2.4, Fig. 1). White blood cell morphology was normal. The number of platelets in the blood film appeared to be normal and platelet morphology was normal.

Differential diagnosis of neonatal microcytic anaemia (see Table 2.12)

- Hereditary pyropoikilocytosis
- Congenital sideroblastic anaemia
- Thalassaemia: α thalassaemia (haemoglobin Bart's hydrops fetalis, haemoglobin H disease) or $\gamma\delta\beta$ thalassemia.

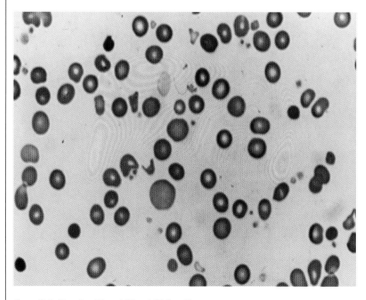

Case 2.4, Fig. 1   Blood film. MGG, ×40.

Although microcytic anaemia is extremely uncommon in the neonatal period, and the disorders associated with microcytic anaemia in this age group are rare or very rare, the likely diagnosis is often fairly easily identified from the blood film. In this case, thalassaemia was considered very unlikely given the family and clinical history, especially given the absence of typical thalassaemic features in the blood film, such as hypochromic red cells, target cells and circulating erythroblasts. Congenital sideroblastic anaemia was also considered unlikely in this female baby as the autosomal recessive forms of this disease cause very severe, transfusion-dependent microcytic anaemia soon after birth (*SLC25A38* mutations) and/or are associated with other major anomalies, including immunodeficiency and developmental delay (*TRNT1* mutations). By contrast, the distinctive red cell morphology was highly suggestive of HPP. Given this, further investigations were arranged, including assessing the blood counts and blood films of both parents for evidence of hereditary elliptocytosis.

Further investigations

Investigations	Results	Normal range/comments
Parental FBCs, including reticulocyte count	All values normal	Bilirubin also normal
Parental blood films	Both normal	The blood film is normal in individuals with common α spectrin variants (polymorphisms) which do not cause disease on their own but may interact with pathogenic spectrin variants inherited *in trans*[85]
HPLC	Patient: normal Parents: normal	
Mass spectrometry for haemoglobin variants	Patient: normal Parents: normal	
Red cell enzyme assays	G6PD (parents): normal	No other red cell enzymes were assayed because the clinical picture did not suggest a red cell enzymopathy and the child was red cell transfusion-dependent.
Functional red cell membrane studies (flow cytometry)	EMA dye binding Patient: reduced Parents: normal	Reduced EMA dye binding is typical of hereditary spherocytosis but can also be seen in HPP[265]
Molecular analysis of red cell membrane proteins	Patient: α spectrin^{LELY}/α spectrin$^{I/174}$ Father: normal Mother: α spectrin^{LELY}/α spectrin^{LELY}	α spectrin^{LELY} is the most frequently recognised hypomorphic variant that can contribute to the phenotype of elliptocytic disorders. *De novo* spectrin variants are common
Bone marrow aspirate	Not done	Not indicated where all investigations are consistent with a diagnosis of HPP

EMA, eosin-5-maleimide; FBC, full blood count; G6PD, glucose-6-phosphate dehydrogenase; HPP, hereditary pyropoikilocytosis; HPLC, high performance liquid chromatography.

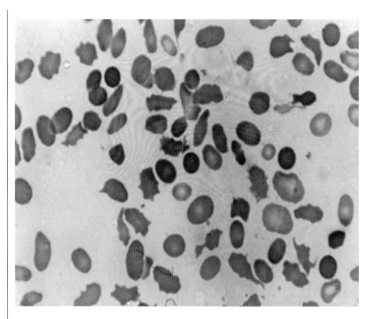

Case 2.4, Fig. 2 Blood film. MGG, ×40.

Management

The infant was started initially treated with a top-up red cell transfusion with rapid symptomatic improvement. However, the Hb gradually dropped over the following few weeks and she proved to be red cell transfusion-dependent. By 6 months of age her blood film showed a much greater proportion of classical elliptocytes, although micro-spherocytes and red cell fragments could still be seen (Case 2.4, Fig. 2). This change in red cell morphology over the first few months of life is characteristic of HPP. A decision was made to place her on regular red cell transfusions every 4 weeks with the introduction of iron chelation by the age of 2 years. She subsequently underwent a splenectomy at the age of 4 years and she remains well and transfusion-independent more than 5 years later.

Diagnostic notes

- The most important clue to the diagnosis is the low MCV in the first blood count. Microcytic anaemia is rare in children less than 3 months of age and HPP should always be considered.
- The age of the baby excludes fetomaternal haemorrhage and HDFN. The ethnic origin makes haemoglobinopathies and G6PD deficiency unlikely (and the child was female).
- Examination of parental blood films is usually helpful in congenital anaemias, particularly where patients have been transfused. Interpretation of family studies may be complex because α spectrin mutations are often clinically silent, as in this case.

For further information see references 18, 70, 85 and 265–268.

Case 2.5   Pyruvate kinase deficiency

Case history

A male neonate born at term to unrelated parents (mother Jamaican, father Scottish) presented with mild hydrops fetalis and severe anaemia (Hb 64 g/l) at birth after a normal pregnancy and delivery. His mother was group O Rh D-negative but routine screening had not detected any red cell alloantibodies in maternal serum during the pregnancy and prophylactic anti-D had been given at 28 weeks' gestation following standard recommendations. He was the first child and there was no family history of note. Six hours after birth he became jaundiced. The jaundice progressed rapidly despite phototherapy and he underwent exchange transfusion at 24 hours of age. At that point he had mild hepatosplenomegaly (1 cm below costal margins) but no other clinical abnormalities and no dysmorphic features were noted.

The diagnoses considered initially were:

- Immune haemolysis (HDFN)
- Haemoglobinopathy (α or γδβ thalassaemia)
- Inherited red cell enzyme deficiency
- Inherited microcytic anaemia: HPP, hereditary elliptocytosis with infantile poikilocytosis or congenital sideroblastic anaemia
- Congenital dyserythropoietic anaemia.

Initial investigations

FBC: WBC 19.5×10^9/l (corrected for NRBC, 24.6×10^9/l), Hb 64 g/l, MCV 128 fl, MCH 30.4 pg, reticulocytes 280×10^9/l, neutrophils 12.3×10^9/l, platelets 168×10^9/l. The serum bilirubin increased from 90 μmol/l at 6 hours to 360 μmol/l at 24 hours of age. As the maternal blood group was O Rh D-negative, the baby's blood group O Rh D-negative and a Coombs test was negative, HDFN was excluded as the cause of the anaemia. No pretransfusion blood film was available but the high MCV virtually excluded a diagnosis of HPP, major haemoglobinopathies and congenital sideroblastic anaemia. Since the baby had been transfused, initial investigations were performed on samples from both parents. Blood counts, blood films, HPLC and G6PD enzyme assays in both parents were normal. A provisional diagnosis of severe non-immune neonatal haemolysis of unknown cause was made and further investigations were planned.

Follow-up

The jaundice gradually improved over the first 2 weeks of life but he continued to be transfusion-dependent, receiving a further four transfusions by the age of 8 months (Hb nadir approximately 50 g/l) with ongoing mild jaundice and variable reticulocytosis. He was otherwise well and growing normally. At this point, the blood film showed occasional circulating erythroblasts and very occasional echinocytes but was largely normochromic and normocytic with no spherocytes (Case 2.5, Fig. 1). The WBC and platelets were also normal in numbers and

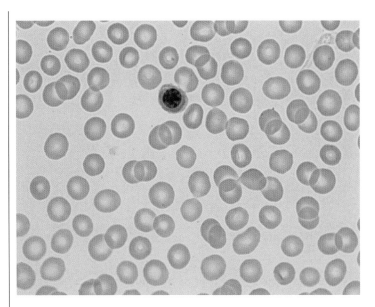

Case 2.5, Fig. 1 Blood film. MGG, ×100.

morphology. A diagnosis of CDA was considered and a bone marrow aspirate was performed, which showed marked erythroid hyperplasia and dyserythropoiesis with 1–2% binucleated forms (Case 2.5, Fig. 2). The findings were considered non-specific and additional investigations were performed on the patient and his parents in order to identify the cause of his haemolytic anaemia (see Table). Molecular analysis using a targeted red cell gene panel showed the child had compound heterozygosity for two known pathogenic variants in the *PKLR* gene, with one inherited from each parent. Repeat enzyme assay just prior to a transfusion confirmed the diagnosis of PK deficiency.

	Patient (age 8 months; pretransfusion)	Mother	Father
Hb (g/l)	50–71	132	143
MCV (fl)	86	89	91
MCH (pg)	29	29	31
Reticulocytes ($\times 10^9$/l)	43–226	57	66
G6PD (U/g Hb) (NR 7–10.4 U/g Hb)	8.8	9.2	7.8
PK (U/g Hb) (NR 6.2–14.2 U/g Hb)	6.2	8.4	7.1
Molecular analysis (targeted NGS panel)	$1529^{G->A}$/$829^{G->A}$	$829^{G->A}$	$1529^{G->A}$

G6PD, glucose-6-phosphate dehydrogenase; Hb, haemoglobin concentration; MCH, mean cell haemoglobin; MCV, mean cell volume; NGS, next generation sequencing; NR, normal range; PK, pyruvate kinase.

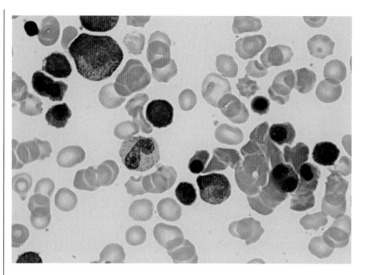

Case 2.5, Fig. 2 Bone marrow aspirate. MGG, ×100.

Diagnostic notes

- Diagnosis of PK deficiency is frequently difficult and therefore delayed.
- PK levels are higher in reticulocytes; this frequently masks PK deficiency both in heterozygotes and homozygotes.
- There is little or no correlation between the PK level and the severity of anaemia unless samples are corrected for the number of reticulocytes.
- Phenotype–genotype studies in PK deficiency are especially difficult in compound heterozygotes because the different mutant enzymes form tetramers with unique properties.
- PK deficiency should be considered in cases of unexplained fetal anaemia and/or hydrops fetalis, atypical 'CDA' and non-spherocytic congenital haemolytic anaemia.
- Management options for PK deficiency include splenectomy, intermittent or regular transfusions, and haemopoietic stem cell transplantation. More recently, clinical trials of an orally administered allosteric activator of PK have begun.

For further information see references 92, 103 and 269–271.

Case 2.6 Infantile pyknocytosis

Case history

A 3-week-old girl born at 30 weeks' gestation, was found to have an unexpectedly low Hb when checked as part of a routine weekly screen in the special care baby unit. She had no abnormalities on examination apart from pallor and mild jaundice. In particular, her birthweight was within the normal range (25th centile), she had no hepatosplenomegaly and no congenital anomalies were noted. Routine FBC at the age of 2 weeks had shown an Hb within the normal range for age (110 g/l). Her neonatal course had been uneventful apart from an episode of presumed sepsis treated with a short course of antibiotics. She was the first born of monochorionic twins delivered uneventfully when her mother went into spontaneous labour. There was no family history of note. Her blood count, including Hb, had been normal at birth (185 g/l). She had developed moderate jaundice on day 4, treated by phototherapy and resolving by day 7. At that time, the blood film was normal and the Coombs test was negative. The baby and her mother were both group O Rh D-positive. The blood count and Hb of her twin sister were normal and almost identical (187 g/l), excluding any significant twin-to-twin transfusion.

The diagnoses considered initially were:

- Anaemia of prematurity
- Infantile pyknocytosis
- Inherited red cell enzyme deficiency.

Preliminary investigations (age 3 weeks)

FBC: WBC 8.5×10^9/l, Hb 66 g/l, MCV 101 fl, MCH 34 pg, reticulocytes 180×10^9/l, neutrophils 2.1×10^9/l, platelets 316×10^9/l. Bilirubin was 120 µmol/l. The blood film showed pyknocytes (irregularly contracted and acanthocytic cells), polychromasia, some red cell fragmentation and occasional spherocytes and NRBC (Case 2.6, Fig. 1). White blood cell and platelet morphology was normal.

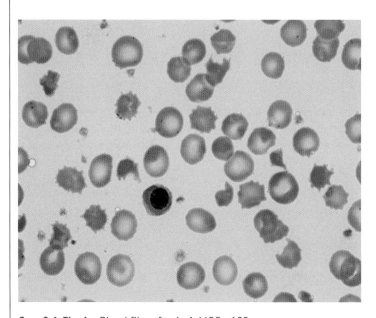

Case 2.6, Fig. 1   Blood film of twin 1. MGG, ×100.

The sudden fall in Hb between week 2 and week 3 of age and the blood film appearances were suggestive of oxidative haemolysis due to an inherited red cell enzyme deficiency or to the self-limiting neonatal-specific condition, infantile pyknocytosis. These features exclude a diagnosis of anaemia of prematurity as the blood film in anaemia of prematurity is normal.

Further investigations

Pretransfusion G6PD assay and PK assays both showed increased levels, consistent with the reticulocytosis (G6PD 19.3 U/g Hb, PK 15.2 U/g Hb). Glutathione peroxidase was 8.5 U/g Hb (normal range 13.0–30.0).

These results exclude a diagnosis of G6PD deficiency and make a diagnosis of PK deficiency unlikely although, as seen in Case 2.5, molecular analysis and parental investigation is needed to fully exclude PK deficiency in cases with persistent haemolysis. Glutathione peroxidase levels are often reduced in infantile pyknocytosis but this finding is not specific for infantile pyknocytosis and no mutations are found in the *GPX* gene.[112]

Clinical course

The baby was given a top-up red cell transfusion, raising her Hb to 120 g/l. Over the next 2 weeks her Hb slowly declined to 100 g/l, but her jaundice and the changes of oxidative haemolysis on her blood film gradually resolved. By the age of 8 weeks her Hb was stable at 95–105 g/l, her blood film was normal, she was gaining weight normally and she was clinically well. One week after initial presentation, the baby's twin sister presented at age 4 weeks with a low Hb (62 g/l) and her blood film showed changes of oxidative haemolysis similar to those of the index case, though milder (Case 2.6, Fig. 2). Both girls continued to do well at follow-up at age 12 months with no further episodes of jaundice or anaemia.

Diagnostic notes

- Infantile pyknocytosis typically presents at the age of 2–4 weeks in otherwise well neonates and resolves by 6–8 weeks of age. Recurrence later in life is not reported.
- There is rarely a family history and there are no congenital anomalies or other associated clinical features. Occasional cases in twins or siblings have been reported previously.[250]
- The blood film is typical of oxidative haemolysis but in addition there are often acanthocytic changes; no evidence of known red cell enzymopathies is found (e.g. no evidence of G6PD deficiency and, where investigated, parental blood counts and blood films are normal).
- The anaemia is often sufficiently severe at presentation to require treatment with red cell transfusion, usually only on a single occasion.
- The diagnosis is made from the combination of the characteristic presentation, blood film and natural history.

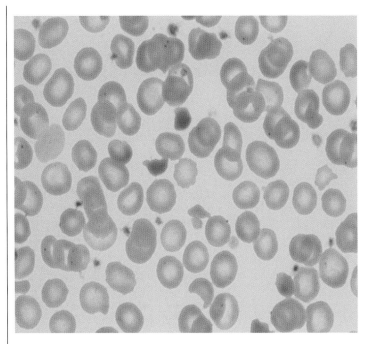

Case 2.6, Fig. 2   Blood film of twin 2. MGG, ×100.

- Transient deficiency of glutathione peroxidase has been implicated as a cause of neonatal oxidative haemolysis[112] and is usually found if enzyme levels are checked prior to transfusion (unpublished data). These levels normalise once the haemolysis resolves.

For further information see references 112 and 272–275.

Case 2.7   Methylene blue-induced haemolytic anaemia

Case history

A preterm male baby was born at 33 weeks' gestation following induction because of abnormal umbilical artery Dopplers suggesting placental insufficiency.[121] A diagnosis of Down syndrome was suspected and confirmed by FISH showing trisomy 21. His FBC was normal (WBC 18.2×10^9/l, Hb 192 g/l, platelets 153×10^9/l) and a blood film showed changes typical of Down syndrome but no evidence of the preleukaemic condition, transient abnormal myelopoiesis (see Chapter 3). He was found to have duodenal atresia and underwent urgent surgery (duodenoduodenostomy) on day 2 of life. During the procedure, methylene blue was used to confirm the integrity of the

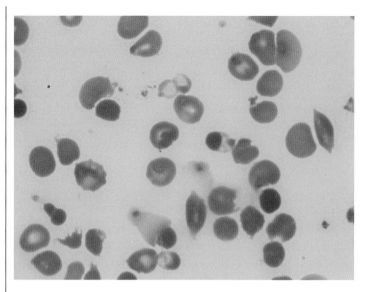

Case 2.7, Fig. 1 Blood film. Based on reference 12. MGG, ×100.

anastomosis. Following this, his skin was noticed to have a bluish tinge, he was noted to pass bluish green urine and over the ensuing 2–3 days he developed rapidly progressive hyperbilirubinaemia.

Investigations

FBC: WBC 25.2 × 10^9/l, Hb 67 g/l, MCV 106 fl, MCH 34 pg, reticulocytes 260 × 10^9/l, neutrophils 14.3 × 10^9/l, platelets 102 × 10^9/l. The blood film showed irregularly contracted red cells, blister cells and ghost cells, some of which contained visible Heinz bodies (Case 2.7, Fig. 1). White blood cell and platelet morphology were normal.

The diagnoses considered initially were:

- Methylene blue-induced haemolysis with or without G6PD deficiency
- Infantile pyknocytosis.

Progress and management

The clinical presentation and blood film findings were considered typical of acute oxidative haemolysis most likely triggered by methylene blue. The G6PD assay showed higher than normal enzyme activity (13.0 U/g Hb), most likely reflecting the reticulocytosis and excluding G6PD deficiency as the underlying diagnosis. The baby was treated by top-up red cell transfusion and made an uneventful recovery.

Diagnostic notes

- A rapid fall in Hb together with increasing jaundice in a neonate is highly suggestive of oxidative haemolysis.
- The blood film in oxidative haemolysis shows distinctive morphological changes in the red cells, including Heinz bodies; these can be confirmed by supravital staining but, as in this baby, are often evident on close examination of a blood film.
- Methylene blue may cause severe oxidative haemolysis in neonates even in the absence of G6PD deficiency;[276,277] one of three previously reported cases also had trisomy 21.[277]

Case 2.8   Haemoglobin Bart's hydrops fetalis

Case history

A neonate born at 28 weeks' gestation was found on the first day of life to have an Hb of 91 g/l. During the pregnancy the routine anomaly scan at 20 weeks' gestation showed polyhydramnios, an enlarged fetal heart and slight oedema around the fetal head and abdomen. The mother was group A Rh D-positive and no red cell alloantibodies were detected in maternal serum. A provisional diagnosis of congenital heart disease was made but detailed scanning the following week showed no structural abnormalities of the heart and no further investigations were performed. After spontaneous onset of labour, the baby was born in very poor condition and required intensive respiratory and cardiovascular support with mechanical ventilation and inotropes. A provisional diagnosis of cardiac failure and severe neonatal sepsis was made and she was started on antibiotics. She was also noted to be pale and jaundiced and had to have marked hepatosplenomegaly. She had no apparent congenital anomalies at birth although subsequent investigations revealed severe pulmonary hypoplasia. She was the second child of parents who originated from southern China. Her older brother (aged 7 years) was well with no history of neonatal jaundice or anaemia. There was no family history of note.

Preliminary investigations (at birth)

FBC: WBC 38.5×10^9/l (corrected for NRBC 10.13×10^9/l), Hb 91 g/l, MCV 97 fl (normal range for gestation 103–130 fl), MCH 23 pg (normal range for gestation 33.5–43 pg), reticulocytes 180×10^9/l, neutrophils 2.1×10^9/l, platelets 98×10^9/l. The blood film showed very marked polychromasia, erythroblastosis and red cell hypochromia, as well as numerous target cells (Case 2.8, Fig. 1). White blood cell and platelet morphology were normal and there was no evidence of sepsis on blood film examination.

The diagnoses considered initially were:

- Thalassaemia: α thalassaemia major, haemoglobin H disease, $\gamma\delta\beta$ thalassaemia
- Congenital sideroblastic anaemia
- Fetomaternal haemorrhage
- Haemolytic disease of the fetus and newborn.

In view of the poor condition of the baby, further investigations to determine the cause of the anaemia were performed on blood samples from both of her parents as well as the baby. The results excluded HDFN as the cause or a contributory factor to the neonatal anaemia in this case and a negative Kleihauer made it very unlikely that significant fetomaternal haemorrhage was the explanation for the anaemia. On the other hand, the striking hypochromia and erythroblastosis was highly suggestive of α thalassaemia major even though this usually results in death *in utero* or within a few hours of birth. Nevertheless, both parental blood films showed mild microcytic anaemia and the presence of haemoglobin H bodies (precipitates of β_4 globin tetramers) consistent

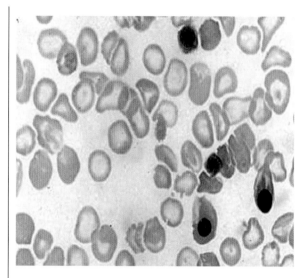

Case 2.8, Fig. 1   Blood film. MGG, ×100.

with α^0 thalassaemia trait. Analysis of the baby's blood prior to transfusion showed mainly haemoglobin Bart's, together with haemoglobin Portland and haemoglobin H, consistent with a diagnosis of α thalassaemia major. Subsequent molecular analysis showed that the baby was homozygous for the most common α globin deletion in southern China ($--^{SEA}$) and that both parents were heterozygous for this deletion ($\alpha\alpha/--^{SEA}$).

Further investigations

	Baby	Mother	Father
Hb (g/l)	91	102	105
MCV (fl)	97	72.7	73
MCH (pg)	23	23.9	22.8
Coombs test	negative	NA	NA
Kleihauer test	NA	Negative	NA
H bodies	Not tested	Present	Present
Haemoglobin HPLC	Haemoglobin Bart's (γ_4) Haemoglobin Portland ($\zeta_2\gamma_2$) Haemoglobin H (β_4)	Haemoglobin A Haemoglobin A_2 (2.6%) Haemoglobin F (1.1%)	Haemoglobin A Haemoglobin A_2 (2.9%) Haemoglobin F (1.3%)
α globin genotype (gap-PCR)	$--^{SEA}/--^{SEA}$	$\alpha\alpha/--^{SEA}$	$\alpha\alpha/--^{SEA}$

Gap-PCR, gap polymerase chain reaction; Hb, haemoglobin concentration; HPLC, high performance liquid chromatography; MCH mean cell haemoglobin; MCV, mean cell volume; NA, not applicable.

Progress and management

Unfortunately, the condition of the baby steadily deteriorated during the second day of life due to increasing difficulty with maintaining normal oxygenation because of pulmonary hypoplasia and she died on day 3 of life. Subsequent review of the case revealed that antenatal counselling had failed to convey the risk of α thalassaemia to the parents and the opportunity for early diagnosis and institution of intrauterine transfusion during the second trimester had been missed.

Diagnostic notes

- Identification of anaemia as microcytic is an important diagnostic clue as microcytic anaemias are rare in neonates; this may be missed in preterm neonates because the MCV in healthy babies is much higher in preterm than term neonates (see Table 1.2).
- Neonates with α thalassaemia major who are born preterm may have sufficient levels of haemoglobin Portland to allow them to survive for several days after birth; however, unless intrauterine transfusion has been instituted by 20/21 weeks' gestation, severe *in utero* hypoxia will cause pulmonary hypoplasia and irreversible neurological damage incompatible with life.
- Evaluation of parental blood counts and blood films is a useful and rapid way of helping to plan the most useful tests for unexplained neonatal anaemia.

For further information see references 154 and 278.

Case 2.9   Fetomaternal haemorrhage

Case history

A male term baby was noted to be very pale at birth with signs of circulatory shock, tachycardia and tachypnoea. He had been born by normal vaginal delivery following a short labour and straightforward pregnancy. The mother was known to be blood group O Rh D-negative and no red cell alloantibodies were noted on antenatal screening. The baby was the third child of unrelated Caucasian parents, both older siblings were well and there was no family history of note. No congenital anomalies were noted on examination, the baby was not clinically jaundiced and there was no hepatosplenomegaly. Urgent blood tests showed severe anaemia (Hb 45 g/l) and he was immediately transfused with group O Rh D-negative red cells.

Preliminary investigations (at birth)

FBC: WBC $56.0 × 10^9$/l (corrected for NRBC $21.5 × 10^9$/l), Hb 45 g/l, MCV 106 fl, MCH 34 pg, reticulocytes $160 × 10^9$/l, neutrophils $12.1 × 10^9$/l, platelets $178 × 10^9$/l. The blood film showed very marked polychromasia and erythroblastosis and red cell anisocytosis with some spherocytes (Case 2.9, Fig. 1). White blood cell and platelet morphology were normal.

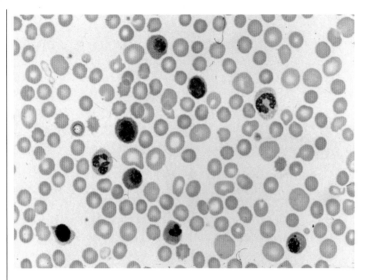

Case 2.9, Fig. 1   Blood film. MGG, ×40.

A provisional diagnosis of an acute fetomaternal haemorrhage was made on the basis of the clinical findings, including the absence of jaundice which made a diagnosis of haemolysis unlikely. The large number of circulating erythroblasts excluded a diagnosis of red cell aplasia.

Further investigations

Serum bilirubin 40 μmol/l, Coombs test negative, Kleihauer test (mother) positive (estimated fetal bleed 120 ml).

Principle of the Kleihauer–Betke test (acid elution) and estimation of the volume of fetomaternal haemorrhage

Haemoglobin F is more resistant to acid elution than adult haemoglobin (haemoglobin A). When a dry blood film is fixed and then immersed in an acid buffer solution, haemoglobin A is denatured and eluted, leaving red cell ghosts, while haemoglobin F-containing red cells, which are resistant, are easily seen against the maternal 'ghost' cells (Case 2.9, Fig. 2 shows a large fetomaternal haemorrhage).

The volume of the fetal blood loss can be estimated by comparing the ratio of haemoglobin F-containing (fetal) cells with ghost haemoglobin A-containing (adult) cells in the maternal blood sample using the following formula:[279]

$$\frac{\text{No. of fetal cells per high power field}}{\text{No. of maternal cells per high power field}} \times 1800^* \times \frac{122^\dagger}{100} \times \frac{100}{92^\ddagger}$$

* Volume of maternal red cells;
† fetal cells are 22% larger than maternal cells;
‡ only 92% of fetal cells stain darkly using this technique.
In the example shown above, 100 fetal cells were seen per 2000 maternal cells and the fetomaternal haemorrhage was estimated as 119.2 ml.

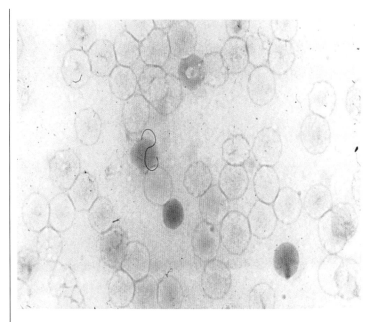

Case 2.9, Fig. 2 Kleihauer test. ×100.

Progress and management

Following emergency red cell transfusion the baby's condition rapidly improved and no further transfusions were necessary during the neonatal period. Follow-up to assess progress against normal developmental milestones was arranged in view of the risk of long-term neurological damage following a major fetomaternal haemorrhage.

Diagnostic notes

- Fetomaternal haemorrhage is one of the commonest causes of severe anaemia at birth.
- It is essential to perform a maternal Kleihauer test within the first few days to make a diagnosis of fetomaternal haemorrhage; later samples will seriously underestimate the size of the haemorrhage and may lead to a missed diagnosis.
- The Coombs test will be negative, ruling out all forms of immune haemolysis apart from very rare cases of severe Coombs-negative ABO haemolytic disease of the newborn.
- The absence of a family history and of specific red cell abnormalities in the blood film makes a rare inherited anaemia unlikely.

For further information see references 279–282.

Abbreviations used in the illustrative cases

CDA	congenital dyserythropoietic anaemia
DBA	Diamond–Blackfan anaemia
FBC	full blood count
FISH	fluorescence *in situ* hybridisation
Gap-PCR	gap polymerase chain reaction
G6PD	glucose-6-phosphate dehydrogenase
Hb	haemoglobin concentration
HDFN	haemolytic disease of the fetus and newborn
HHV-6	human herpesvirus-6
HPLC	high performance liquid chromatography
HPP	hereditary pyropoikilocytosis
Ig	immunoglobulin
MCH	mean cell haemoglobin
MCV	mean cell volume
MGG	May–Grünwald–Giemsa
MMR	measles, mumps, rubella
NR	normal range
NRBC	nucleated red blood cells
PK	pyruvate kinase
RBC	red blood cell count
TEC	transient erythroblastopenia of childhood
WBC	white blood cell count

References

1 Brugnara C and Platt OS (2009) The neonatal erythrocyte and its disorders. In: Orkin SH, Nathan DG, Ginsburg D, Look AT, Fisher DE and Lux SE (eds), *Nathan and Oski's Hematology of Infancy and Childhood*, 7th edn. Saunders, Philadelphia, pp. 21–66.

2 Linderkamp O, Nelle M, Kraus M and Zilow EP (1992) The effect of early and late cord clamping on blood viscosity and other hemorheological parameters in full-term infants. *Acta Paediat*, **81**, 745–750.

3 Roy NBA, Wilson, EA, Henderson, S, Wray, K, Babbs, C, Okoli, S *et al.* (2016) A novel 33-Gene targeted resequencing panel provides accurate, clinical-grade diagnosis and improves patient management for rare inherited anaemias. *Br J Haematol*, **175**, 318–330.

4 Rets A, Clayton AL, Christensen RD and Agarwal AM (2019) Molecular diagnostic update in hereditary hemolytic anemia and neonatal hyperbilirubinemia. *Int J Lab Hematol*, **41** (Suppl 1), 95–101.

5 Brown K (2000) Haematological consequences of parvovirus B19 infection. *Baillière's Best Pract Res Clin Haematol*, **13**, 245–259.

6 Ronchi A, Zeray F, Lee LE, Owen KE, Shoup AG, Garcia F et al. (2020) Evaluation of clinically asymptomatic high risk infants with congenital cytomegalovirus infection. *J Perinatol*, **40**, 89–96.

7 Crane J, Mundle W and Boucoiran I; Maternal Fetal Medicine Committee (2014) Parvovirus B19 infection in pregnancy. *J Obstet Gynaecol Can*, **36**, 1107–1116.

8 Bellini C, Donarini G, Paladini D, Calevo MG, Bellini T, Ramenghi KA and Hennekam RC (2015) Etiology of non-immune hydrops fetalis: an update. *Am J Med Genet Part A*, **167A**, 1082–1088.

9 Bascietto F, Liberati M, Murgano D, Buca D, Iacovelli A, Flacco ME *et al.* (2018) Outcome of fetuses with congenital parvovirus B19 infection: systematic review and meta-analysis. *Ultrasound Obstet Gynecol*, **52**, 569–576.

10 Lejeune A, Cremer M, von Bernuth H, Edelmann A, Modrow S and Bührer C (2014) Persistent pure red cell aplasia in dicygotic [sic] twins with persistent congenital parvovirus B19 infection- remission following high dose intravenous immunoglobulin. *Eur J Pediatr*, **173**, 1723–1726.

11 Brown KE, Green SW, Antunez de Mayolo J, Bellanti JA, Smith SD, Smith TJ and Young NS (1994) Congenital anaemia after transplacental B19 parvovirus infection. *Lancet*, **343**, 895–896.

12 Janssen O and Lin J (2021) Postnatal IVIG treatment for persistent anaemia in neonate due to congenital parvovirus infection. *BMJ Case Rep*, **14**, e237393.

13 Dabboubi R, Amri Y, Yahyaoui S, Mahjoub R, Sahli CA, Sahli C *et al.* (2020) A new case of congenital atransferrinemia with a novel splice mutation: c.293-63del. *Eur J Med Genet*, **63**, 103874.

14 Ulirsch JC, Verboon JM, Kazerounian S, Guo MH, Yuan D, Ludwig LS *et al.* (2018) The genetic landscape of Diamond-Blackfan anemia. *Am J Hum Genet*, **103**, 930–947.

15 Gerrard G, Volganon M, Foong HE, Kasperaviciute D, Iskander D, Game L *et al.* (2013) Target enrichment and high-throughput sequencing of 80 ribosomal protein genes to identify mutations associated with Diamond-Blackfan anaemia. *Br J Haematol*, **162**, 530–536.

16 Vlachos A, Ball S, Dahl N, Alter BP, Sheth S, Ramenghi U *et al.* Participants of Sixth Annual Daniella Maria Arturi International Consensus Conference (2008) Diagnosing and treating Diamond Blackfan anaemia: results of an international clinical consensus conference. *Br J Haematol*, **142**, 859–876.

17 Da Costa L, Leblanc T and Mohandas N (2020) Diamond-Blackfan anemia. *Blood*, **136**, 1262–1273.

18 Da Costa L, Chanoz-Poulard G, Simansour M, French M, Bouvier R, Prieur F *et al.* (2013) First *de novo* mutation in *RPS19* gene as the cause of hydrops fetalis in Diamond-Blackfan anemia [published correction appears in *Am J Hematol*, 2013, 160]. *Am J Hematol*, **88**, 340–341.

19 Wlodarski MW, Da Costa L, O'Donohue MF, Gastou M, Karboul N, Montel-Lehry N *et al.* (2018) Recurring mutations in *RPL15* are linked to hydrops fetalis and treatment independence in Diamond-Blackfan anemia. *Haematologica*, **103**, 949–958.

20 Sankaran VG, Ghazvinian R, Do R, Thiru P, Vergilio JA, Beggs AH *et al.* (2012) Exome sequencing identifies GATA1 mutations resulting in Diamond-Blackfan anemia. *J Clin Invest*, **122**, 2439–2443.

21 Gripp KW, Curry C, Olney AH, Sandoval C, Fisher J, Chong JX *et al.*; and UW Center for Mendelian Genomics (2014). Diamond-Blackfan anemia with mandibulofacial dystostosis is heterogeneous, including the novel DBA genes TSR2 and RPS28. *Am J Med Genet A*, **164A**, 2240–2249.

22 Mirabello L, Khincha PP, Ellis SR, Giri N, Brodie S, Chandrasekharappa SC *et al.* (2017) Novel and known ribosomal causes of Diamond-Blackfan anaemia identified through comprehensive genomic characterisation *J Med Genet*, **54**, 417–425

23 Bartels M and Bierings M (2019) How I manage children with Diamond-Blackfan anaemia. *Br J Haematol*, **184**, 123–133.

24 Broomfield A, Sweeney MG, Woodward CE, Fratter C, Morris AM, Leonard JV *et al.* (2015) Paediatric single mitochondrial DNA deletion disorders: an overlapping spectrum of disease. *J Inherit Metab Dis*, **38**, 445–457.

25 Akesson LS, Eggers S, Love CJ, Chong B, Krzesinski EI, Brown NJ *et al.* (2019) Early diagnosis of Pearson syndrome in neonatal intensive care following rapid mitochondrial genome sequencing in tandem with exome sequencing. *Eur J Hum Genet*, **27**, 1821–1826.

26 Gagne KE, Ghazvinian R, Yuan D, Zon RL, Storm K, Mazur-Popinska M *et al.* (2014) Pearson marrow pancreas syndrome in patients suspected to have Diamond-Blackfan anemia. *Blood*, **124**, 437–440.

27 Iolascon A, Andolfo I and Russo R (2019) Congenital dyserythropoietic anaemias. *Blood*, **136**, 1274–1283.

28 Fermo E, Bianchi P, Notarangelo LD, Binda S, Vercellati C, Marcello A *et al.* (2010) CDAII presenting as hydrops foetalis: molecular characterization of two cases. *Blood Cells Mol Dis*, **45**, 20–22.

29 Meznarich JA, Draper L, Christensen RD, Yaish HM, Luem ND, Pysher TJ *et al.* (2018) Fetal presentation of congenital dyserythropoietic anemia type 1 with novel compound heterozygous CDAN1 mutations. *Blood Cells Mol Dis*, **71**, 63–66.

30 Ravindranath Y, Johnson RM. Goyette G, Buck S, Gadgeel M and Gallagher PG (2018) KLF1 E325K-associated Congenital Dyserythropoietic Anemia Type IV: insights into the variable clinical severity. *J Pediatr Hematol Oncol*, **40**, e405–e409.

31 Tangsricharoen T, Natesirinilkul R, Phusia A, Fanhchaksai K, Ittiwut C, Chetruengchai W *et al.* (2021) Severe neonatal haemolytic anaemia caused by compound heterozygous *KLF1* mutations: report of four families and literature review. *Br J Haematol*, **194**, 626–634.

32 Roy NBA and Babbs C (2019) The pathogenesis, diagnosis and management of congenital dyserythropoietic anaemia type I. *Br J Haematol*, **185**, 436–449.

33 Shalev H, Tamary H, Shaft D, Reznitsky P and Zaizov R (1997) Neonatal manifestations of congenital dyserythropoietic anemia type 1. *J Pediatr*, **131**, 95–97.

34 Parez N, Dommergues M, Zupan V, Chambost H, Fieschi JB, Delaunay J *et al.* (2000) Severe congenital dyserythropoietic anaemia type 1: prenatal management, transfusion support and alpha-interferon therapy. *Br J Haematol*, **110**, 420–423.

35 Kato K, Sugitani M, Kawataki M, Ohyama M, Aida N, Koga N *et al.* (2001) Congeni-tal dyserythropoietic anemia type 1 with fetal onset of severe anemia. *J Pediatr Hematol Oncol*, **23**, 63–66.

36 Lin SM, Chen M, Ma ES, Lam YH, Wong KY andTang MH (2014) Intrauterine therapy in a fetus with congenital dyserythropoietic anaemia type I. *J Obstet Gynaecol*, **34**, 352–353

37 García-Zamora E, Naz-Villalba E, Pampín-Franco A, García-Iñigo FJ and López-Estebaranz JL (2020) Congenital dyserythropoietic anemia type 1 with nails and bone abnormalities. *Clin Exp Dermatol*, **45**, 515–517.

38 Russo R, Gambale A, Langella C, Andolfo I, Unal S AND Iolascon A (2014) Retrospective cohort study of 205 cases with congenital dyserythropoietic anemia type II: definition of clinical and molecular spectrum and identification of new diagnostic score. *Am J Hematol*, **89**, E169–E175.

39 Braun M, Wölfl M, Wiegering V, Winkler B, Ertan K, Bald R *et al.* (2014) Successful treatment of an infant with CDA type II by intrauterine transfusions and postnatal stem cell transplantation. *Pediatr Blood Cancer*, **61**, 743–745.

40 Nichols KE, Crispino JD, Poncz M, White JG, Orkin SH, Maris JM and Weiss MJ (2000) Familial dyserythropoietic anaemia and thrombocytopenia due to an inherited mutation in GATA1. *Nat Genet*, **24**, 266–270.

41 Viprakasit V, Ekwattanakit S, Riolueang S, Chalaow N, Fisher C, Lower K *et al.* (2014) Mutations in Kruppel-like factor 1 cause transfusion-dependent hemolytic anemia and persistence of embryonic globin gene expression. *Blood*, **123**, 1586–1595.

42 Magor GW, Tallack MR, Gillinder KR, Bell CC, McCallum N, Williams B *et al.* (2015) KLF1-null neonates display hydrops fetalis and a deranged erythroid transcriptome. *Blood*, **125**, 2405–2417.

43 Steiner LA, Ehrenkranz RA, Peterec SM, Steiner RD, Reyes-Múgica M and Gallagher PG (2011) Perinatal onset mevalonate kinase deficiency. *Pediatr Dev Pathol*, **14**, 301–306.

44 Shteyer E, Saada A, Shaag A, Al-Hijawi FA, Kidess R, Revel-Vilk S and Epeleg O (2009) Exocrine pancreatic insufficiency, dyserythropoeitic anemia, and calvarial hyperostosis are caused by a mutation in the *COX4I2* gene. *Am J Hum Genet*, **84**, 412–417.

45 Seu KG, Trump LR, Emberesh S, Lorsbach RB, Johnson C, Meznarich J *et al.* (2020) *VPS4A* mutations in humans cause syndromic congenital dyserythropoietic anemia due to cytokinesis and trafficking defects. *Am J Hum Genet*, **107**, 1149–1156.

46 Tormey CA and Hendrickson JE (2019) Transfusion-related red blood cell alloantibodies: induction and consequences. *Blood*, **133**, 1821–1830.

47 Simmons DP and Savage WJ (2015) Hemolysis from ABO incompatibility. *Hematol Oncol Clin North Am*, **29**, 429–443.

48 de Haas M, Thurik FF, Koelewijn JM and van der Schoot CE (2015) Haemolytic disease of the fetus and newborn. *Vox Sang*, **109**, 99–113.

49 Vaughan JI, Manning M, Warwick RM, Letsky E, Murray NA and Roberts IAG (1998) Inhibition of erythroid progenitor cell growth by anti-Kell (K): a mechanism for fetal anemia in K-immunized pregnancies *N Engl J Med*, **338**, 798–803.

50 Bu X, Sun P and Wan Y (2021) ABO haemolytic disease of the newborn in a blood group AB neonate due to maternal immunoglobulin G anti-A and anti-B antibodies. *Br J Haematol*, **192**, 416.

51 Geaghan SM (2011) Diagnostic laboratory technologies for the fetus and neonate with isoimmunization. *Semin Perinatol*, **35**, 148–154.

52 Delaney M and Matthews DC (2015) Hemolytic disease of the fetus and newborn: managing the mother, fetus and newborn. *Hematology Am Soc Hematol Educ Program*, **2015**, 146–151.

53 Ziprin JH, Payne E, Hamidi L, Roberts I and Regan F (2005) ABO Incompatibility due to IgG anti-B antibodies presenting with severe fetal anaemia. *Tranfus Med*, **15**, 57–60.

54 Sherer DM, Abramowicz JS, Ryan RM, Sheils LA, Blumberg N and Woods JR (1991) Severe fetal hydrops resulting from ABO incompatibility. *Obstet Gynecol*, **78**, 897–899.

55 Smith HM, Shirey RS, Thoman SK and Jackson JB (2013) Prevalence of clinically significant red blood cell alloantibodies in pregnant women at a large tertiary-care facility. *Immunohematology*, **29**, 127–130.

56 Bowden JB, Hebert AA and Rapini RP (1989) Dermal hematopoiesis in neonates: report of five cases. *J Am Acad Dermatol*, **20**, 1104–1110.

57 Bennardello F, Coluzzi S, Curciarello G, Todros T and Villa S (2015) Recommendations for the prevention and treatment of haemolytic disease of the the foetus and newborn. *Blood Transfus*, **13**, 109–134.

58 White J, Qureshi H, Massey E, Needs M, Byrne G, Daniels G and Allard S; British Committee for Standards in Haematology (2016) Guideline for blood grouping and red cell antibody testing in pregnancy. *Transfus Med*, **26**, 246–263.

59 Zwiers C, van Kamp I, Oepkes D and Lopriore E (2017) Intrauterine transfusion and non-invasive treatment options for hemolytic disease of the newborn- review on current management and outcomes. *Expert Rev Hematol*, **10**, 337–344.

60 Rath ME, Smits-Wintjens VE, Walther FJ and Lopriore E (2011) Hematological morbidity and management in neonates with hemolytic disease due to red cell alloimmunization. *Early Hum Dev*, **87**, 583–588.

61 New HV, Berryman J, Bolton-Maggs PHB, Cantwell C, Chalmers EA, Davies T *et al.* on behalf of the British Committee for Standards in Haematology (2016) Guidelines on transfusion for fetuses, neonates and older children. http://www.b-s-h.org.uk/media/2884/2016-neonates-final-v2.pdf

62 Zwiers C, Scheffer-Rath ME, Lopriore E, de Haas M and Liley HG (2018) Immunoglobulin for alloimmune hemolytic disease in neonates. *Cochrane Database Syst Rev*, **3**, CD003313.

63 Ree IMC, de Haas M, Middleburg RA, Zwiers C, Oepkes D, van der Bom JG and Lopriore E (2019) Predicting anaemia and transfusion dependency in severe alloimmune haemolytic disease of the fetus and newborn in the first 3 months after birth. *Br J Haematol*, **186**, 565–573.

64 Ree IMC, Lopriore E, Zwiers C, Böhringer S, Janssen MWM, Oepkes D and de Haas M (2020) Suppression of compensatory erythropoiesis in hemolytic disease of the fetus and newborn due to intrauterine transfusions. *Obstet Gynecol*, **223**, 119.e1–119.e10

65 Leonard A, Hittson Boal L, Pary P, Mo YD, Jacquot C, Luban NL *et al.* (2019) Identification of red blood cell antibodies in maternal breast milk implicated in prolonged hemolytic disease of the fetus and newborn. *Transfusion*, **59**, 1183–1189.

66 Zuppa AA, Alighieri G, Calabrese V, Visintini F, Cota F, Carducci C *et al.* (2010) Recombinant human erythropoietin in the prevention of late anemia in intrauterine transfused neonates with Rh-isoimmunization. *J Pediatr Hematol Oncol*, **32**, e95–e101.

67 Rath ME, Smits-Wintjens VE, Oepkes D, Walther FJ and Lopriore E (2013) Iron status in infants with alloimmune haemolytic disease in the first three months of life. *Vox Sang*, **105**, 328–333.

68 del Giudice EM, Perrotta S, Nobili B, Specchia C, d'Urzo G and Iolascon A (1999) Coinheritance of Gilbert syndrome increases the risk for developing gallstones in patients with hereditary spherocytosis. *Blood*, **94**, 2259–2262.

69 Christensen R, Yaish HM and Gallagher PG (2015) A pediatrician's guide to diagnosing and treating hereditary spherocytosis in neonates. *Pediatrics*, **135**, 1107–1114.

70 Iolascon A, Andolfini I and Russo R (2019) Advances in understanding the pathogenesis of red cell membrane disorders. *Br J Haematol*, **187**, 13–24.

71 Fermo E, Vercellati C and Bianchi P (2021) Screening tools for hereditary hemolytic anemia: new concepts and strategies. *Expert Rev Hematol*, **14**, 281–292.

72 Da Costa L, Galimand J, Fenneteau O and Mohandas N (2013) Hereditary spherocytosis, elliptocytosis, and other red cell membrane disorders. *Blood Rev*, **27**, 167–178.

73 Grace RF and Lux SE (2009) Disorders of the red cell membrane. In: Orkin SH, Nathan DG, Ginsburg D, Look AT, Fisher DE and Lux SE (eds), *Nathan and Oski's Hematology of Infancy and Childhood*, 7th edn. Saunders, Philadelphia, pp. 659–837.

74 Yaish HM, Christensen RD and Agarwal A (2013) A neonate with Coombs-negative hemolytic jaundice with spherocytes but normal erythrocyte indices: a rare case of autosomal-recessive hereditary spherocytosis due to alpha-spectrin deficiency. *J Perinatol*, **33**, 404–406.

75 Hannah DM, Tressler TB and Taboada CD (2017) Nonimmune hydrops fetalis due to autosomal recessive hereditary spherocytosis. *Case Rep Womens Health*, **16**, 4–7.

76 Donepudi R, Wesyerfield L, Stonecipher A, Nassr A, Cortes MS, Espinosa J et al. (2020) A family affair – severe fetal and neonatal hemolytic anemia due to novel alpha-spectrin mutations in two siblings. *Am J Med Genet A*, **182**, 561–564.

77 Iolascon A, Faienza MF, Moretti A, Perrotta S and Miraglia del Giudice E (1998) UGT1 promoter polymorphism accounts for increased neonatal appearance of hereditary spherocytosis. *Blood*, **91**, 1093.

78 Berardi A, Lugli L, Ferrari F, Gargano G, D'Apolito M, Marrone A and Iolascon A (2006) Kernicterus associated with hereditary spherocytosis and UGT1A1 promoter polymorphism. *Biol Neonate*, **90**, 243–246.

79 Delhommeau F, Cynober T, Schischmanoff PO, Rohrlich P, Delaunay J, Mohandas N and Tchernia G (2000) Natural history of hereditary spherocytosis during the first year of life. *Blood*, **95**, 393–397.

80 Schröter W and Kahsnitz E (1983) Diagnosis of hereditary spherocytosis in newborn infants. *J Pediatr*, **103**, 460.

81 Bianchi P, Fermo E, Vercellati C, Marcello AP, Porretti L, Cortelezzi A et al. (2012) Diagnostic power of laboratory tests for hereditary spherocytosis: a comparison study in 150 patients grouped according to molecular and clinical characteristics. *Haematologica*, **97**, 516–523.

82 Christensen RD, Agarwal AM, Nussenzveig RH, Heikal N, Liew MA and Yaish HM. (2015) Evaluating eosin-5-maleimide binding as a diagnostic test for hereditary spherocytosis in newborn infants. *J Perinatol*, **35**, 357–361.

83 Glele-Kakai C, Garbarz M, Lecomte MC, Leborgne S, Galand C, Bournier O et al. (1996) Epidemiological studies of spectrin mutations related to hereditary elliptocytosis and spectrin polymorphisms in Benin. *Br J Haematol*, **95**, 57.

84 An X and Mohandas N (2008) Disorders of red cell membrane. *Br J Haematol*, **141**, 367–375.

85 Niss O, Chonat S, Dagaonkar N, Almansoori MO, Kerr K, Rogers ZR et al. (2016) Genotype-phenotype correlations in hereditary elliptocytosis and hereditary pyropoikilocytosis. *Blood Cell Mol Dis*, **61**, 4–9.

86 Al-Riyami AZ, Iolascon A, Al-Zadjali S, Andolfo I, Al-Mammari S, Manna F *et al.* (2017) Targeted next generation sequencing identifies a novel b-spectrin gene mutation A2059P in two Omani children with hereditary pyropoikilocytosis. *Am J Hematol*, **92**, E607– E609.

87 Dhermy D, Galand C., Bournier O, King MJ, Cynober T, Roberts I *et al.* (1998) Co-inheritance of alpha-and beta-spectrin gene mutations in a case of hereditary elliptocytosis. *Blood*, **92**, 4481–4482.

88 Christensen RD, Nussenzveig RH, Reading NS, Agarwal AM, Prchal JT and Yaish HM (2014) Variations in both alpha-spectrin (SPTA1) and beta-spectrin (SPTB) in a neonate with prolonged jaundice in a family where nine individuals had hereditary elliptocytosis. *Neonatology*, **105**, 1–4.

89 Sivaguru G, Simini G and Bain BJ (2021) Persistent neonatal jaundice resulting from hereditary pyropoikilocytosis. *Am J Hematol*, Sep 22, doi: 10.1002/ajh.26358

90 Laosombat V, Dissaneevate S, Wongchanchailert M and Satayasevanaa B (2005) Neonatal anemia associated with Southeast Asian ovalocytosis. *Int J Hematol*, **82**, 201–205.

91 Picard V, Proust A, Eveillard M, Flatt JF, Couec ML, Caillaux G *et al.* (2014) Homozygous Southeast Asian ovalocytosis is a severe dyserythropoietic anemia associated with distal renal tubular acidosis. *Blood*, **123**, 1963–1965.

92 Grace RF and Glader B (2018) Red blood cell enzyme disorders. *Pediatr Clin North Am*, **65**, 579–595.

93 Luzzatto L, Ally M and Notaro R (2020) Glucose-6-phosphate dehydrogenase deficiency. *Blood*, **136**, 1225–1240.

94 Worlledge S, Luzzatto L, Ogiemudia SE, Luzzatto P and Edington GM (1968) Rhesus immunization in Nigeria. *Vox Sang*, **14**, 202–211.

95 Doxiadis SA and Valaes F (1964) The clinical picture of glucose 6-phosphate dehydrogenase deficiency in early childhood. *Arch Dis Child*, **39**, 545–553.

96 Meloni T, Costa S and Cutillo S (1975) Haptoglobin, hemopexin, hemoglobin and hematocrit in newborns with erythrocyte glucose-6-phosphate dehydrogenase deficiency. *Acta Haematol*, **54**, 284–290.

97 Luzzatto L and Poggi V (2009) Glucose-6-phosphate dehydrogenase deficiency. In: Orkin SH, Nathan DG, Ginsburg D, Look AT, Fisher DE and Lux SE (eds), *Nathan and Oski's Hematology of Infancy and Childhood*, 7th edn. Saunders, Philadelphia, pp. 883–907.

98 Kaplan M, Muraca M, Vreman HJ, Hammerman C, Vilei MT, Rubantelli FF and Stevenson DK (2005) Neonatal bilirubin production-conjugation imbalance: effect of glucose- 6-phosphate dehydrogenase deficiency and borderline prematurity. *Arch Dis Child*, **90**, F123–F127.

99 de Gurrola GC, Araúz JJ, Durán E, Aguilar-Medina M, Ramos-Paván R, García-Magallanes N *et al.* (2008) Kernicterus by glucose-6-phosphate dehydrogenase deficiency: a case report and review of the literature. *J Med Case Rep*, **2**, 146.

100 Kaplan M, Vreman HJ, Hammerman C, Schimmel MS, Abrahamov A and Stevenson DK (1998) Favism by proxy in nursing glucose-6-phosphate dehydrogenase-deficient neonates. *J Perinatol*, **18**, 477–479.

101 Bichali S, Brault D, Masserot C, Boscher C, Couec ML, Deslandes G *et al.* (2017) Maternal consumption of quinine-containing sodas may induce G6PD crises in breastfed children. *Eur J Pediatr*, **176**, 1415–1418.

102 Roos D, van Zwieten R, Wijnen JT, Gómez-Gallego F, de Boer M, Stevens D *et al.* (1999) Molecular basis and enzymatic properties of glucose 6-phosphate dehydrogenase Volendam, leading to chronic nonspherocytic anemia, granulocyte dysfunction, and increased susceptibility to infections. *Blood*, **94**, 2955–2962.

103 Grace RF, Bianchi P, van Beers EJ, Eber SW, Glader B, Yaisg HM *et al.* (2018) Clinical spectrum of pyruvate kinase deficiency: data from the Pyruvate Kinase Deficiency Natural History Study. *Blood*, **131**, 2183–2192.

104 Bianchi P, Fermo E, Lezon-Geyda K, van Beers EJ, Morton HD, Barcellini W *et al.* (2020) Genotype-phenotype correlation and molecular heterogeneity in pyruvate kinase deficiency. *Am J Hematol*, **95**, 472–482.

105 Voit RA and Grace RF (2020) Pyruvate kinase deficiency in a newborn with extramedullary hematopoiesis in the skin. *Blood*, **136**, 770.

106 Olivier F, Wiekowska A, Piedboeuf B and Alvarez F (2015) Cholestasis and hepatic failure in a neonate: a case report of severe pyruvate kinase deficiency. *Pediatrics*, **136**, e1366–e1368.

107 Chonat S, Eber SW, Holzhauer S, Kollmar N, Morton DH, Glader B *et al.* (2021) Pyruvate kinase deficiency in children. *Pediatr Blood Cancer*, **68**, e21948.

108 Grace RF, Rose C, Layton DM, Galacteros F, Barcellini W, Morton DH *et al.* (2019) Safety and efficacy of mitapivat in pyruvate kinase deficiency. *N Engl J Med*, **381**, 933–944.

109 Eyssette-Guerreau S, Bader-Meunier B, Garcon L, Guitton C and Cynober T (2006) Infantile pyknocytosis: a cause of haemolytic anaemia of the newborn. *Br J Haematol*, **133**, 439–442.

110 Tuffy P, Brown AK and Zuelzer WW (1959) Infantile pyknocytosis: a common erythrocyte abnormality of the first trimester. *Am J Dis Child*, **98**, 227.

111 Spoorenberg ME, Wachters-Hagedoorn RE, van Wijk R and de Kok JBJ (2021) Infantile pyknocytosis in a premature dichorionic diamniotic twin. *J Pediatr Hematol Oncol*, **43**, e1037–e1039.

112 Rees C, Lund K and Bain BJ (2019) Infantile pyknocytosis. *Am J Hematol*, **94**, 489–490.

113 Kanno H (2000) Hexokinase: Gene structure and mutations. *Bailliere's Clin Haematol*, **13**, 83–88.

114 Whitelaw AGL, Rogers PA, Hopkinson DA, Gordon H, Emerson PM, Darley JH *et al.* (1979) Congenital haemolytic anaemia resulting from glucose phosphate isomerase deficiency: genetics, clinical picture, and prenatal diagnosis. *J Med Genet*, **16**, 189–196.

115 Ravindranath Y, Paglia DE, Warrier I, Valentine W, Nakatani M and Brockway RA (1987) Glucose phosphate isomerase deficiency as a cause of hydrops fetalis. *N Engl J Med*, **316**, 258–261.

116 See W-SQ, So C-CJ, Cheuk DK-L, van Wijk R and Ha S-Y (2019) Congenital hemolytic anemia because of glucose phosphate isomerase deficiency: identification of 2 novel missense mutations in the *GPI* gene. *J Pediatr Hematol Oncol*, **42**, 696–e697.

117 Zanella A, Bianchi P, Fermo E and Valentini G (2006) Hereditary pyrimidine-5-nucleotidase deficiency: from genetics to clinical manifestations. *Br J Haematol*, **113**, 113–123.

118 Servidei S, Bonilla E, Diedrich RG, Kornfeld M, Oates JD, Davidson M *et al.* (1986) Fatal infantile form of phosphofructokinase deficiency. *Neurology*, **36**, 1465–1470.

119 Beutler E (2007) PGK deficiency. *Br J Haematol*, **136**, 3–11.

120 Aissa K, Kamoun F, Sfahi L, Ghedira ES, Aloulou H, Kamoun T *et al.* (2014) Hemolytic anemia and progressive neurologic impairment: think about triosephosphate isomerase deficiency. *Pediatr Pathol*, **33**, 234–238.

121 Vanhinsbergh L, Uthaya S and Bain BJ (2018) Methylene blue-induced Heinz body hemolytic anemia in a premature neonate. *Am J Hematol*, **93**, 716–717.

122 Woods CR (2009) Congenital syphilis–persisting pestilence. *Pediatr Infect Dis J*, **28**, 536–537.

123 Bulova SI, Schwartz E and Harrer WV (1972) Hydrops fetalis and congenital syphilis. *Pediatrics*, **49**, 285–287.

124 Nelson LG and Hodgman JE (1966) Congenital toxoplasmosis with hemolytic anemia. *Calif Med*, **105**, 454–457.

125 Ramaswamy VV, Rao GV, Suryanarayana N, Darisi PK and Gummadapu S (2019) Case 3: Hydrops fetalis, pancytopenia and hemolytic jaundice in a preterm neonate: a diagnosis made after 3 months. *Neoreviews*, **20**, e597–e599.

126 Coll O, Menendez C, Botet F, Dayal R and the WAPM Perinatal Infections Working Group (2008) Treatment and prevention of malaria in pregnancy and newborn. *J Perinatol*, **36**, 15–29.

127 Prior AR, Prata F, Mouzinho A and Marques JG (2012) Congenital malaria in a European country. *BMJ Case Rep*, 2012:bcr2012007310.

128 Riley EM, Wagner GE, Akanmori BD and Koram KA (2001) Do maternally acquired antibodies protect infants from malaria infection? *Parasite Immunol*, **23**, 51–59.

129 Punta VD, Gulletta M, Matteeli A, Spinioni V, Reggazzoli A and Castoli F (2010) Congenital Plasmodium vivax malaria mimicking neonatal sepsis: a case report. *Malar J*, **9**, 63.

130 Sanchez PJ, Patterson JC and Ahmed A (2012) Toxoplasmosis, syphilis, malaria and tuberculosis. In: Gleason CA, Devasker SU (eds), *Avery's Diseases of the Newborn*. Elsevier Saunders, Philadelphia, pp. 522–529.

131 Murray JC, Bernini JC, Bijou HL, Rossmann SN, Mahoney DH and Morad AB (2001) Infantile cytomegalovirus-associated autoimmune hemolytic anemia. *J Pediatr Hematol Oncol*, **23**, 318–320.

132 Humberg A, Leienbach V, Fortmann MI, Rausch TK, Buxmann H and Mueller A (2018) Prevalence of congenital CMV infection and antiviral therapy in very-low-birthweight infants: observations of the German Neonatal Network. *Klin Pediatr*, **230**, 257–262.

133 Yamamoto S, Shiraishi A, Ishimura M, Motomura Y, Yada Y, Moriuchi H and Ohga S (2021) Cytomegalovirus-associated hemolytic anemia in an infant born to a mother with lupus. *Neonatology*, **118**, 368–372.

134 Todd RM and O'Donohoe NV (1958) Acute acquired haemolytic anaemia associated with herpes simplex infection. *Arch Dis Child*, **33**, 524–526.

135 Fa F, Laup L, Mandelbrot L, Sibiude J and Picone O (2020) Fetal and neonatal abnormalities due to congenital herpes simplex virus infection: a literature review. *Prenat Diagn*, **40**, 408–414.

136 Reef SE, Plotkin S, Cordero JF, Katz M, Cooper L, Schwartz B *et al.* (2000) Preparing for elimination of congenital rubella syndrome (CRS): summary of a workshop on CRS elimination in the United States. *Clin Infect Dis*, **31**, 85–95.

137 Koenig A, Schabel A, Sugg U, Brand U and Roelcke D (2001) Autoimmune hemolytic anaemia caused by IgG lambda-monocytic cold agglutinins of anti-Pr specificity after rubella infection. *Transfusion*, **41**, 488–492.

138 Siddiqui A, Journeycake JM, Borogovac A and George JN (2021) Recognizing and managing hereditary and acquired thrombotic thrombocytopenic purpura in infants and children. *Pediatr Blood Cancer*, **68**, e28949.

139 Kremer Hovinga JA and George JN (2019) Hereditary thrombotic thrombocytopenic purpura. *N Engl J Med*, **381**, 1653–1662.

140 Fujimura Y, Lämmle B, Tanabe S, Sakai K, Kimura T, Kokame K *et al.* (2019) Patent ductus arteriosus generates neonatal hemolytic jaundice with thrombocytopenia in Upshaw-Schulman syndrome. *Blood Adv*, **3**, 3191–3195.

141 Pollack S, Eisenstein I, Mory A, Paperna T, Ofir A, Baris-Feldman H *et al.* (2021) A novel homozygous deletion in Complement Factor 3 underlies early-onset autosomal recessive atypical hemolytic uremic syndrome- case report. *Front Immunol*, **12**, 608604.

142 Sharma S, Pradhan M, Meyers KE, Le Palma K and Laskin BL (2015) Neonatal atypical hemolytic uremic syndrome from a factor H mutation treated with ecluzimab. *Clin Nephrol*, **84**, 181–185.

143 Gomes SM, Teixeira RP, Rocha G, Soares P, Guimaraes H, Santos P *et al.* (2021) Neonatal atypical hemolytic uremic syndrome in the excluzimab era. *AJP Rep*, **11**, e95–e98.

144 Bahr T, Judkins AJ, Baer VL, Henry E, Grubb PH, Hulse W, Pysher TJ *et al.* (2020) The fragmented red cell count can support the diagnosis of a microangiopathic neonatal condition. *J Perinatol*, **40**, 354–355.

145 Zukerberg LR, Nickoloff BJ and Weiss SW (1993) Kaposiform hemangioendothelioma of infancy and childhood: an aggressive neoplasm associated with Kasabach-Merritt syndrome and lymphangiomatosis. *Am J Surg Pathol*, **17**, 321–328.

146 Croteau SE, Liang MG, Kozakewich HP, Alomari AI, Fishman SJ, Mulliken JB and Trenor CR (2013) Kaposiform hemangioendothelioma: atypical features and risks of Kasabach-Merritt phenomenon in 107 referrals. *J Pediatr*, **162**, 142–147.

147 O'Rafferty C, O'Regan GM, Irvine AD and Smith OP (2015) Recent advances in the pathobiology and management of Kasabach–Merritt phenomenon. *Br J Haematol*, **171**, 38–51.

148 Tribolet S, Hoyoux C, Boon LM, Cheruy C, Demarche M, Jamblin P *et al.* (2019) A not so harmless mass: Kaposiform hemangioendothelioma complicated by a Kasabach–Merritt phenomenon. *Arch Pediatr*, **26**, 365–369.

149 Higgs DR (2009) The pathophysiology and clinical features of alpha-thalassemia. In: Steinberg MH, Forget BG, Higgs DR and Weatherall DJ (eds), *Disorders of Hemoglobin*, Vol. 1. Cambridge University Press, New York, pp. 266–295.

150 Piel FB and Weatherall DJ (2014) The alpha-thalassemias. *N Engl J Med*, **371**, 1908–1916.

151 Goh LPW, Chong ETJ and Lee PC (2020) Prevalence of alpha(α)-thalassemia in Southeast Asia (2010–2020): a meta-analysis involving 83,674 subjects. *Int J Environ Res Public Health*, **17**, 7354.

152 Giardine B, Borg J, Viennas E, Pavlidis C, Moradkhani K, Joly P *et al.* (2014) Updates of the HbVar database of human hemoglobin variants and thalassemia mutations. *Nucleic Acids Res*, **42** (database issue), D1063–D1069.

153 Li TKT, Leung KY, Lam YH, Tang MHY and Chan V (2010) Haemoglobin level, proportion of haemoglobin Bart's and haemoglobin Portland in fetuses affected by homozygous α0-thalassemia from 12 to 40 weeks' gestation. *Prenat Diagn*, **30**, 1126–1130.

154 Songdej D, Babbs C and Higgs DR, BHFS International Consortium (2017) An international registry of survivors with Hb Bart's hydrops fetalis syndrome. *Blood*, **129**, 1251–1259.

155 King AJ and Higgs DR (2018) Potential new approaches to the management of the Hb Bart's hydrops fetalis syndrome: the most severe form of α-thalassemia. *Hematology Am Soc Hematol Educ Program*, **2018**, 353–360.

156 Jatavan P, Chattipakorn N and Tongsong T (2018) Fetal hemoglobin Bart's hydrops fetalis: pathophysiology, prenatal diagnosis and possibility of intrauterine treatment. *J Matern Fetal Neonatal Med*, **31**, 946–957.

157 MacKenzie TC, Amid A, Angastiniotis M, Butler C, Gilbert S, Gonzalez J *et al.* (2021) Consensus statement for the perinatal management of patients with alpha thalassemia major. *Blood Adv*, 2021 Nov 8; bloodadvances.2021005916.

158 Galanello R, Pirastu M, Melis MA, Paglietti E, Moi P and Cao A (1983) Phenotype-genotype correlation in haemoglobin H disease in childhood. *J Med Genet*, **20**, 425–429.

159 Harteveld CL and Higgs DR (2010) Alpha-thalassaemia. *Orphanet J Rare Dis*, **5**, 13.

160 Chan V, Chan TK, Liang ST, Ghosh A, Kan YW and Todd D (1985) Hydrops fetalis due to an unusual form of Hb H disease. *Blood*, **66**, 224–228.

161 Chan V, Chan VW, Tang M, Lau K, Todd D and Chan TK (1997) Molecular defects in Hb H hydrops fetalis. *Br J Haematol*, **96**, 224–228.

162 Lorey F, Charoenkwan P, Witkowska HE, Lafferty J, Patterson M, Eng B *et al.* (2001) Hb H hydrops foetalis syndrome: a case report and review of literature. *Br J Haematol*, **115**, 72–78.

163 Viprakasit V, Green S, Height S, Ayyub H and Higgs DR (2002) Hb H hydrops fetalis syndrome associated with the interaction of two common determinants of alpha thalassaemia (--MED/(alpha)TSaudi(alpha). *Br J Haematol*, **117**, 759–762.

164 Luewan S, Charoenkwan P, Sirichotiyakul S and Tongsong T (2020) Fetal haemoglobin H-Constant Spring disease: a role for intrauterine management. *Br J Haematol*, **190**, e233–e236.

165 Levine RL and Lincoln DR (1975) Hemoglobin Hasharon in a premature infant with hemolytic anemia. *Pediatr Res*, **9**, 7–11.

166 Mavilio F, Marinucci M, Guerriero R, Cappellozza G and Tentori L (1980) Post-translational control of human hemoglobin synthesis: the role of differential affinity between globin chains in the control of mutated globin gene expression. *Biochim Biophys Acta*, **610**, 339–351.

167 Giardine BM, Joly P, Pissard S, Wajcman H, Chui DHK, Hardison RC and Patrinos GP (2021) Clinically relevant updates of the HbVar database of human hemoglobin variants and thalassemia mutations. *Nucleic Acids Res*, **49**, D1192–D1196.

168 Lee-Potter JP, Deacon-Smith RA, Simkiss MJ, Kamuzora H and Lehmann H (1975) A new cause of haemolytic anaemia in the newborn: a description of an unstable fetal haemoglobin: F Poole, $\alpha_2{}^{G}\gamma_2 130$ tryptophan → glycine. *J Clin Pathol*, **28**, 317–320.

169 Van den Driessch M, Moerman J, Moens M, Van Eldere S, Derclaye I and Philippe M (2005) Severe hereditary haemolytic anaemia in a Caucasian newborn: a new fetal haemoglobin variant Hb F-Bonheiden ($^G\gamma$ 38(C4) Thr→Pro), *Eur J Pediatr*, **164**, 261–262.

170 Arnon S, Tamary H, Dgany O, Litmanovitz I, Regev R, Bauer S *et al.* (2004) Hydrops fetalis associated with homozygosity for hemoglobin Taybe (a 38/39 THR deletion) in newborn triplets. *Am J Hematol*, **76**, 263–266.

171 Bain BJ, Haynes A, Prentice AG, Luckit J, Swirsky D, Williams Y *et al.* (1999) British Society for Haematology Slide Session, Annual Scientific Meeting, Brighton, 1999. *Clin Lab Haematol*, **21**, 417–425.

172 Pirastu M, Kan YW, Lin CC, Baine RM and Holbrook CT (1983) Hemolytic disease of the newborn caused by a new deletion of the entire beta-globin cluster. *J Clin Invest*, **72**, 602–609.

173 Driscoll MC, Dobkin CS and Alter BP (1989) Gamma delta beta-thalassemia due to a de novo mutation deleting the 5′ beta-globin gene activation-region hypersensitive sites. *Proc Natl Acad Sci U S A*, **86**, 7470–7474

174 Game L, Bergounioux J, Close JP, Marzouka BE and Thein SL (2003) A novel deletion causing $(\varepsilon\gamma\delta\beta)^0$ thalassaemia in a Chilean family. *Br J Haematol*, **123**, 154–159.

175 Erlandson ME and Hilgartner M (1959) Hemolytic disease in the neonatal period. *J Pediatr*, **54**, 566–585.

176 Hegyi T, Delphin ES, Bank A, Blanc WA and Polin RA (1977) Sickle cell anemia in the newborn. *Pediatrics*, **60**, 213–216.

177 Fouquet C, Le Rouzic M-A, Leblanc T, Fouyssac F, Leverger G, Hessissen L *et al.* (2011) Genotype/phenotype correlations of childhood-onset congenital sideroblastic anaemia in a European cohort. *Br J Haematol*, **187**, 530–542.

178 Kannengiesser C, Sanchez M, Sweeney M, Hetet G, Kerr B, Moran E *et al.* (2011) Missense SLC25A38 variations play an important role in autosomal recessive inherited sideroblastic anemia. *Haematologica*, **96**, 808– 813.

179 Ravindra N, Athiyarath R, Eswari S, Sumithra S, Kulkarni U, Fouzia NA *et al.* (2021) Novel frameshift variant (c.409dupG) in SLC25A38 is a common cause of congenital sideroblastic anaemia in the Indian subcontinent. *J Clin Pathol*, **74**, 157–162.

180 Wiseman DH, May A, Jolles S, Connor P, Powell C, Heeney MH *et al.* (2013) A novel syndrome of congenital sideroblastic anemia, B-cell immunodeficiency, periodic fevers, and developmental delay (SIFD). *Blood*, **122**, 112–123.

181 Barton C, Kausar S, Kerr D, Bitetti S and Wynn R (2018) SIFD as a novel cause of severe fetal hydrops and neonatal anaemia with iron loading and marked extramedullary haemopoiesis. *J Clin Pathol*, **71**, 275–278.

182 Wylie BJ, D'Alton ME (2010) Fetomaternal hemorrhage. *Obstet Gynecol*, **115**, 1039-1051.

183 Loureiro B, Martinez-Biarge M, Foti F, Papadaki M, Cowan FM and Wusthoff CJ (2017) MRI patterns of brain injury and neurodevelopmental outcomes in neonates with severe anemia at birth. *Early Hum Dev*, **105**, 17–22.

184 Carr NR, Henry E, Bahr T, Ohls RK, Page JM, Ilstrup SJ *et al.* (2022) Fetomaternal hemorrhage: evidence from a multihospital healthcare system that up to 40% of severe cases are missed. *Transfusion*, **62**, 60–70.

185 Stefanovic V (2016) Fetomaternal hemorrhage complicated pregnancy: risks, identification, and management. *Curr Opin Obstet Gynecol*, **28**, 86–94.

186 Balasubramanian H, Malpani P, Sindhur M, Kabra NS, Ahmed J and Srinivasan L (2019) Effect of umbilical cord sampling versus admission blood sampling on requirement of blood transfusion in extremely preterm infants: a randomized controlled trial. *J Pediatr*, **211**, 39–45.

187 Fisk NM, Duncombe DJ and Sullivan MH (2009) The basic and clinical science of twin-to-twin transfusion syndrome. *Placenta*, **30**, 379–390.

188 Zhao D, Lipa M, Wielgos M, Cohen D, Middeldorp JM, Oepkes D and Lopriore E (2016) Comparison between monochorionic and dichorionic placentas with special attention to vascular anastomoses and placental share. *Twin Res Hum Genet*, **19**, 191–196.

189 Verbeek L, Slaghekke F, Sueters M, Middeldorp JM, Klumper FJ, Haak CM *et al.* (2017) Hematological disorders at birth in complicated monochorionic twins. *Exp Rev Hematol*, **10**, 525–532.

190 Baschat A, Chmait RH, Deprest J, Gratacós E, Hecher K, Kontopoulos E *et al.* WAPM Consensus Group on Twin-to-Twin Transfusion (2011) Twin-to-twin transfusion syndrome (TTTS). *J Perinat Med*, **39**, 107–112.

191 Berghella V and Kaufmann M (2001) Natural history of twin-twin transfusion syndrome. *J Reprod Med*, **46**, 480–484.

192 Verbeek L, Middeldorp JM, Hulzebos CV, Oepkes D, Walther FJ and Lopriore E (2013) Hypoalbuminemia in donors with twin-twin transfusion syndrome. *Fetal Diagn Ther*, **33**, 98–102.

193 Spruijt MS, Lopriore E, Steggerda S, Salghekke F and Van Klink JMM (2020) Twin-to-twin transfusion syndrome in the era of fetoscopic laser surgery: antenatal management, neonatal outcome and beyond. *Expert Rev Hematol*, **13**, 259–267.

194 Robyr R, Lewi L, Salomon LJ, Yamamoto M, Bernard J-P, Deprest J and Ville Y (2006) Prevalence and management of late fetal complications following successful selective laser coagulation of chorionic plate anastomoses in twin-to-twin transfusion syndrome. *Am J Obstet Gynecol*, **194**, 796–803.

195 Lopriore E, Middeldorp JM, Oepkes D, Kanhai HH, Walther FJ and Vandenbussche FPHA (2007) Twin anemia-polycythemia sequence in two monochorionic twin pairs without oligo-polyhydramnios sequence. *Placenta*, **28**, 47–51.

196 Tollennar LSA, Lopriore E, Middelthorp JM, Haak MC, Klumper FJ, Oepkes D *et al.* (2019) Improved prediction of twin anemia-polycythemia sequence by delta middle cerebral artery peak systolic velocity: new antenatal classification system. *Ultrasound Obstet Gynecol*, **53**, 788–793.

197 Tollenaar LS, Slaghekke F, Middelthorp JM, Klumper FJ, Haak MC, Oepkes D and Lopriore E (2016) Twin anemia polycythemia sequence: current views on pathogenesis, diagnostic criteria, perinatal management, and outcome. *Twin Res Hum Genet*, **19**, 222–233.

198 Mabuchi A, Ishii K, Yamamoto R, Taguchi T, Murata M, Hayashi S and Mitsuda N (2014) Clinical characteristics of monochorionic twins with large hemoglobin level discordance at birth. *Ultrasound Obstet Gynecol*, **44**, 311–315.

199 Yarci E, Alyamac DE, Oncel MY, Kose Cetinkaya A, Derme T, Canpolat FE *et al.* (2014) Successful management of twin anemia/polycythemia sequence by syngeneic partial exchange transfusion. *Fetal Diagn Ther*, **36**, 251–254.

200 Ashwal E, Yinon Y, Fishel-Bartal M, Tsur A, Chayen B, Weisz B and Lipitz S (2016) Twin anemia-polycythemia sequence: perinatal management and outcome. *Fetal Diagn Ther*, **40**, 28–34.

201 Straňák Z, Korček P, Hympánová L, Kynčl M and Krofta L (2017) Prenatally acquired multiple limb ischemia in a very low birth weight monochorionic twin. *Fetal Diagn Ther*, **41**, 237–238.

202 Lopriore E, Holtkamp N, Sueters M, Middeldorp JM, Walther FJ and Oepkes D (2014) Acute peripartum twin-twin transfusion syndrome: incidence, risk factors, placental characteristics and neonatal outcome. *J Obstet Gynaecol Res*, **40**, 18–24.

203 Meleti D, DeOliveira LG, Araujo E, Caetano ACR, Boute T, Nardozza LMM and Moron AF (2013) Evaluation of passage of fetal erythrocytes into maternal circulation after invasive obstetric procedures. *J Obstet Gynaecol Res*, **39**, 1374–1382.

204 O'Leary BD, Walsh CA, Fitzgerald JM, Downey P and McAuliffe FM (2015) The contribution of massive fetomaternal hemorrhage to antepartum stillbirth: a 25-year cross-sectional study. *Acta Obstet Gynecol Scand*, **94**, 1354–1358.

205 Oxford CM and Ludmir J (2009) Trauma in pregnancy. *J Clin Obstet Gynecol*, **52**, 611–629.

206 Christensen RD, Lambert DK, Baer VL, Richards DS, Bennett ST, Ilstrup SJ and Henry E (2013) Severe neonatal anemia from fetomaternal hemorrhage: records from a multihospital healthcare system. *J Perinatol*, **33**, 429–434.

207 Maier JT, Schalinski E, Schneider W, Gottschalk U and Hellmeyer L (2015) Fetomaternal hemorrhage (FMH), an update: review of literature and illustrative case. *Arch Gynecol Obstet*, **292**, 595–602.

208 Kim YA and Makar RS (2012) Detection of fetomaternal hemorrhage. *Am J Hematol*, **87**, 417–423.

209 Porra V, Bernaud J and Gueret P (2007) Identification and quantification of fetal red blood cells in maternal blood by a dual-color flow cytometric method: Evaluation of the fetal cell count kit. *Transfusion*, **47**, 1281–1289.

210 Patton WN, Nicholson GS and Sawers AH (1990) Assessment of fetal-maternal haemorrhage in mothers with hereditary persistence of fetal haemoglobin. *J Clin Pathol*, **43**, 728–731.

211 Goldman M, Blajchman MA and Ali MA (1991) Overestimation of fetomaternal haemorrhage by the acid-elution technique in mothers with beta-thalassaemia minor. *Transfus Med*, **1**, 129–132.

212 Davis BH (2019) Enumeration of fetal red blood cells, hemoglobin-specific RBC and F-reticulocytes in human blood. *Curr Protoc Cytom*, **90**, e56.

213 Troia L, Al-Kouatly HB, McCurdy R, Konchak PS, Weiner S and Berghella V (2019) The recurrence risk of fetomaternal hemorrhage. *Prenatal Diagn Ther*, **45**, 1–12.

214 den Besten G, van der Weide K, Schuerman F, Michael Cotten C and Rondeel JMM (2018) Establishing the cause of anemia in a premature newborn infant. *Lab Med*, **49**, e74–e77.

215 Bahr TM, DuPont TL, Christensen TR, Rees T, O'Brien EA, Ilstrup SJ et al. (2019) Evaluating emergency-release blood transfusion of newborn infants at the Intermountain Healthcare hospitals. *Transfusion*, **59**, 3113–3119.

216 Simões M, Vale G, Lacerda C, Pais P and Pignatelli D (2021) Fetomaternal hemorrhage: a clue to intraplacental choriocarcinoma and neonatal malignancy. *J Matern Fetal Neonatal Med*, May 4; 1–3. doi: 10.1080/14767058.2021.1918665 online ahead of print.

217 Ryu N, Ogawa M, Matsui H, Usui H and Shozu M (2015) The clinical characteristics and early detection of postpartum choriocarcinoma. *Int J Gynecol Cancer*, **25**, 926–930.

218 Sebire NJ, Lindsay I, Fisher RA and Seckl MJ (2005) Intraplacental choriocarcinomas: experience from a tertiary referral center and relationship with infantile choriocarcinoma. *Fetal Pediatr Pathol*, **24**, 21–29.

219 Ngan HYS, Seckl MJ, Berkowitz RS, Xiang Y, Golfier F, Sekharan PK *et al.* (2018) Update on the diagnosis and management of gestational trophoblastic disease. *Int J Gynaecol Obstet*, **143** (Suppl 2), 79–85.

220 Melcer Y, Maymon R and Jauniaux E (2018) Vasa Previa: prenatal diagnosis and management. *Curr Opin Obstet Gynecol*, **30**, 385–391.

221 Melcer Y, Jauniaux E, Maymon S, Tsviban A, Pekar-Zlotin M, Betser M and Maymon R (2018) Impact of targeted scanning protocols on perinatal outcomes in pregnancies at risk of placenta accreta spectrum or vasa previa. *Am J Obstet Gynecol*, **218**, 443.e1–443.e8.

222 Carroll PD and Widness JA (2012) Nonpharmacological, blood conservation techniques for preventing neonatal anemia – effective and promising strategies for reducing transfusion. *Semin Perinatol*, **36**, 232–243.

223 Rao R and Georgieff MK (2002) Perinatal aspects of iron metabolism. *Acta Paediatr*, **91**, 124–129.

224 Whyte RK, Kirpalani H, Asztalos EV, Andersen C, Blajchman M, Heddle N *et al.* (2009) Neurodevelopmental outcome of extremely low birthweight infants randomly assigned to restrictive or liberal thresholds for blood transfusion. *Pediatrics*, **123**, 207–213.

225 Patel RM, Knezevic A, Shenvi N, Hinkes M, Keene S, Roback JD *et al.* (2016) Association of red blood cell transfusion, anemia, and necrotizing enterocolitis in very low-birth-weight infants. *JAMA*, **315**, 889–897.

226 Lust C, Vesoulis Z, Jackups R, Liao S, Rao R and Mathur AM (2019) Early red cell transfusion is associated with development of severe retinopathy of prematurity. *J Perinatol*, **39**, 393–400.

227 Whitehead HV, Vesoulis ZA, Maheshwari A, Rambhia A and Mathur AM (2019) Progressive anemia of prematurity is associated with a critical increase in cerebral oxygen extraction. *Early Human Dev*, **140**, 104891.

228 Ohlsson A and Aher SM (2020) Early erythropoiesis-stimulating agents in preterm or low birth weight infants. *Cochrane Database Syst Rev*, **2**, CD004863.

229 Aher SM and Ohlsson A (2020) Late erythropoiesis-stimulating agents to prevent blood transfusion in preterm or low birth weight infants. *Cochrane Database Syst Rev*, **1**, CD004868.

230 Saito-Benz M, Flanagan P and Berry MJ (2019) Management of anemia in pre-term infants. *Br J Haematol*, **188**, 354–366.

231 Lin JC, Strauss RG, Kulhavy JC, Johnson KL, Zimmerman MB, Cress GA *et al.* (2000) Phlebotomy overdraw in the neonatal intensive care nursery. *Pediatrics*, **106**, E19.

232 Widness JA, Madan A, Grindeanu LA, Zimmerman MB, Wong DK and Stevenson DK (2005) Reduction in red cell transfusions among preterm infants: results of a randomized trial with an in-line blood gas and chemistry monitor. *Pediatrics*, **115**, 1299–1306.

233 Ballin A, Livshiz V, Mimouni FB, Dolllberg S, Kohelet D, Oren A *et al.* (2009) Reducing blood transfusion requirements in preterm infants by a new device: a pilot study. *Acta Paediatr*, **98**, 247–250.

234 McCarthy EK, Dempsey EM and Kiely ME (2019) Iron supplementation in preterm and low-birth-weight infants: a systematic review of intervention studies. *Nutr Rev*, **77**, 865–877

235 Fogarty M, Osborn DA, Askie L, Seidler AL, Hunter K, Lui K *et al.* (2018) Delayed vs early umbilical cord clamping for preterm infants: a systematic review and meta-analysis. *Am J Obstet Gynecol*, **218**, 1–18.

236 Nagano N, Saito M, Sugiura T, Miyahara F, Namba F and Ota E (2018) Benefits of umbilical cord milking versus delayed cord clamping on neonatal outcomes in preterm infants: a systematic review and meta-analysis. *PLoS ONE*, **13**, e0201528.

237 Kumar J and Yadhav A (2019) Umbilical cord milking in preterm infants: time to act. *J Perinatol*, **39**, 889–890.

238 Juul SE, Comstock BA, Wadhawan R, Maycock DE, Courtney SE, Robinson T *et al.* (2020) A randomised trial of erythropoietin for neuroprotection in preterm infants. *N Engl J Med*, **382**, 233–243.

239 Bechensteen M and Stutchfield PR (2001) Severe congenital myotonic dystrophy and severe anaemia of prematurity in an infant of Jehovah's Witness parents. *Dev Med Child Neurol*, **43**, 346–349.

240 Bechensteen AG, Hågå P, Halvorsen S, Whitelaw A, Liestøl K, Lindemann R *et al.* (1993) Erythropoietin, protein, and iron supplementation and the prevention of the anaemia of prematurity. *Arch Dis Child*, **69**, 19–23.

241 Rapetti-Mauss R, Lacoste C, Picard V, Guitton C, Lombard E, Loosveld M *et al.* (2015) A mutation in the Gardos channel is associated with hereditary xerocytosis. *Blood*, **126**, 1273–1280.

242 Lucewicz A, Fisher K, Henry A and Welsh AW (2016) Review of the correlation between blood flow velocity and polycythemia in the fetus, neonate and adult: appropriate diagnostic levels need to be determined for twin anemia-polycythemia sequence. *Ultrasound Obstet Gynecol*, **47**, 152–157.

243 Watts T and Roberts I (1999) Haematological abnormalities of the growth-restricted infant. *Semin Neonatol*, **4**, 41–54.

244 Kirkham FJ, Zafeiriou D, Howe D, Czarpran P, Harris A, Gunny R and Vollmer B (2018) Fetal stroke and cerebrovascular disease: advances in understanding from lenticulostriate venous imaging, alloimmune thrombocytopenia and monochorionic twins. *Eur J Pediatr Neurol*, **22**, 989–1005.

245 Roberts I, Alford K, Hall G, Juban G, Richmond H, Norton A *et al.* (2013) *GATA1*-mutant clones are frequent and often unsuspected in babies with Down syndrome: identification of a population at risk of leukemia. *Blood*, **122**, 3908–3917.

246 Hooven TA, Hooper EN, Wonkatal SN, Francis RO, Sahni R and Lee MT (2016) Diagnosis of a rare fetal haemoglobinopathy in the age of next-generation sequencing. *BMJ Case Rep*, 10.1136/bcr-2016-215193.

247 Keir AK, New H, Robitaille N, Crichton GL, Wood EM and Stanworth SJ (2019) Approaches to understanding and interpreting the risks of red blood cell transfusion in neonates. *Transfus Med*, **29**, 231–238.

248 Howarth C, Bannerjee J and Aladangady N (2018) Red blood cell transfusion in preterm infants: current evidence and controversies. *Neonatology*, **114**, 7–16.

249 Carson JL, Stanworth SJ, Dennis JA, Trivella M, Roubinian N, Fergusson DA *et al.* (2021) Transfusion thresholds for guiding red blood cell transfusion. *Cochrane Database Syst Rev*, **12**, CD002042.

250 Franz AR, Engel C, Bassler D, Rüdiger M, Thome UH, Maier RF *et al.* (2020) Effects of liberal vs restrictive transfusion thresholds on survival and neurocognitive outcomes in extremely low-birth-weight infants: the ETTNO randomized clinical trial. *JAMA*, **324**, 560–570.

251 Vlachos A and Muir E (2010) How I treat Diamond-Blackfan anemia. *Blood*, **116**, 3715–3723.

252 Vlachos A, Rosenberg PS, Atsidaftos E, Alter BP and Lipton JM (2012) Incidence of neoplasia in Diamond Blackfan anemia: a report from the Diamond Blackfan Anemia Registry. *Blood*, **119**, 3815–3819.

253 Raiser DM, Narla A and Ebert BL (2013) The emerging importance of ribosomal protein dysfunction in hematologic disorders. *Leuk Lymphoma*, **55**, 491–500.

254 van der Akker M, Dror Y and Odame I (2014) Transient erythroblastopenia of childhood is an underdiagnosed and self-limiting disease. *Acta Paediatr*, **103**, e288–e294.

255 Prassouli A, Papadakis V, Tsakris A, Stefanaki K, Garoufi A, Haidas S *et al.* (2005) Classic transient erythroblastopenia of childhood with human parvovirus B19 genome detection in the blood and bone marrow. *J Pediatr Hematol Oncol*, **27**, 333–336.

256 Ogawa A and Yanagisawa R (2016) Deformation of erythroblasts in transient erythroblastopenia of childhood caused by HHV-6. *Blood*, **127**, 2776.

257 Dgany O, Avidan N, Delaunay J, Krasnov T, Shalmon L, Shalev H *et al.* (2002) Congenital dyserythropoietic anemia type I is caused by mutations in codanin-1. *Am J Hum Genet*, **71**, 1467–1474.

258 Woesner S, Trujillo M, Florsensa L, Mesa MC and Wickramasinghe SN (2003) Congenital dyserythropoietic anaemias other than type I–III with a peculiar erythroblastic morphology. *Eur J Haematol*, **71**, 211–214.

259 Schwarz K, Iolascon A, Verissimo F, Trede NS, Horsley W, Chen W *et al.* (2009) Mutations affecting the secretory COPII coat component SEC23B cause congenital dyserythropoietic anemia type II. *Nat Genet*, **41**, 936–940.

260 Heimpel H, Matuschek A, Ahmed M, Bader-Meunier B, Colita A, Delaunay J *et al.* (2010) Frequency of congenital dyserythropoietic anemias in Europe. *Eur J Haematol*, **85**, 20–28.

261 Iolascon A, Heimpel H, Wahlin A and Tamary H (2013) Congenital dyserythropoietic anemias: molecular insights and diagnostic approach. *Blood*, **122**, 2161–2166.

262 Keir A, Agpalo M, Lieberman L and Callum J (2015) How to use: the direct antiglobulin test in newborns. *Arch Dis Child Educ Pract Ed*, **100**, 198–203.

263 McGillivray A, Polverino J, Badawi N and Evans N (2016) Prospective surveillance of extreme neonatal hyperbilirubinemia in Australia. *J Pediat*, **168**, 82–87.

264 Waldron P and de Alarcon P (1999) ABO hemolytic disease of the newborn: a unique constellation of findings in siblings and review of protective mechanisms in the fetal-maternal system. *Am J Perinatol*, **16**, 391–398.

265 King M-J, Jepson MA, Guest A and Mushens R (2011) Detection of hereditary pyropoikilocytosis by the eosin-5-maleimide (EMA)-binding test is attributable to a marked reduction in EMA-reactive transmembrane proteins. *Int J Lab Hematol*, **33**, 205–211.

266 Bolton-Maggs PHB, Langer JC, Iolascon A, Tittensor P and King M-J (2011) Guidelines for the diagnosis and management of hereditary spherocytosis – 2011 update. *Br J Haematol*, **156**, 37–49.

267 Coetzer TL, Sahr K, Prchal J, Blacklock H, Peterson L, Koler R *et al*. (1991) Four different mutations in codon 28 of alpha spectrin are associated with structurally and functionally abnormal spectrin alpha I/74 in hereditary elliptocytosis. *J Clin Invest*, **88**, 743–749.

268 Chakravorty S, King M-J and Bain BJ (2012) Unexpectedly bizarre blood film in hemoglobin H disease. *Am J Hematol*, **87**, 1104.

269 Christensen RD, Nussenzveig RH, Yaish HM, Henry E, Eggert LD and Agarwal AM (2014) Causes of hemolysis in neonates with extreme hyperbilirubinemia. *J Perinatol*, **34**, 616–619.

270 Gallagher PG and Glader B (2016) Diagnosis of pyruvate kinase deficiency. *Pediatr Blood Cancer*, **63**, 771–772.

271 Kung C, Hixon J, Kosinski PA, Cianchetta G, Histen G, Chen Y *et al*. (2017) AG-348 enhances pyruvate kinase activity in red blood cells from patients with pyruvate kinase deficiency. *Blood*, **130**, 1347–1356.

272 El Nabouch M, Rakotoharinandrasana I, Ndayikeza A, Picard V and Kayemba-Kay's S (2015) Infantile pyknocytosis, a rare cause of hemolytic anemia in newborns: report of two cases in twin girls and literature overview. *Clin Case Rep*, **3**, 535–538.

273 Eyssette-Guerreau S, Bader-Meunier B, Garcon L, Guitton C and Cynober T (2006) Infantile pyknocytosis: a cause of hemolytic anemia of the newborn. *Br J Haematol*, **133**, 439–442.

274 Necheles TF, Boles TA and Allen DM (1968) Erythrocyte glutathione-peroxidase deficiency and hemolytic disease of the newborn infant. *J Pediatr*, **72**, 319–324.

275 Necheles TF, Steinberg MH and Cameron D (1970) Erythrocyte glutathione-peroxidase deficiency. *Br J Haematol*, **19**, 605–612.

276 Vincer MJ, Allen AC, Evans JR, Nwaesei C and Stinson DA (1987) Methylene-blue-induced hemolytic anemia in a neonate. *Can Med Assoc J*, **136**, 503–504.

277 Sills MR and Zinkham WH (1994) Methylene blue induced Heinz body haemolytic anaemia. *Arch Pediatr Adolesc Med*, **148**, 306–310.

278 Higgs DR (2009) The pathophysiology and clinical features of alpha-thalassemia. In: Steinberg MH, Forget BG, Higgs DR and Weatherall DJ (eds), *Disorders of Hemoglobin*, 2nd edn. Cambridge University Press, Cambridge, pp. 266–295.

279 Austin E, Bates S, de Silva N, Howarth D, Lubenko A et al. (2011) Guidelines for the estimation of fetomaternal haemorrhage. https://b-s-h.org.uk/media/15705/transfusion-austin-the-estimation-of-fetomaternal-haemorrhage.pdf

280 Kumpel B, Hazell M, Guest A, Dixey J, Mushens R, Bishop D, Wreford-Bush T and Lee E (2014) Accurate quantitation of D+ fetomaternal hemorrhage by flow cytometry using a novel reagent to eliminate granulocytes from analysis. *Transfusion*, **54**, 1305–1316.

281 Bain BJ and Chapple L (2015) Interpreting a post-partum Kleihauer test. *Am J Hematol*, **90**, 77.

282 Den Besten G, van der Weide K, Schuerman FABA, Michael Cotten C and Rondeel JMM (2018) Establishing the cause of anemia in a premature newborn infant. *Lab Med*, **49**, e74–e77.

3

Neonatal infection and leucocyte disorders

Leucocyte abnormalities in neonatal systemic disease

Increases in leucocyte numbers

Increases in leucocyte numbers secondary to systemic disease are very common in neonates, particularly in association with infection. Careful examination of the blood film often provides additional clues to the underlying cause and is a rapid and sensitive way of identifying likely bacterial or viral infection (Table 3.1).

Causes and significance of neonatal neutrophilia

The principal causes of neutrophilia are shown in Table 3.2. In the hospital setting the two most common causes of neonatal neutrophilia are maternal chorioamnionitis and acute bacterial infection. The haematological features of acute bacterial infection are usually marked and distinctive and are described in detail below. It is worth noting that infection with *Bordetella pertussis* during the neonatal period may be accompanied by marked neutrophilia as well as lymphocytosis.[1] Neutrophilia is also seen after a number of specific types of viral infection, particularly chikungunya virus.[2,3] Most studies suggest that the neutrophil count is reduced in neonatal coronavirus disease 19 (COVID-19), although a recent study has shown that the presence of neutrophilia is a predictive factor for severe disease.[4] By contrast, the haematological features of chronic bacterial infection in neonates are usually much more subtle. Typically, there is a moderate neutrophilia, often persisting for several weeks, and the majority of neutrophils are mature and lack toxic granulation. This pattern of chronic neutrophilia is seen in association with osteomyelitis or localised skin or wound infections.

Neutrophilia also occurs in neonates with constitutional trisomies, including Down syndrome, trisomy 13 and trisomy 18; this suggests that aneuploidy itself might perturb neutrophil development during fetal life, but if so the mechanism of this is completely unknown.[5,6] The clinical significance of neutrophilia in neonates with constitutional aneuploidies lies with recognising that neutrophilia is not a useful sign on its own, either of acute infection or of transient abnormal myelopoiesis (TAM) seen in neonates with Down syndrome (discussed in detail below). Neutrophilia secondary to constitutional trisomies is confined to the neonatal period, although follow-up data for trisomy 13 and

Neonatal Haematology: A Practical Guide, First Edition. Irene Roberts and Barbara J. Bain.
© 2022 John Wiley & Sons Ltd. Published 2022 by John Wiley & Sons Ltd.

Table 3.1 Haematological features of infection in neonatal blood films

Features of infection on neonatal blood film	Differential diagnosis	Pitfalls/comments
Band cells	Acute bacterial infection Congenital viral infection Rare congenital causes (e.g. Pelger–Huët anomaly)	Band cells in the absence of other leucoerythroblastic features are not a normal feature in preterm babies
Toxic granulation of neutrophils	Acute bacterial infection Chronic bacterial infection (e.g. osteomyelitis) HIE (toxic granulation may persist for up to 2 weeks after birth) Maternal chorioamnionitis without acute infection in the baby (may persist for up to 1 week after birth) Meconium aspiration (may persist for up to 1 week after birth)	Toxic granulation after the first week of life is usually due to infection (apart from cases of severe HIE) Neonates born to mothers with severe chorioamnionitis may have very marked leucocytosis (WBC up to 80×10^9/l), even in the absence of acute neonatal infection (normal or minimally raised CRP and lack of band cells being the most helpful distinguishing features)
Vacuolation of neutrophils	*Staphylococcus epidermidis* infection (typically line infections) *Candida* spp. infection NEC Other acute bacterial infections, e.g. due to Gram-negative species	Neonates with NEC nearly always have neutrophil vacuolation Acute bacterial infection and NEC often co-exist; neutrophil vacuolation is not specific to NEC but the absence of neutrophil vacuolation makes NEC unlikely
Leucoerythroblastic features	Normal feature in the first week of life in preterm babies ($\leq$28 weeks' gestation at birth) HIE (features present at birth and may persist for up to 2 weeks) Neonates with Down syndrome in the first 2 weeks of life	Neonates with leucoerythroblastic features due to infection nearly always have a peak in band cells as well

CRP, C-reactive protein; HIE, hypoxic ischaemic encephalopathy; NEC, necrotising enterocolitis; WBC, white cell count.

trisomy 18 are extremely limited because fewer than 20% of affected neonates survive for more than 12 months.[7]

Although rare, certain inherited immunodeficiency syndromes classically present with persistent neutrophilia, which is often first evident in the neonatal period. These disorders are important to recognise promptly because of the high frequency of severe

Table 3.2   Causes of neutrophilia in neonates

Condition	Diagnostic notes
Infection	
Acute bacterial infection*	Often preceded by transient neutropenia and with an increased proportion of band cells
	Usually accompanied by toxic granulation of the neutrophils
Chronic bacterial infection (e.g. osteomyelitis)	Toxic granulation often mild
	Neutrophil left shift usually absent
Some viral infections (e.g. chikungunya virus)	Neutrophilia, usually mature; occasional cases with severe thrombocytopenia
Maternal chorioamnionitis*	Mature neutrophilia with toxic granulation
Constitutional trisomies	
Trisomy 21 (Down syndrome)	Neutrophilia is commonly seen in neonates with Down syndrome even in the absence of infection or TAM
Trisomy 13 (Patau syndrome)	
Trisomy 18 (Edwards syndrome)	
Transient abnormal myelopoiesis associated with Down syndrome	Blast cells are >10%
	Leucocytosis (WBC >30 × 10^9/l) is common
Inherited immunodeficiency disorders	
LAD syndromes, IRF8 deficiency	Persistent neutrophilia; delayed separation of the cord (LAD syndromes); hypofunctional/dysplastic neutrophils (IRF8 deficiency)
Other	
Benign altitude-related neutrophilia	Neutrophilia without left shift in neonates born at altitude (≥1550 m above sea level) who have no clinical or laboratory evidence of infection
Drugs (e.g. corticosteroids, G-CSF)	

* Common causes of neonatal neutrophilia.
TAM, transient abnormal myelopoiesis; WBC, white cell count; G-CSF, granulocyte colony-stimulating factor.

infection, which may be fatal.[8,9] These include the leucocyte adhesion deficiency (LAD) syndromes caused by bi-allelic mutations in the *ITGB2*, *SLC35C1* and *FERMT3* genes in LAD-I, LAD-II and LAD-III, respectively;[10,11] and interferon regulatory factor 8 (IRF8) deficiency caused by bi-allelic mutations in *IRF8*.[9,12] The co-occurrence of persistent neutrophilia with delayed separation of the umbilical cord is highly suggestive of a LAD syndrome.[11]

Finally, treatment of neonates with corticosteroids or recombinant granulocyte colony-stimulating factor (G-CSF) causes neutrophilia that begins a few days after therapy is started and lasts for several days after discontinuation. Another benign cause of neutrophilia, with no neutrophil left shift and no other clinical or laboratory signs of infection, has been reported in neonates born at altitude (≥1550 m).[13] The duration of the

Table 3.3   Causes of lymphocytosis in neonates

Congenital infection

Cytomegalovirus
Coxsackievirus

Acquired neonatal infection

Cytomegalovirus
Respiratory syncytial virus
SARS-CoV-2 (COVID-19)
Bordetella pertussis
Malaria

Immunodeficiency disorders

Omenn syndrome
Autoimmune lymphoproliferative syndrome

COVID-19, coronavirus disease 19; SARS-CoV-2, severe
acute respiratory syndrome coronavirus 2.

neutrophilia is not clear as all the neonates in this study were discharged before day 4 of life and the mechanism was not investigated. However, these data suggest that, in relevant countries, care should be taken not to rely on the neutrophil count alone as a marker of infection.

Causes and significance of neonatal lymphocytosis

The main causes of lymphocytosis during the neonatal period are shown in Table 3.3. Lymphocytosis is not very common in neonates and is usually associated with congenital or nosocomially acquired viral infection, particularly with cytomegalovirus (CMV), respiratory syncytial virus (RSV) or coxsackievirus.[14–16] However, it is important to note that the majority of neonates with congenital CMV infection have no clinical findings at birth and that thrombocytopenia is the most common haematological feature of infection (see Chapter 4).[15] Neonatal COVID-19 is also associated with lymphocytosis, in contrast to adults, who tend to have lymphopenia.[17] Neonatal infection with *Bordetella pertussis*, although uncommon, can be associated with very severe infection and a dramatic lymphocytosis.[18] In addition, both transplacentally acquired and neonatally acquired malaria cause atypical lymphocytosis similar to that seen in neonatal CMV infection.[19] Finally, lymphocytosis may be seen in association with certain inherited immunodeficiency syndromes, in particular Omenn syndrome[20] and autoimmune lymphoproliferative syndrome (ALPS).[21,22]

Causes and significance of neonatal eosinophilia

Eosinophilia is common during the neonatal period, occurring in about 10% of all babies admitted to neonatal intensive care units[23] and in up to 75% of the most preterm neonates (<27 weeks' gestation).[24,25] The principal causes are shown in Table 3.4 and a typical example in a preterm neonate is shown in Fig. 3.1. The most common causes of eosinophilia in neonates are bacterial infection and necrotising enterocolitis (NEC) with the eosinophilia

Table 3.4 Causes of eosinophilia in neonates

Condition	Diagnostic notes
Infection Bacterial, particularly due to Gram-negative organisms Viral, e.g. RSV	Usually mild and transient Develops 1–2 days after the onset of infection Average duration 6 days
Necrotising enterocolitis	Seen in ~50% of cases Develops within 24 hours of the diagnosis of NEC
Allergic/inflammatory conditions Food protein-induced enterocolitis Eosinophilic oesophagitis[26] Neonatal eosinophilic pustulosis[27]	Eosinophilia is persistent and may be marked Clinical features of the underlying condition will be present
Transient abnormal myelopoiesis in neonates with Down syndrome	Seen in up to 23% of cases but not usually prominent May be a later feature (median age at presentation 41 days)

NEC, necrotising enterocolitis; RSV respiratory syncytial virus.

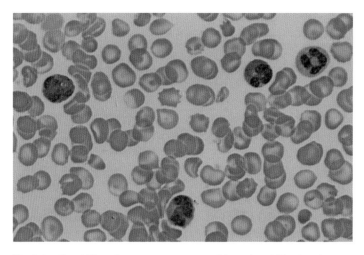

Fig. 3.1 Blood film of a preterm neonate with eosinophilia showing two eosinophils and two neutrophils. May–Grünwald–Giemsa (MGG), ×100 objective.

developing 1 or 2 days after the onset of these complications.[23,24] The eosinophilia is usually mild and transient, but early, persistent eosinophilia in NEC has been found to predict for late complications.[28] Eosinophilia is also found secondary to allergic conditions in neonates, such as food protein-induced enterocolitis, a condition presenting with bloody stools and eosinophilia in breastfed or formula-fed neonates.[29] Finally, eosinophilia is seen in up to 23% of cases of TAM where the eosinophils are part of mutant *GATA1* clone[30] and may contribute to the liver fibrosis seen in severe cases.[31]

Causes and significance of abnormalities in monocyte number in neonates

Monocytosis is fairly common in neonates, occurring most often in association with infection (Table 3.5). In general, monocytosis is a non-specific early feature of acute bacterial infection, the number of monocytes rising with the neutrophil count but usually falling more quickly as the infection resolves. Monocytosis is particularly associated with congenital syphilis, protozoal infections and *Candida* infections.[32–34] More recently, monocytosis together with neutropenia has been noted as a presenting finding in neonates with COVID-19[35] and in neonatal varicella infection.[36] There is often a compensatory monocytosis in neonates with either inherited or acquired neutropenia, including neonatal alloimmune neutropenia,[37] as discussed later. The other major group of conditions associated with monocytosis are neonatal preleukaemic and leukaemic conditions, including TAM in neonates with Down syndrome, juvenile myelomonocytic leukaemia (JMML) due to inherited rasopathies, and congenital leukaemia. Differentiation of these conditions from infection may be difficult, especially in JMML where the monocytic component of the disease is very prominent.[38–42] Neonates with Wiskott–Aldrich syndrome may also present with monocytosis and diagnostic confusion with JMML is increasing recognised.[43–45]

Table 3.5 Causes of monocytosis in neonates

Condition	Diagnostic notes
Infection	Particularly seen in congenital protozoal infections, congenital syphilis and *Candida* infections
	Common early feature of bacterial infection which resolves within a few days
	Blasts nearly always <8%
Transient abnormal myelopoiesis/ transient myeloproliferative disorder associated with Down syndrome	Acquired mutations in the *GATA1* gene always present
	Peripheral blood blasts variable (1–90%)
	Also occurs in neonates with mosaic Down syndrome and no other clinical features of Down syndrome
	Other features usually present (see Table 3.10)
Transient juvenile myelomonocytic leukaemia associated with congenital rasopathies	Most commonly seen in association with Noonan syndrome (*PTPN11* mutations)
	Peripheral blood blasts variable
	Increased numbers of abnormal monocytes always present
	Family history may be helpful (e.g. of neurofibromatosis)
Congenital neutropenia	Isolated severe neutropenia from birth,
Inherited (e.g. Kostmann syndrome)	recurrent bacterial infection, family history monocytosis increases during infections
Neonatal alloimmune neutropenia	Isolated severe neutropenia at birth,
	No family history; recovers in 1–2 months
Wiskott–Aldrich syndrome	Other features of WAS (e.g. eczema, microthrombocytopenia, recurrent infections) in a male infant

WAS, Wiskott–Aldrich syndrome.

Neonatal monocytopenia is rare but may be a useful clue to a diagnosis of certain inherited immunodeficiency disorders, particularly IRF8 deficiency, which is associated with severe and potentially fatal infection in the neonatal period.[9]

Circulating blast cells in neonates

In contrast to infants and older children, neonates have increased numbers of circulating immature 'blast cells', most commonly resembling the myeloblasts seen in acute leukaemia (Table 3.6). The numbers of circulating blasts are generally inversely proportional to gestational age and tend to increase in the early stages of acute infection (Fig. 3.2). Most reported cases of increased blast cells are in preterm neonates, are transient and occur as part of a general hyperleucocytosis, often without an underlying cause being identified.[46–48] Even in extremely preterm neonates with severe sepsis the percentage of blasts almost always remains below 8%.[6] The term 'neonatal leukaemoid reaction' (NLR) has been used to describe a white blood cell count $\geq 50 \times 10^9$/l in a neonate. NLR was shown to be associated with sepsis, bronchopulmonary dysplasia, intraventricular haemorrhage (IVH) and a high mortality rate when gestation-matched neonates with and without NLR were compared.[49] Neonates with Down syndrome almost always have circulating blast cells, even in the absence of TAM (discussed later in this chapter).[6] Blast cells are also a feature of neonatal JMML seen in some patients with inherited rasopathies.[38,39] The main significance of the

Table 3.6 Causes of increased blast cells in neonatal blood films

Condition	Diagnostic notes
Non-specific normal feature in preterm neonates, particularly if unwell due to infection or other causes	Transient feature which resolves within a few days Blasts nearly always <8%
Transient abnormal myelopoiesis/ transient myeloproliferative disorder associated with Down syndrome	Acquired mutations in the *GATA1* gene always present Peripheral blood blasts variable (1–90%) Also occurs in neonates with mosaic Down syndrome and no other clinical features of Down syndrome Other features usually present (see Table 3.10)
Transient juvenile myelomonocytic leukaemia associated with congenital rasopathies	Most commonly seen in association with Noonan syndrome Peripheral blood blasts variable Increased numbers of abnormal monocytes always present Family history may be helpful (e.g. of neurofibromatosis)
Congenital leukaemia (in neonates without Down syndrome)	40% acute myeloid leukaemia 60% acute lymphoblastic leukaemia Peripheral blood blasts usually >20% Characteristic molecular and cytogenetic abnormalities (e.g. *KMT2A* rearrangements in ALL and t(1;22) in AML)

ALL, acute lymphoblastic leukaemia; AML, acute myeloid leukaemia.

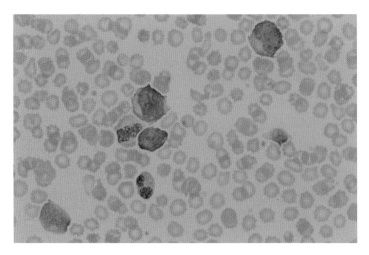

Fig. 3.2 Blood film of a preterm neonate born at 24 weeks' gestation showing blast cells and promyelocytes. Note the large number of echinocytes typical of a neonate born at this gestation. MGG, ×40.

presence of circulating blast cells is to be able to distinguish the very rare neonates with congenital leukaemia from the vast majority with self-limiting benign or preleukaemic or spontaneously remitting leukaemic disorders.

Neonatal infection and its differential diagnosis: clues from the blood count and blood film

The typical haematological changes associated with bacterial infection at any age are neutrophilia, an increased proportion of immature forms (usually referred to as neutrophil 'left shift' or increased band forms) and toxic granulation of the neutrophils. In neonates, one of the most important diagnostic considerations is the postnatal age of the baby at the time that the blood sample is collected as this is crucial to the correct interpretation of the findings.

The detection of neutrophil left shift in neonatal blood films is straightforward when the vast majority of circulating neutrophils are non-segmented 'band' forms (Fig. 3.3). However, in many cases the changes are less clear cut; many studies have described attempts to measure the extent of neutrophil left shift in a reproducible and reliable manner. The most sensitive approach is to calculate the ratio of immature band cells to total neutrophils, the (I/T) neutrophil ratio, on the basis of a manual differential count.[50,51] In many hospitals this has been superseded by automated counts of immature neutrophils/granulocytes reported as the immature granulocyte percentage (IG%) although both manual and automated approaches appear to give broadly similar results and neither is 100% reliable.[52] All of these approaches are greatly affected both by gestational age and by postnatal age and close liaison between the haematology laboratory and the clinical team is crucial to interpreting the significance of the results.

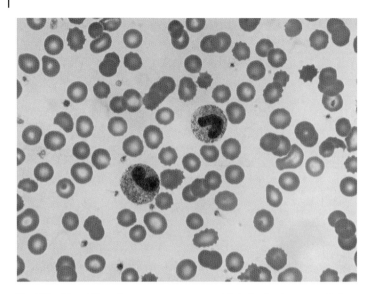

Fig. 3.3   Blood film of a preterm neonate with infection by group B *Streptococcus* showing two band cells with toxic granulation. MGG, ×100.

Acute bacterial infection

Neonatal infection remains a major cause of morbidity and mortality throughout the world, accounting for approximately 22% of global annual neonatal deaths.[53] The haematological findings can be very useful in making a prompt diagnosis both in well-resourced counties and in low and middle-income countries.[53–55] Indeed, in our experience, it is often possible to identify the most likely pathogen by integrating the clinical and haematological findings.

Neonatal sepsis is often categorised as either early-onset sepsis (EOS) or late-onset sepsis (LOS), with EOS variably defined but generally indicating sepsis within the first 3–7 days after birth. This reflects the mode of infection (during labour and delivery for most cases of EOS and nosocomial for LOS). Historically, the most frequent cause of acute bacterial infection presenting at or within 24 hours of birth is group B *Streptococcus*. This remains a very important cause of EOS but has been overtaken in some countries by nosocomially acquired Gram-negative infections.[56] The blood film appearances of group B *Streptococcus* infection on day 1 of life are highly characteristic (see Fig. 3.3); the proportion of band cells to mature neutrophils is markedly increased, toxic granulation is minimal and the total neutrophil and leucocyte counts are frequently reduced (for normal ranges, see Table 1.2). By day 2–3 of life, there is typically a neutrophilia with toxic granulation and less marked neutrophil left shift as the neonate responds appropriately to the infection.

The presence of increased band cells, in the absence of a more generalised left shift of myeloid cells including myelocytes, promyelocytes and blast cells, is not a normal feature in a neonate at any gestation and is a very sensitive indicator of acute bacterial infection. The only other causes of increased band cells typically seen in neonates are congenital viral infection, such as CMV or coxsackievirus infection, and inherited causes such as the autosomal dominant Pelger–Huët anomaly due to inherited mutations in *LBR*, which

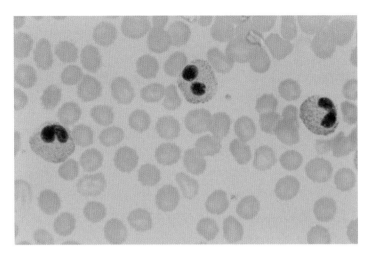

Fig. 3.4 Blood film of a term neonate with Pelger–Huët anomaly showing three neutrophils with typical dumbbell-shaped nuclei. MGG, ×100.

encodes the lamin B receptor.[57,58] In heterozygous cases, the neutrophils have unsegmented, dumbbell-shaped or bilobed nuclei (Fig. 3.4) and the eosinophils have round nuclei (Fig. 3.5), whereas in homozygotes the neutrophil nuclei are also round.[59]

After group B *Streptococcus*, the most common cause of acute bacterial infection at birth is a Gram-negative organism, most often *Haemophilus influenzae*. In such cases, in our experience, the neutrophils often show cytoplasmic vacuolation as well as toxic granulation and atypical mononuclear cells (i.e. atypical lymphocytes) may also be seen (Fig. 3.6). The presence of atypical mononuclear cells, with or without monocytosis, is also a feature of congenital infection with *Listeria monocytogenes* (Fig. 3.7), *Toxoplasma gondii* (Fig. 3.8) and *Mycoplasma pneumoniae* (Fig. 3.9).

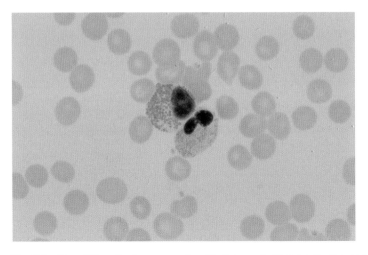

Fig. 3.5 Blood film of a term neonate with Pelger–Huët anomaly showing a Pelger eosinophil with a rounded nucleus as well as a neutrophil with a typical dumbbell-shaped nucleus. MGG, ×100.

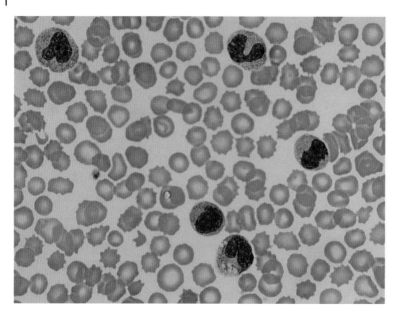

Fig. 3.6 Blood film of a preterm neonate showing typical features of a Gram-negative bacterial infection: neutrophil toxic granulation, marked left shift and vacuolation. Note the thrombocytopenia and some red cell fragments consistent with concomitant disseminated intravascular coagulation (DIC). MGG, ×100.

(a) (b)

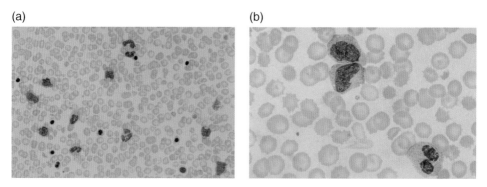

Fig. 3.7 Blood film of a neonate with congenital *Listeria monocytogenes* infection showing peripheral blood monocytosis. Note the erythroblastosis secondary to intrauterine growth restriction (IUGR) which is also a feature of neonatal listeriosis: (a) ×40; (b) ×100, MGG.

Although with experience, examination of neonatal blood films is a rapid and useful way of helping to establish the presence of infection in a neonate, there are two important limitations. First, the assessment is fairly subjective and, in our experience, is most accurate when serial daily blood films are available for review as the change in the blood film appearance are often more important than the magnitude of those changes. Secondly, it is important to be aware of a number of pitfalls. In particular, two of the cardinal signs of acute bacterial infection, neutrophilia and toxic granulation, can also be seen in a number

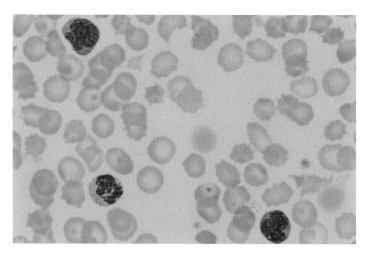

Fig. 3.8 Blood film of a neonate with congenital toxoplasmosis showing atypical mononuclear cells. Note the presence of target cells, which may reflect the liver involvement also present in this neonate. MGG, ×100.

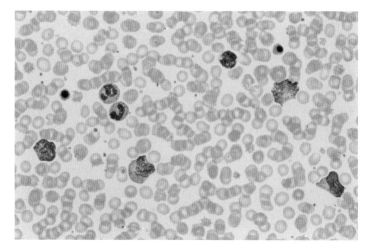

Fig. 3.9 Blood film of a preterm neonate born at 26 weeks' gestation with congenital pneumonia caused by *Mycoplasma pneumoniae* infection showing neutrophils and atypical mononuclear cells. Note the large number of echinocytes typical of a neonate born at this gestation. MGG, ×40.

of other conditions that are unique to neonates, including meconium aspiration, hypoxic ischaemic encephalopathy (Fig. 3.10) and maternal chorioamnionitis (see Table 3.1). All of these complications cause transient haematological changes, which gradually resolve over the first few days of life.

There have been many attempts to develop more objective ways of identifying acute neonatal infection based on the haematological findings available from the full blood count and blood film review. While most of these rely on various combinations of the white cell count (WBC) and the proportion of immature neutrophils, one of the best developed is the

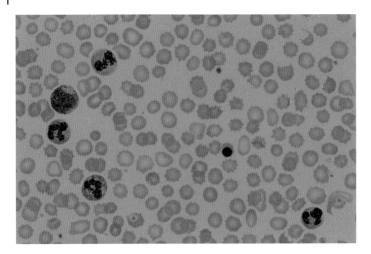

Fig. 3.10 Blood film of a preterm neonate born at 27 weeks' gestation and found to have hypoxic ischaemic encephalopathy showing toxic granulation of the neutrophils, a promyelocyte and nucleated red blood cells (NRBC). Note also the thrombocytopenia and occasional schistocyte consistent with DIC. MGG, ×60.

Hematologic Scoring System, which includes neutrophil morphology.[60] The developers, Rodwell and colleagues, assigned a score of 1 for each of seven findings: abnormal WBC, abnormal total neutrophil count, elevated immature polymorphonuclear (PMN) count, elevated immature to total PMN ratio, immature to mature PMN ratio greater than or equal to 0.3, platelet count less than or equal to 150×10^9/l and 'degenerative' changes in the neutrophils (defined as toxic granulation, vacuolation and/or Döhle bodies). Using a score of ≥3, they could identify almost 100% of neonates with definite or probable infection with a false positive rate of 14%, while with a score of ≤2 the likelihood that sepsis was absent was 99%. They subsequently reported that the scoring system could also be used to identify sepsis in neutropenic neonates when a score of ≥3 was combined with a neutrophil count of $<0.5 \times 10^9$/l.[61] This approach was found to be still valuable in a more recent study[54] and, although it is highly reliant on the availability of skilled laboratory staff, expensive equipment is not required. It seems likely that the application of more sophisticated automated methods, including artificial intelligence (AI)/machine learning, will soon provide an alternative approach.[55]

Maternal chorioamnionitis
Many babies, particularly those who are born before term, have marked neutrophilia and toxic granulation at birth with very few band forms. In the vast majority of cases, these changes are not a sign of acute bacterial infection in the baby but instead are due to maternal chorioamnionitis (Fig. 3.11), which is a very common trigger of preterm delivery. These changes likely reflect the passage of maternal cytokines, such as interleukin-6 (IL-6) and IL-8, across the placenta during labour and delivery.[62] In such cases, neonatal blood cultures are negative and C-reactive protein levels are normal or mildly increased.[63] The leucocyte count is usually high and may even exceed 100×10^9/l despite the absence of acute infection in the baby.[49] These changes in the blood film are maximal in the first 24 hours

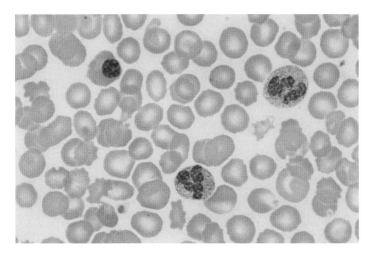

Fig. 3.11 Impact of maternal chorioamnionitis on the blood film at birth showing that toxic granulation of the neutrophils is already present. MGG, ×100.

after birth and gradually resolve over the first 3–4 days of life. It is important to note that identical findings appearing in a blood film after this time are almost always indicative of acute bacterial infection in the baby.

Leucocyte vacuolation

Prominent vacuolation of the cytoplasm of neutrophils, monocytes and sometimes eosinophils can also be a useful diagnostic finding in neonatal blood films (see Table 3.1). As well as a fairly common finding in Gram-negative infections, this can also be a feature of neonatal *Staphylococcus epidermidis* infections in association with indwelling vascular catheters (Fig. 3.12). In some cases the organism is visible within these vacuoles (Fig. 3.13); however, systematic evaluation of neonatal blood films or buffy coats suggests that this is not a very sensitive way of detecting bacteraemia and is seen only in very severe sepsis.[64] Systemic fungal infection with *Candida* or *Aspergillus* species, which are major causes of morbidity and mortality in preterm neonates less than 28 weeks' gestation at birth,[65] also often causes neutrophil and monocyte vacuolation which typically produces a 'motheaten' appearance of the cells (Fig. 3.14). Many cases also have thrombocytopenia.[65] Blood film evaluation can be a useful diagnostic tool in neonates at high risk of fungal infection as the leucocyte changes may be an early diagnostic sign.

One of the most serious complications seen in neonates, particularly preterm neonates, is necrotising enterocolitis, an inflammatory intestinal disease of uncertain aetiology. In the early stages of the disease, the clinical signs are often non-specific (abdominal distension and feeding intolerance) and the haematological features at this stage include neutropenia and often a fall in the platelet count, initially not to thrombocytopenic levels.[66] This is rapidly followed by neutrophil and monocyte vacuolation and thrombocytopenia (Fig. 3.15). In our experience, neutrophil and monocyte vacuolation are almost always present in neonates with NEC and are a very useful early indicator of the diagnosis. Machine learning approaches based on the full blood count are now being developed in order to generate predictive models for diagnosis of the cases of NEC that are best treated by early surgery.[66]

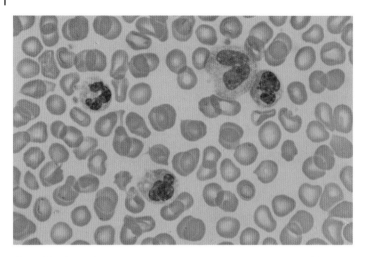

Fig. 3.12 Blood film of a 3-week-old preterm neonate born at 29 weeks' gestation who developed infection of an indwelling intravascular catheter with *Staphylococcus epidermidis*. The film shows three vacuolated neutrophils as well as a giant monocyte. MGG, ×100.

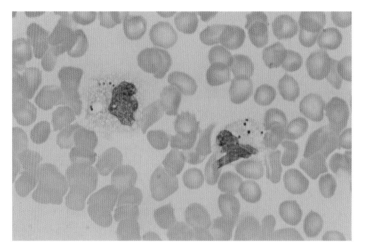

Fig. 3.13 Blood film of a preterm neonate with *Staphylococcus epidermidis* infection showing the presence of the organisms within two monocytes. Note also the cytoplasmic vacuolation. MGG, ×100.

Viral infection

Neonates with congenital viral infection, most commonly CMV but also enteroviruses and rubella, usually have circulating atypical lymphocytes that can be readily seen in blood films for the first few weeks of life, providing a useful clue to the underlying diagnosis (Figs 3.16 and 3.17) (see Cases 4.1 and 4.2, pages 227 and 230). Similar cells are also seen in neonates who develop nosocomial viral infection, for example due to CMV or RSV. Virus-associated lymphocytosis in neonates is usually transient and mild. As the viraemia resolves, the numbers of circulating atypical lymphocytes fall. In occasional cases of congenital CMV infection, the viraemia and thrombocytopenia persist for several months and

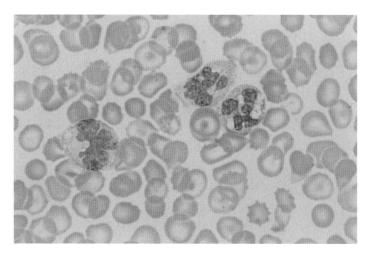

Fig. 3.14 Blood film of a neonate with *Candida* infection showing neutrophil and monocyte vacuolation. Note the large number of target cells, which likely reflect systemic infection involving the liver. MGG, ×100.

(a)   (b)

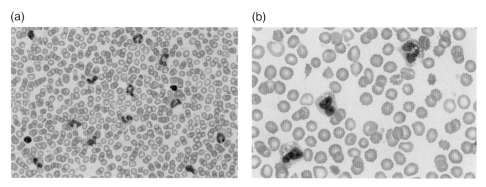

Fig. 3.15 Blood film of a preterm neonate with necrotising enterocolitis showing vacuolation of the neutrophils and monocytes, which usually appears as one or more rounded punched out 'holes' in the cytoplasm of these cells: MGG, (a) ×40, (b) ×100.

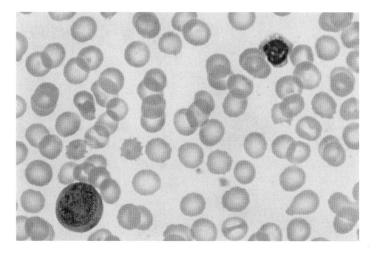

Fig. 3.16 Blood film of a neonate with congenital cytomegalovirus (CMV) infection showing the presence of typical activated lymphocytes. MGG, ×100.

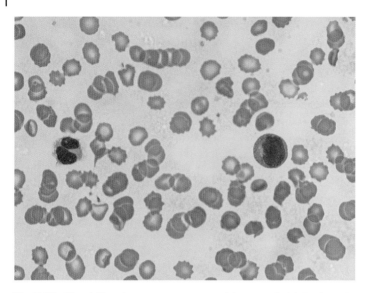

Fig. 3.17 Blood film of a preterm neonate with congenital infection with coxsackievirus showing a large lymphocyte with deeply basophilic cytoplasm and a second cell that may be a binucleated reactive lymphocyte. MGG, ×100.

in such cases the ongoing presence of atypical lymphocytes in the blood film is a useful marker of active infection. Adults with COVID-19 have also been reported to have atypical lymphocytes[67] but their presence in neonates has not yet been reported.

Storage disorders: diagnostic clues from the blood film

A number of storage disorders cause morphological abnormalities of the white blood cells (reviewed in reference 68). In particular, vacuolation of lymphocytes is seen in two of the most severe of these disorders, Wolman disease (lysosomal acid lipase deficiency) and GM1-gangliosidosis (β-galactosidase deficiency).

Wolman disease is an extremely rare lysosomal storage disease caused by bi-allelic mutations in the *LIPA* gene.[69] Deficiency of the lysosomal acid lipase enzyme leads to accumulation of intracellular lipids in the liver, spleen, lymph nodes, intestine and bone marrow, the lipid being visible as vacuoles within the circulating lymphocytes[68,70] (Fig. 3.18a). Wolman disease typically presents in the first few months of life with hepatosplenomegaly, jaundice, failure to thrive and malabsorption.[71] Although the diagnosis is established using enzymatic analysis and/or deoxyribonucleic acid (DNA) sequencing, evaluation of a neonatal blood film for the typical appearances of lymphocyte vacuolation is a useful screening test in neonates with unexplained hepatosplenomegaly. Prompt diagnosis is important as the disease is fatal by 12 months of age (median age at death 3.7 months)[71,72] and effective enzyme replacement therapy with sebelipase alfa is available.[70] Type I (infantile) GM1 gangliosidosis is a rare, very severe sphingolipidosis caused by mutations in the *GLB1* gene that cause decreased activity of β-galactosidase and storage of GM1 ganglioside. The disease may present as hydrops fetalis or with severe central nervous system (CNS) dysfunction,

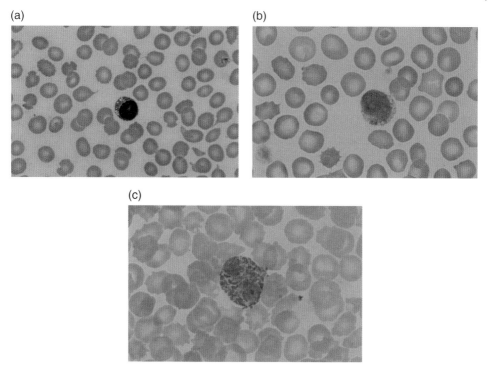

Fig. 3.18 Blood films in storage disorders: (a) lymphocyte vacuolation in Wolman disease; (b) lymphocyte vacuolation in β-galactosidase deficiency; (c) Alder–Reilly bodies in a neutrophil in Sly disease. MGG, ×100.

developmental delay and hepatosplenomegaly.[73] Unfortunately, the disease is uniformly fatal in the first few years of life but the presence of lymphocyte vacuolation on a fetal or neonatal blood film (Fig. 3.18b) may be a useful screening test to guide the specific biochemical and molecular tests for confirmation of the diagnosis.[74]

Leucocyte abnormalities can be seen in the blood film of neonates or infants with a number of other inherited storage disorders (Table 3.7). In several of the mucopolysaccharidoses, metachromatic staining of granules known as the Alder–Reilly anomaly is apparent in the neutrophils (Fig. 3.18c). In other storage disorders, such as perinatally lethal Gaucher disease, due to mutations in the *GBA* gene, the disease manifests with thrombocytopenia or as a 'blueberry muffin' skin rash rather than with leucocyte abnormalities.[75]

Neonatal neutropenia

Definition and causes of neutropenia

Neutropenia is classically defined as a blood neutrophil concentration more than 2 standard deviations below the reference range. However, as discussed in Chapter 1, the neutrophil count varies widely with postnatal age, and different considerations therefore need to

Table 3.7 Cytological abnormalities in metabolic and storage disorders and other constitutional abnormalities that may present in the neonatal period

Cytological features	Possible diagnoses	Diagnostic clues
Large, brightly staining granules, which can also be larger than normal, in neutrophils and other granulocytes (Alder–Reilly anomaly); abnormal lymphocyte and monocyte granules are sometimes also present	As an isolated anomaly or associated with one of the mucopolysaccharidoses (e.g. Sly syndrome, Sanfilippo syndrome, Hurler syndrome, Hunter disease), mucosulphatidosis, infantile type neuronal ceroid lipofuscinosis	Family history, features of a storage disorder – dysmorphism, hepatomegaly, slow development
Giant and aberrantly staining granules in all granulocytes, monocytes and lymphocytes	Chédiak–Higashi anomaly	Family history, pancytopenia, infection, jaundice, albinism and neurological abnormalities
Cytoplasmic inclusions in granulocytes (Döhle body-like)	*MYH9*-related disorders including May–Hegglin anomaly	Family history, macrothrombocytopenia; other disease features (e.g. deafness and nephropathy) are absent in the neonatal period
Cytoplasmic vacuolation	Carnitine deficiency, neutral lipid storage disease, Pearson syndrome	Pancytopenia in Pearson syndrome
Lymphocyte vacuolation	Mucopolysaccharidoses (e.g. Hunter disease), mucosulphatidosis, mucolipidosis type II (I-cell disease) and type IV, Niemann–Pick disease type A, Wolman disease, GM1-gangliosidosis, mannosidosis, fucosidosis, Pompe disease, sialic acid storage disease	Family history, features of a storage disorder – dysmorphism, hepatosplenomegaly, CNS dysfunction, developmental delay

be made in interpreting the significance of the neutrophil count in neonates. Although clinicians often worry when a routine blood count reveals a neutrophil count below the normal range (see Table 1.2) because of anxiety about missing cases of severe congenital neutropenia (SCN), in practice, most neutropenia in neonates is mild, transient and of no clinical significance. A pragmatic approach is to consider a neutrophil count at birth of less than 2×10^9/l as abnormal and worth monitoring, and a neutrophil count during the first month of life of $<0.7 \times 10^9$/l as significant enough to merit further investigation.

Causes of neonatal neutropenia are summarised in Table 3.8. The commonest cause of neutropenia at birth in preterm neonates is transiently reduced neutrophil production secondary to intrauterine growth restriction (IUGR) or maternal hypertension.[76,77] Most affected neonates also have thrombocytopenia and increased erythropoiesis, manifest as polycythaemia and/or increased circulating nucleated red blood cells (NRBC) (Fig. 3.19). Similar haematological abnormalities (transient neutropenia and thrombocytopenia

Table 3.8 Causes of neonatal neutropenia*

Chronic *in utero* hypoxia

Maternal hypertension
Intrauterine growth restriction
Maternal diabetes

Infection

Acute, perinatal bacterial infection, e.g. group B *Streptococcus*
Congenital viral infections, e.g. cytomegalovirus
Neonatal bacterial infections
Neonatal viral infections, e.g. cytomegalovirus

Necrotising enterocolitis

Immune

Autoimmune (maternal or neonatal)
Alloimmune

Chromosomal anomalies

Trisomy 21
Trisomy 18
Trisomy 13

Metabolic disorders

Hyperglycinaemia
Isovaleric acidaemia
Propionic acidaemia
Methylmalonic acidaemia
3-Methylglutaconic aciduria type II (Barth syndrome)
Pearson syndrome

Marrow replacement

Congenital leukaemia (see Table 3.11)
Congenital primary myelofibrosis

*Causes of inherited severe congenital neutropenia (SCN) are
shown in Table 3.9.

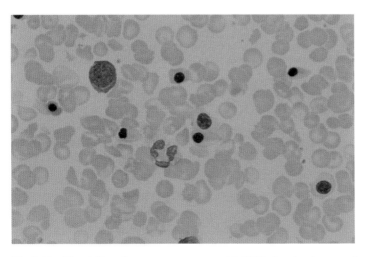

Fig. 3.19 Blood film of a preterm neonate with IUGR showing increased numbers of normoblasts
and a basophilic erythroblast. MGG, ×60.

together with polycythaemia) are seen in the infants born to mothers with diabetes.[76] It is important to note that the neutrophils in neonates with IUGR or those with neutropenia secondary to maternal hypertension or diabetes are not left shifted, helping to differentiate this form of neutropenia from sepsis-associated neutropenia. A retrospective study in 200 neonates with IUGR noted that the NRBC count correlated inversely with the neutrophil count during the first days after birth and also that the most severely weight-restricted neutropenic neonates had a trend toward higher NRBC counts.[77] This suggests that the underlying driver for these haematological abnormalities may be chronic fetal hypoxia, although the precise mechanisms have not been identified. This form of neutropenia resolves spontaneously, usually within a few days of birth and does not persist beyond the first 2 weeks of life.[76,77]

The commonest cause of neutropenia in term infants is bacterial or viral infection. Neutropenia in the first few hours of life is typically associated with group B *Streptococcus* infection and can be severe ($<0.5 \times 10^9$/l) but, in contrast to inherited SCN, the neutropenia is transient and replaced by increasing neutrophilia within 1–2 days. Neutropenia is also an important early sign of NEC and of LOS (i.e. sepsis developing after the first 7 days of life). As infection- and NEC-associated neutropenia is self-limiting, persistent neutropenia in a term or preterm baby should always be investigated. This includes looking carefully for evidence of other acquired causes, such as congenital or nosocomial viral infection and immune neutropenia (see later). Other important causes of neutropenia are SCN due to a selective failure of neutrophil production (e.g. Kostmann syndrome) (see Table 3.9), marrow replacement due to congenital leukaemia or congenital myelofibrosis, and a number of rare metabolic disorders that are listed in Table 3.8. Finally, severe neutropenia may also be one of the manifestations of rare bone marrow failure syndromes, such as Pearson syndrome and Fanconi anaemia, although in most cases anaemia or thrombocytopenia is more prominent (see Chapter 2). Note that neonates with the Pelger–Huët anomaly are not neutropenic unless they have concomitant infection, although typically automated neutrophil counts are unreliable in these cases (Case 3.1, see page 169).

Immune neutropenia

The majority of cases of immune neutropenia in the neonatal period are caused by alloantibodies in the mother directed against neutrophil antigens lacking in the fetus/newborn. Occasional cases arise where the mother herself has autoimmune neutropenia and transplacental maternal autoantibodies cause neonatal neutropenia. True autoimmune neutropenia almost always develops after the age of 6 months but occasional cases presenting in the newborn have been reported.[78]

Alloimmune neonatal neutropenia

This condition is the neutrophil equivalent of haemolytic disease of the fetus and newborn (HDFN) and fetal/neonatal alloimmune thrombocytopenia (FNAIT). In contrast to HDFN and FNAIT, it is not clear whether neutropenia causes any clinically significant disease prior to birth. Alloimmune neutropenia occurs when fetal neutrophils express paternally derived antigens of the human neutrophil antigen (HNA) system that are absent on

Table 3.9 Inherited causes of severe congenital neutropenia that present in neonates (see also Online Mendelian Inheritance in Man, https://www.omim.org/)

Nature of condition	Cytogenetic or genetic abnormality implicated (inheritance)
Isolated severe congenital neutropenia	*ELANE* (AD)
	HAX1 (AR)
	CSF3R (AR)
	GFI1 (AD)
	VPS45 (AR)
	JAGN1 (AR)
	TCIRG1 (AD)
	SRPS4 (AD)
	CSF3R (AR or AD)
Congenital neutropenia associated with immunodeficiency or syndromic features	
Shwachman syndrome*	*SBDS* (AR) or *DNAJC21* (AR)
Reticular dysgenesis	*AK2* (AR)
Dursun syndrome	*G6PC3* (AR)
Barth syndrome	*TAFAZZIN* (XLR)
CLPB syndrome**	*CLPB* (AD)
Wiskott–Aldrich syndrome	*WAS* (XLR)

* Neutropenia is often intermittent and may be missed in the neonatal period.
** Some cases have isolated severe congenital neutropenia without syndromic features.
AD autosomal dominant; AR, autosomal recessive; XLR, X-linked recessive.
Based on references 89 and 90.

maternal neutrophils and against which the mother produces immunoglobulin G (IgG) neutrophil alloantibodies.

Five HNA systems have been recognised as targets for maternal alloantibodies: HNA-1, HNA-2, HNA-3, HNA-4 and HNA-5 (reviewed in reference 79). The most common causative antibodies are directed against HNA-1a and HNA-1b, followed by HNA-2. Antibodies directed against HNA-1c, HNA-1d, HNA-3a, HNA-3b, HNA-4a, HNA-4b and HNA-5a are rare.[79] No cases of neonatal alloimmune neutropenia due to anti-HNA-5b have yet been reported. Recent data suggest that although anti-HNA antibodies can be detected in approximately 1% of mothers, only 1 in 10 women with antibodies will deliver babies with documented neonatal alloimmune neutropenia (0.1% of all live births).[80] Other studies have reported an even lower frequency of neonatal alloimmune neutropenia, 0.01%[81] or even 0.001% (reviewed in reference 80), perhaps because most milder cases are missed unless screening is performed as part of a research study. Like FNAIT, neonatal alloimmune neutropenia can occur in the first pregnancy.[82]

The full range of clinical presentations of neonatal alloimmune neutropenia is not known as most asymptomatic cases will be missed, given that routine full blood counts are not performed unless neonates are admitted to hospital. Severe cases present in the first few days of life with fever and infections of the respiratory tract, urinary tract and skin, including omphalitis. Retrospective series have identified many cases of neonatal alloimmune neutropenia where there is no evidence of infection and the diagnosis has been made because of an incidental finding of severe neutropenia where a full blood count has been performed for another reason or because of a previously affected sibling.[81,82] The majority of cases of neonatal alloimmune neutropenia are diagnosed in term babies but occasional cases in preterm neonates have been reported.[83]

The main diagnostic clue to neonatal alloimmune neutropenia is a history of unexplained neutropenia that persists for several weeks or months with or without concomitant bacterial infection. The neutropenia is self-limiting and usually resolves in 1–2 months although occasional cases where the neutropenia has persisted for more than 6 months have been reported.[81,84] The reason for prolonged neutropenia and the mechanism by which this occurs is very unclear. The haemoglobin and platelet count are normal and there are no specific features in the blood film. The diagnosis is made by demonstrating antineutrophil antibodies in the mother and baby, which react against paternal, but not maternal, neutrophil antigens. Investigation typically includes maternal HNA antibody screening, HNA genotyping of the baby and both parents and cross-matching of maternal serum against paternal neutrophils if possible.[80] Serological investigation of neonatal alloimmune neutropenia requires particular expertise and is usually performed in specialist laboratories that are often national reference centres. The mainstay of treatment of neonatal alloimmune thrombocytopenia is antibiotics.[84] The morbidity and mortality of neonatal alloimmune neutropenia is low but G-CSF may be useful to boost the neutrophil count in cases with resistant infection and/or prolonged neutropenia,[85] although the response is variable[86,87] and there are no controlled trials to confirm the benefit of G-CSF in this setting.

Neonatal neutropenia due to maternal autoantibodies

This rare condition is caused by the transfer of maternal IgG antibodies across the placenta from mothers with autoimmune neutropenia.[88] The clinical manifestations are very similar to those of neonatal alloimmune neutropenia as the neutropenia may be severe. It is therefore important to consider this diagnosis by checking the blood count and blood film in all infants born to mothers with a history of autoimmune neutropenia. The neutropenia is self-limiting and management is as for neonatal alloimmune neutropenia.

Inherited congenital or neonatal neutropenia

Severe congenital neutropenias are a group of inherited diseases characterised by selective failure of neutrophil differentiation. Although the neutrophil count is extremely low (by definition $<0.5 \times 10^9$/l) and neutrophils are often almost completely absent in the peripheral blood (Fig. 3.20), the bone marrow typically shows maturation arrest of granulopoiesis at the promyelocyte stage of differentiation. Although the disorders are all very rare (estimated incidence 3–8.5 cases per million individuals),[89] it is important to identify SCN in the neonatal period because these babies are at high risk of life-threatening infection from birth. Indeed, the majority of affected infants present with infections in the first few days or weeks of life.[89]

Typical presentations of neutropenia-associated infections in the neonatal period include omphalitis, pneumonia, septicaemia, cellulitis and, occasionally, deep tissue abscesses. Infections are often more severe and/or prolonged than in neonates who are able to mount a normal neutrophil response. In most cases, the neutrophil count at diagnosis of SCN is $<0.2 \times 10^9$/l (see Fig. 3.20), often with a compensatory monocytosis (Fig. 3.21). However, investigations are indicated in all neonates where the neutropenia is severe ($<0.5 \times 10^9$/l), particularly when this persists beyond the first 2 weeks of life despite resolution of infection and/or if there is a relevant family history.[89,90]

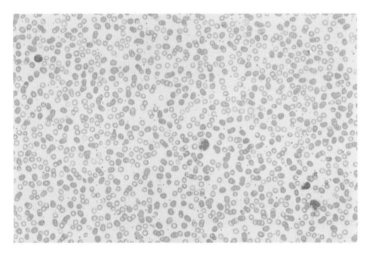

Fig. 3.20   Blood film of a 3-week-old term neonate with severe congenital neutropenia (SCN) showing two monocytes and two lymphocytes (note the absence of neutrophils on this low power view). MGG, ×20.

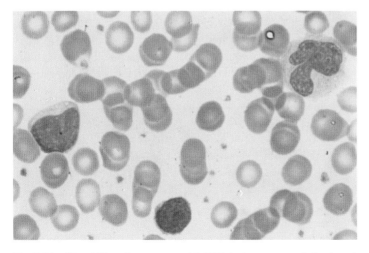

Fig. 3.21   Blood film of a neonate with SCN during an acute infection showing a monocyte and promonocyte, as well as a lymphocyte, but no neutrophils. MGG, ×100.

The main causes of SCN that present in the neonatal period are shown in Table 3.9. While most cases present with isolated neutropenia, SCN is also seen in a number of immunodeficiency and multisystem disorders where the presence of the other features may provide clues to the underlying diagnosis. Increasingly, next generation sequencing is used to provide a rapid diagnosis based on gene panels containing known SCN-associated genes. The most common genetic cause of SCN is mutation of *ELANE* (previously known as *ELA2*), the gene that encodes neutrophil elastase, which explains 45–60% of all cases of SCN. The next most frequent causative genes are: the *SBDS* gene, which causes Shwachman–Diamond syndrome; the *G6PT* gene, which encodes glucose-6-phosphate translocase and causes glycogen storage disease type 1b; and *HAX1*, which is now known to explain the SCN in the original Kostmann family.[89] The number of genes known to cause SCN is steadily increasing with increasing use of whole genome and whole exome sequencing; those that have been reported to present in the neonatal period are shown in Table 3.9 and include mutations in *GFI1* (growth factor-independent protein 1), *JAGN1*, *CSF3R*, *TCIRG1*, *SRP54*, *SRP68*, *DNAJC21* and several genes affecting the endosomal-lysosomal system, such as *VPS45*.[89–93]

To date the causative genes in SCN have been shown to be important for normal neutrophil differentiation, survival and function, although their role in neutrophil development was sometimes unsuspected prior to the identification of the underlying defects in cases presenting as SCN. In about one-third of cases no causative gene is identified.[90] In that situation, bone marrow examination may be useful in helping to pinpoint the pathophysiology of the disease, for example by demonstrating differentiation arrest, and whole exome sequencing may reveal new candidate causes of SCN, which must always be validated by family and functional studies. Establishing a molecular diagnosis is extremely important, not only for identification of current or future family members, but also because patients with SCN have an increased risk of developing leukaemia of up to 60% in certain subtypes.[94,95] The long-term outlook for patients with SCN has been transformed by the introduction of G-CSF as the mainstay of treatment. Overall survival is now >80%, although around 10% of patients still die from sepsis or severe bacterial infections.[95,96]

Severe congenital neutropenia due to *ELANE* mutation

Up to 60% of cases of SCN are due to heterozygous mutations in *ELANE*.[97] To date, more than 200 different *ELANE* mutations, either inherited or *de novo*, have been described.[98] The autosomal dominant pattern of inheritance in *ELANE*-mutated SCN means that the majority of cases will have a family history. A second clue to the presence of an *ELANE* mutation as the underlying cause is the absence of congenital anomalies or other syndromic features, which are common in other types of SCN. The treatment of SCN in the neonatal period is a combination of antibiotics for infection and G-CSF to maintain the absolute neutrophil count above 1×10^9/l, usually starting with a dose of 5 µg/kg/day subcutaneously and titrating according to the neutrophil count.[84,89,90]

Shwachman–Diamond syndrome

Shwachman–Diamond syndrome is an autosomal recessive disorder caused by bi-allelic mutations in the *SBDS* gene.[89,90] The syndrome is characterised by the triad of exocrine pancreatic insufficiency, skeletal dysplasia and neutropenia. Although the

Shwachman–Diamond syndrome typically presents later in infancy with failure to thrive, severe disease has been reported in term and preterm neonates.[99,100] For those cases that do present in the neonatal period, the diagnosis is suggested by the presence of neutropenia in a neonate with IUGR with or without skeletal abnormalities.[101] Importantly, Shwachman–Diamond syndrome may present in the neonatal period with severe thoracic dystrophy. Indeed, there are several reports of misdiagnosis of the syndrome as the skeletal disease Jeune syndrome (asphyxiating thoracic dystrophy [ATD]), where the delay in identifying the correct diagnosis as Shwachman–Diamond syndrome, and the associated bone marrow and gastrointestinal failure, may have contributed to the risk of early neonatal death from this condition.[101,102] Although neutropenia is almost always present, many cases also have anaemia and/or thrombocytopenia, including in the neonatal period.[99,101] The diagnosis is based on the clinical history together with the blood count, evidence of exocrine pancreatic insufficiency, the presence of the distinctive skeletal abnormalities (metaphyseal dysplasia, thoracic dystrophy, short and splayed ribs) and molecular analysis using a targeted next generation sequencing panel or whole exome sequencing to identify the causative mutation in the *SBDS* gene. Most patients respond well to treatment with pancreatic enzyme replacement, G-CSF to prevent recurrent infections and antibiotics as necessary. Unfortunately, these patients appear to have a particularly high risk of developing leukaemia later in life.[103] It is also worth noting that other very rare bone marrow failure syndromes, such as bi-allelic mutations in the *DNAJC21* or *SRP54* genes, may present with a Shwachman–Diamond-like syndrome.[91,92] It is therefore important to perform DNA analysis to establish the correct molecular diagnosis and plan appropriate management.

Severe congenital neutropenia due to glucose-6-phosphate transporter (*SLC37A4*) mutation

Glycogen storage disease 1b is caused by bi-allelic mutations in the *SLC37A4* gene and deficiency of the glucose-6-phosphate transporter (G6PT1).[89] Although the clinical presentation may be delayed until later in infancy, the disease has been reported to present in the neonatal period with hepatomegaly, hypoglycaemia, seizures and persistent neutropenia, most likely due to apoptosis of developing and mature neutrophils.[104] The diagnosis is based on the clinical history together with the blood count and molecular analysis by targeted next generation sequencing or whole exome sequencing. As with other causes of SCN, treatment with G-CSF corrects the neutropenia but these patients also have an increased risk of developing leukaemia later in life.[105]

Severe congenital neutropenia due to *HAX1* mutation

Although first described more than 60 years ago, the cause of Kostmann syndrome was only identified in 2007 as being due to homozygous mutations of the *HAX1* gene.[106] In the original series of patients, all from the same large pedigree, the patients presented at birth or shortly thereafter with omphalitis, skin infections, abscesses or sepsis and all of the children died during the first year of life.[107] It is now clear that mutations in exon 2 of *HAX1* solely affect expression of isoform A of the HAX1 protein and manifest as SCN, while mutations in other exons of *HAX1* affect expression of both isoform A and isoform B, resulting in both neurological problems (cognitive dysfunction, developmental delay, seizures) and SCN.[108,109] In both types of disease HAX1 deficiency causes ineffective neutrophil production and maturation arrest at the promyelocyte stage. The diagnosis is based on the clinical history together with the blood count and molecular analysis using a targeted next generation sequencing panel or whole exome sequencing. As for other forms of SCN, treatment with G-CSF is effective in boosting the neutrophil count and preventing infection but these patients are also at risk of developing leukaemia later in life.[110]

Haematological features of neonates with Down syndrome

Several retrospective studies have reported an increased frequency of haematological abnormalities in neonates with Down syndrome,[111,112] including a markedly increased risk of leukaemia in early childhood and of a neonatal condition known as transient abnormal myelopoiesis (TAM), which may be best regarded as a transient leukaemia rather than as a preleukaemic condition (reviewed in reference 113). The high frequency of other haematological abnormalities in neonates with Down syndrome has only been recognised fairly recently after a prospective study of blood counts and blood films in 200 unselected neonates with Down syndrome documented the haematological findings in detail (see reference 6). This study showed that all neonates with Down syndrome had haematological abnormalities (Table 3.10). Importantly, these abnormalities were seen in the absence of TAM (discussed later). In particular, neonates with Down syndrome had higher haemoglobin concentrations compared with other neonates of the same gestation, increased circulating erythroblasts and abnormal red cell morphology, including macrocytosis, target cells and basophilic stippling (Fig. 3.22). In addition, in the absence of TAM, neonates with Down syndrome had lower median platelet counts than neonates without Down syndrome and 51% had thrombocytopenia (platelets $<150 \times 10^9$/l). Neonates with Down syndrome had higher numbers of neutrophils and monocytes than neonates without Down syndrome, while the total lymphocyte count was reduced, consistent with previous studies in older children with Down syndrome.[114–116] Importantly, circulating blast cells were seen on the blood film in virtually all neonates with Down syndrome (98%).[6] In our experience, blast cells are usually <10% of peripheral blood leucocytes in these neonates but they may be as high as 15%, even when very sensitive methods are used to exclude the mutations in the *GATA1* gene that define TAM (reviewed in reference 117). The presence of blast cells in the blood film in such a high proportion of neonates with Down syndrome means that making a definitive diagnosis of TAM may be very difficult and mutational analysis of the *GATA1* gene is often required to confirm the diagnosis (see later).

Congenital leukaemia

Leukaemia is rare in neonates, with the exception of neonates with Down syndrome. While congenital leukaemia affects approximately three non-Down syndrome neonates per million live births, for those with Down syndrome approximately 200 neonates per million live births will have the congenital syndrome known as TAM.[118,119] Transient abnormal myelopoiesis, also known as transient myeloproliferative disorder or transient leukaemia,

Table 3.10 Haematological abnormalities in neonates with Down syndrome

Condition	Acquired *GATA1* mutation	Haematological features	Clinical features
Transient abnormal myelopoiesis	Yes 100% of cases	Hb usually normal (anaemia rare) Platelet count may be increased, in the normal range or reduced Leucocytosis usual but WBC range overlaps with DS neonates without TAM Blasts >10% Megakaryocyte fragments usually present in blood film BM blasts usually not increased (BM examination unhelpful)	Hepatosplenomegaly 40% Skin rash 20% Pleural/pericardial effusion ± ascites 10% Jaundice 70–80%
Silent transient abnormal myelopoiesis	Yes 100% of cases	Hb increased or normal Platelets normal or reduced WBC normal Blasts <10%	No increase in frequency of hepatosplenomegaly, jaundice, skin rash, pleural/pericardial effusions or ascites compared to neonates with DS who lack *GATA1* mutations
Trisomy 21 (no evidence of TAM or silent TAM)	No	Compared with neonates without DS: Hb increased (24% polycythaemic, Hct >0.65) Platelets lower (40% thrombocytopenic) WBC counts higher due to increased neutrophils, basophils and monocytes 98% have peripheral blood blasts (<15%)	No clinical features are specific for TAM as ~60% of neonates with trisomy 21 have jaundice and up to 10% have hepatosplenomegaly, rash, pleural/pericardial effusion or ascites secondary to medical complications in the absence of *GATA1* mutations

BM, bone marrow; DS, Down syndrome; Hb, haemoglobin concentration; Hct, haematocrit; TAM, transient abnormal myelopoiesis.

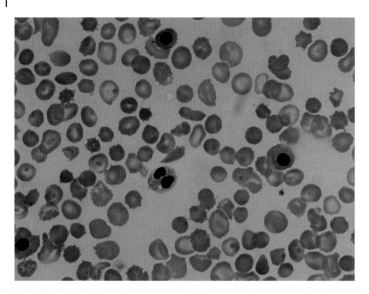

Fig. 3.22 Blood film of a neonate with Down syndrome showing increased erythroblasts, target cells and macrocytes as well as some spherocytes and echinocytes. A pseudo-Pelger neutrophil and giant platelet can also be seen. All of these abnormalities are frequent in neonates with Down syndrome even in the absence of a diagnosis of transient abnormal myelopoiesis (TAM) due to acquired *GATA1* mutations (see Fig. 3.23). MGG, ×60.

affects around 10% of neonates with Down syndrome while a further 15–20% have a clinically silent form of the disease (silent TAM). As the estimated incidence of Down syndrome worldwide is between 1 in 500 and 1 in 1100 live births, TAM is the commonest leukaemia in neonates. The rarity of neonatal leukaemia suggests that, with the exception of neonates with Down syndrome, fetal haemopoietic stem and progenitor cells are not inherently susceptible to leukaemic transformation. Finally, children with congenital rasopathies, in particular Noonan syndrome, may develop a neonatal leukaemia resembling JMML which, like TAM, is usually transient and resolves without treatment.[120]

Leukaemia and preleukaemia in neonates with Down syndrome

Overview and definition

Transient abnormal myelopoiesis is a clonal disorder almost unique to Down syndrome, which presents in fetal life, at birth or within the first few weeks of life. The characteristic features are the presence of circulating blast cells, most often resembling megakaryo-blasts, as well as dysplastic changes in other peripheral blood cells.[6,121] TAM is now known to be caused by mutations in the haemopoietic transcription factor gene *GATA1*, and is only seen in conjunction with trisomy 21, including cases of mosaicism where some or all of the haemopoietic cells are trisomic for chromosome 21. Somatic mutations in exon 2 or 3 of *GATA1* cause production of shorter GATA1 protein (GATA1s) that is leukaemogenic solely in fetal or neonatal blood cells that harbour trisomy 21 and only causes TAM in Down syndrome newborns, including mosaic Down syndrome.[122–125] GATA1s protein disrupts fetal blood cell development, causing blast cell accumulation in blood, liver and other tissues and associated fibrosis in severe cases. Importantly, in a proportion of neonates with Down syndrome who have *GATA1* mutations at birth, the *GATA1*-mutant cells persist and acquire additional mutations, leading to a specific form of acute myeloid leukaemia known as myeloid leukaemia of Down syndrome (ML-DS) within the first 4 years of life.[122,125] In contrast to leukaemias in children without Down syndrome, acute lymphoblastic leukaemia (ALL) has not yet been reported in neonates with Down syndrome.[118,119]

Clinical features

The clinical findings in TAM vary from life-threatening disease to an asymptomatic incidental finding. Most cases present within 7 days of birth. All symptomatic cases have increased blast cells in the peripheral blood.[6] Severe disease manifests with one or more of: hepatomegaly (40%), splenomegaly (30%), vesiculopapular skin rash, which may give the appearance of a 'blueberry muffin' baby (11%), and pleural and/or pericardial effusion (9%).[126] Cholestatic jaundice is common (70%) but is not specific for TAM. Mortality in severe cases approaches 20%, usually from progressive liver failure and coagulopathy. Asymptomatic disease may be clinically silent (increased blasts only) or clinically and haematologically silent (silent TAM; blasts not increased but *GATA1* mutation present).[6] Although the majority of cases of TAM present at or just after birth, later presentations of TAM sometimes occur when the neonate had no relevant clinical features at birth and a blood count and blood film were not performed at that time. However, a small proportion of cases present several weeks after birth with severe conjugated hyperbilirubinaemia, hepatomegaly, liver failure and coagulopathy. In this situation, there may be very few blast cells in the peripheral blood. The reasons for this are not clear but, at least in some cases, it is associated with diffuse blast cell infiltration of the liver and progressive fibrosis.[125–129] Finally, around 4% of neonates with TAM present with hydrops fetalis, intrauterine death or death during labour.[130,131]

Haematological features

Leucocytosis is common in neonates with TAM and may be extreme (WBC $>100 \times 10^9$/l). In contrast to congenital leukaemia in neonates without Down syndrome, anaemia is uncommon. The platelet count in TAM is extremely variable and may be normal, reduced or increased.[6,125,127] It is now clear that thrombocytopenia is not useful in the diagnosis of TAM as there is no significant difference in platelet counts between Down syndrome neonates with and without TAM.[6] In some cases of TAM not only is the platelet count increased but the thrombocytosis is extreme.[132] The most important haematological finding supporting a diagnosis of TAM is the presence of increased blasts (>10%) in the peripheral blood of a neonate with Down syndrome (Case 3.2, see page 171). It is important to point out that blast cells usually disappear quickly from the peripheral blood over the first 2 weeks of life and therefore blood films should be requested as soon as possible after birth since their detection will not be reliable during and beyond the second week of life. Blast morphology varies from undifferentiated myeloblasts to typical small megakaryoblasts with cytoplasmic blebbing or large, partially differentiated megakaryoblasts (Fig. 3.23). TAM blasts usually express CD117 and variable proportions express CD34, CD7, CD36 and/or CD41/42b.[133] Some may express CD235a (glycophorin A).[133,134]

(a)

(b)

(c)

(d)

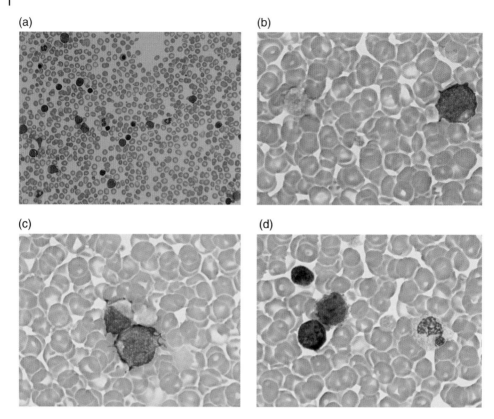

Fig. 3.23 Blood films of neonates with Down syndrome with TAM: (a) severe TAM with large numbers of pleomorphic circulating blast cells; (b) megakaryoblast, giant platelet and megakaryocyte cytoplasmic fragment; (c) a megakaryoblast, a megakaryocyte and a giant platelet; (d) typical megakaryoblast with cytoplasmic blebbing, two erythroblasts and giant platelets. MGG, (a) ×40, (b–d) ×100.

In contrast to congenital leukaemia in neonates without Down syndrome, the blast cells are often very pleomorphic in TAM (Fig. 3.23a,d). In addition, megakaryocytes and giant platelets are often present (Fig. 3.23a–d). This finding, together with the presence of normal or increased platelet counts, in many cases, suggests that the blast cells are able to differentiate into megakaryocytes and platelets, at least to some extent. There are also sporadic reports suggesting that in other cases of TAM there is differentiation into erythroblasts,[134] eosinophils[30,135] or basophils[136] (Fig. 3.24).

Molecular genetics

The current standard for a specific diagnosis of TAM is detection of an exon 2 or 3 *GATA1* mutation by DNA sequencing of peripheral blood leucocytes.[126] More than 95% of mutations are in exon 2 of the gene.[137] As small mutant *GATA1* clones may transform to ML-DS, sensitive next generation sequencing is necessary to avoid false negative results. To avoid false negatives, *GATA1* mutation analysis should be performed in the first week after birth while there are circulating peripheral blood blast cells.[126] Even using next generation

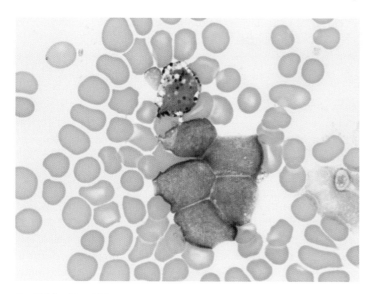

Fig. 3.24 Blood film of a term neonate with Down syndrome and TAM showing six blast cells including one with basophilic granules and prominent vacuoles. MGG, ×100.

sequencing, large or complex deletions in exon 2 or 3 of the *GATA1* gene may be missed or difficult to assess.[138] For this reason *GATA1* analysis should always be performed in conjunction with a full blood count and morphological review of a peripheral blood film in order to determine the blast cell percentage.[126] As the presence of *GATA1* mutations in neonatal blood cells in Down syndrome is specific for TAM, blast cell immunophenotyping and bone marrow examination are unnecessary in the neonatal period although both are useful for diagnosis of ML-DS. An alternative approach to identifying neonates with TAM is to use a flow cytometric method to identify the short GATA1 protein (GATA1s) that is produced by the leukaemic blast cells.[139] This is reported to be just as sensitive as next generation sequencing methods although the specific mutation is not identified and the value of this approach has not yet been tested in large series.

Natural history and prognosis

Transient abnormal myelopoiesis is known to develop in fetal life although the majority of cases only present at or just after birth.[130] It does not present after the age of 3 months. More than 90% of cases of TAM resolve spontaneously within 2–3 months. For the small proportion of neonates with severe disease (5–20%), progressive multiorgan failure carries a high risk of early death due to widespread infiltration of the tissues by *GATA1*-mutant blast cells. Risk factors for early death in severe TAM include: preterm delivery, ascites, leucocyte count $>100 \times 10^9$/l, hepatomegaly and coagulopathy.[126,127,133] For such cases, the mainstay of treatment is supportive care and the judicious use of cytarabine as recommended in recent guidelines.[126]

Importantly, because 20% of cases of clinical TAM later develop ML-DS, it is important to keep cases of TAM under regular clinical and haematological review until the age of 4 years, the specific time window these children are at risk of this disease.[118,121,125,127] At present, no clinical, haematological or molecular features at birth reliably predict which cases of TAM will develop ML-DS, so any change in the blood count during follow-up, especially the development of thrombocytopenia, should prompt careful review of the blood film.

Fetal presentation of transient abnormal myelopoiesis

Although TAM is known to develop during fetal life, the majority of cases do not present until after birth and there have been relatively few detailed case reports describing the findings of fetal disease. A recent systematic review identified 38 cases of which just over half survived beyond the neonatal period: 12 (32%) resulted in stillbirth and 4 (11%) in neonatal death.[130] Diagnosis *in utero* was usually prompted by abnormal ultrasound findings, particularly hepatomegaly, with or without splenomegaly ($n = 31$; 79.5%), hydrops fetalis ($n = 12$; 30.8%) and pericardial effusion ($n = 9$; 23.1%); a smaller number of cases had cardiac abnormalities ($n = 5$; 12.8%), fetal ascites ($n = 4$; 10.3%), pleural effusion ($n = 3$; 7.69%) or peripheral oedema ($n = 1$; 2.56%). Where fetal blood sampling was performed, this showed leucocytosis and large numbers of circulating blast cells. There is currently insufficient evidence to determine the most effective way of managing TAM *in utero*. The majority of cases have been managed using supportive therapy (for example red cell transfusion, if indicated for anaemia) or early delivery and no cases have been treated *in utero* with cytarabine. In the index case described by Tamblyn and colleagues[130] the clinical and haematological features of TAM were already largely resolved before birth, despite the absence of treatment, suggesting that even severe fetal TAM should be very carefully monitored rather than treated with chemotherapy before birth.

Acute leukaemia in neonates without Down syndrome

In neonates without Down syndrome, acute leukaemia may present with a range of immunophenotypes, including acute myeloid leukaemia (AML), ALL, mixed phenotype acute leukaemia (MPAL) or, rarely, blastic plasmacytoid dendritic cell neoplasm. The majority of cases of neonatal leukaemia are AML rather than ALL (Fig. 3.25a). However, there appears to be no family history of leukaemia or childhood cancer in most cases.

Neonatal AML differs from AML later in childhood in several ways. First, in a recent review of published cases, we found a striking predominance of monocytic, megakaryocytic and erythroid leukaemias in the neonatal setting compared with any other time of life[119] (Fig. 3.25b). Secondly, there have been many well-documented examples of spontaneous remission of neonatal AML, although in some cases this is transient (discussed in more detail later). Finally, the spectrum of genetic abnormalities associated with neonatal AML differs from that in older children. Of the 110 cases we identified in our recent review, just over half had one of three molecular genetic abnormalities: rearrangement of the *KMT2A* gene (formerly known as the *MLL* gene) on the long arm of chromosome 11; a translocation between chromosome 8 and chromosome 16, t(8;16)(p11.21;p13.3), creating a *KAT6A-CREBBP* fusion; and t(1;22)(p13.3;q13.1), creating an *RBM15-MRTFA* (previously *RBM15-MKL1*) fusion gene (see Fig. 3.25).

Neonatal ALL also differs from ALL later in childhood. First, cases are nearly all CD10-negative B-lineage (Pro-B) leukaemias. Secondly, virtually all cases are associated with

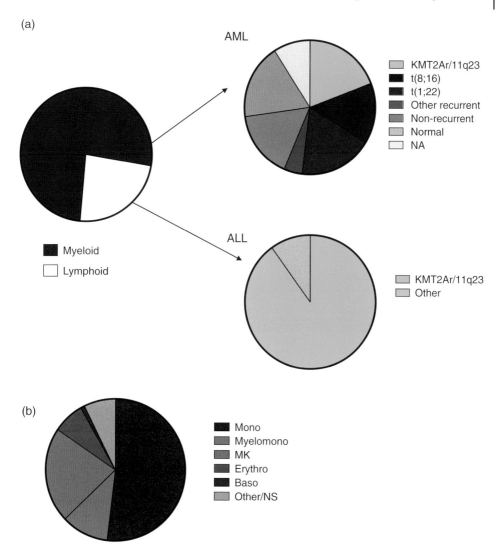

Fig. 3.25 Summary of the phenotypic, immunophenotypic and genetic features of neonatal acute leukaemia. (a) The majority of leukaemias in neonates without Down syndrome are acute myeloid leukaemias (AML). Of these, the three most common genetic subtypes are cause by rearrangements of the *KMT2A* (previously *MLL*) gene (*KMT2A* rearranged) or translocations between chromosome 8 and 16 (t(8;16); *KAT6A-CREBBP* fusion gene) or chromosomes 1 and 22 (t(1;22); *RBM15-MRTFA* fusion gene). In contrast, acute lymphoblastic leukaemia (ALL) in neonates is almost always associated with rearranged *KMT2A*. (b) The majority of neonatal AML have monoblastic characteristics but acute megakaryoblastic (MK) and erythroblastic leukaemias also occur and are proportionately more common in neonates than in older children or adults. Almost all neonatal ALL has B-lineage characteristics. These data are summarised from Roberts *et al.* (2018)[119] and are based on a literature review of 144 cases of neonatal acute leukaemia.

KMT2A gene rearrangement (see Fig 3.25). Thirdly, there appears to be a low frequency of additional mutations, suggesting that expression of a *KMT2A* fusion gene alone is sufficient to cause ALL in fetal/neonatal cells. The role of *KMT2A* in neonatal leukaemia is therefore of particular interest. It is only in this age group that a single molecular abnormality is responsible for the majority of leukaemias. Furthermore, it is only in neonates that *KMT2A* rearrangement causes such a wide spectrum of leukaemias: ALL in about 60% of cases and AML in about 40%, as well as a small number of MPAL or, even more rarely, blastic plasmacytoid dendritic cell neoplasm (Table 3.11).[119]

Table 3.11 Congenital leukaemias excluding those associated with Down syndrome)*

Condition	Molecular abnormality	Characteristic features
AML	**With rearrangement of *KMT2A* at 11q23.3**	
	t(4;11)(q21;q23.3); *KMT2A-AFF1*	Acute myelomonocytic or monoblastic leukaemia
	t(9;11)(p21.3;q23.3); *KMT2A-MLLT3*	Mainly acute monoblastic leukaemia
	t(10;11)(p12.31;q23.3); *KMT2A-MLLT10*	Acute myelomonocytic, monocytic or monoblastic leukaemia
	t(11;19)(q23.3;p13.11); *KMT2A-ELL*	Acute myelomonocytic or monoblastic leukaemia
	t(11;19)(q23.3;q13.3); *KMT2A-MLLT1*	Acute monocytic leukaemia
	t(1;11)(p36;q23); *KMT2A* rearranged	Acute monoblastic leukaemia
	t(1;11)(q21;q23); *KMT2A* rearranged	AML not further specified
	Other	
	t(1;22)(p13.3;q13.1); *RBM15-MRTFA* (previously *RBM15-MKL1*)	Acute megakaryoblastic leukaemia
	t(8;16)(p11.2;p13.3); *KAT6A-CREBBP* and variants	Mainly acute monoblastic leukaemia[†]
	t(8;21)(q22;q22.1); *RUNX1-RUNX1T1*	
	Miscellaneous including: t(5;6)(q31;q21)[‡] *RUNX1* duplication	Acute monocytic/monoblastic leukaemia
ALL	t(4;11)(q21;q23.3); *KMT2A-AFF1* and variants	Pro-B (early precursor) ALL
	t(11;19)(q23.3;p13)	ALL (pro-B or common/pre-B)
MPAL	t(4;11)(q21;q23.3); *KMT2A-AFF1*	Pro-B/acute monoblastic leukaemia
BPDCN	t(2;17;8)(p23;q23;p23); *CLTC-ALK1*	Blastic plasmacytoid dendritic cell neoplasm

* For a more exhaustive list and supporting references, see reference 119.
† Spontaneous remission is common.
‡ Spontaneous remission occurred in the one reported case.
ALL, acute lymphoblastic leukaemia; AML, acute myeloid leukaemia; BPDCN, blastic plasmacytoid dendritic cell neoplasm; MPAL, mixed phenotype acute leukaemia.
Based on reference 119.

Clinical features

The most common clinical signs of neonatal leukaemia are hepatosplenomegaly and skin lesions (leukaemia cutis), which are seen in two-thirds of congenital AML and 50% of congenital ALL cases,[140] as well as in the even rarer blastic plasmacytoid dendritic cell neoplasm.[141,142] Leukaemia cutis characteristically manifests as a generalised red, brown or purple nodular rash, leading to the term 'blueberry muffin' baby (see Fig. 3.27).[143] Skin involvement is a particular feature of neonatal leukaemias compared with leukaemia in older children and may be the sole sign of neonatal leukaemia, without any apparent peripheral blood or bone marrow involvement.[144,145] However, neonates who present with leukaemia cutis need to be monitored carefully as the disease often evolves to systemic disease over the following months.[146] It is therefore important to consider a diagnosis of leukaemia in any neonate who presents with a 'blueberry muffin' rash even if the blood count and blood film are normal. Other causes of a 'blueberry muffin' rash in the newborn are shown in Table 3.12.

The majority of affected neonates have systemic disease and are unwell at presentation.[148] As well as hepatomegaly and/or splenomegaly, many will present with or develop jaundice, progressive pallor, pleural effusions and/or ascites and some have lymphadenopathy. In the most severe cases, this is followed by hepatic failure which can lead to rapid death even if the leukaemia regresses.[149] Although CNS disease has been reported to occur in around 50% of cases of neonatal leukaemia overall, a recent series of 12 neonates with

Table 3.12   Causes of a 'blueberry muffin' rash in a neonate

Malignant and premalignant disorders

Leukaemia cutis

Transient abnormal myelopoiesis

Haemophagocytic lymphohistiocytosis

Langerhans cell histiocytosis

Metastatic neuroblastoma

Disseminated juvenile xanthogranuloma[147]

Congenital infections

Syphilis

Toxoplasmosis

Rubella

Cytomegalovirus

Coxsackievirus

Severe fetal anaemia

Haemolytic disease of the fetus and newborn

Hereditary spherocytosis

εγδβ thalassaemia

Twin-to-twin transfusion

Fetomaternal haemorrhage

AML found only two cases with CNS disease.[148] The signs of CNS involvement include a bulging fontanelle, reduced level of consciousness, papilloedema and retinal haemorrhages. As the leucocyte count is often very high (see Fig. 3.25), affected neonates may develop signs of leucostasis, including increasing respiratory distress, cardiac failure, renal failure and severe acidosis.[150–153]

Haematological features

The haematological features of neonatal leukaemia include hyperleucocytosis due to large numbers of circulating blast cells (Fig. 3.26), with leucocyte counts as high as $830 \times 10^9/l$ being reported,[150] as well as anaemia and thrombocytopenia, which often worsen very quickly over the first few days or hours of life. Some neonates develop coagulation abnormalities secondary to hepatic infiltration or disseminated intravascular coagulation (DIC).[148] In the majority of cases of AML, immunophenotyping of peripheral blood or bone marrow blasts or immunohistochemistry of biopsied skin nodules shows monocytic/ monoblastic or megakaryoblastic features (Fig. 3.27). Occasional cases of acute basophilic leukaemia[154] and erythroleukaemia are also reported in neonates.[149,153,155–158] Neonatal ALL (Fig. 3.28) is nearly always of B-lineage, usually with a pro-B immunophenotype ($CD19^+$, $CD45^{low}$, $CD22^{low}$, $CD79a^+$, $CD10^-$, $CD20^-$) and often with co-expression of CD33 or CD15.[159–161] However, rare cases of T-lineage ALL have been reported.[162] Importantly, a number of cases have been reported where neonates present with B-lineage ALL but at relapse, often soon afterwards, are found to have 'switched' lineage, relapsing as AML, almost always with a monoblastic immunophenotype.[163]

The dramatic clinical presentation and haematological features, particularly the presence of very large numbers of circulating blast cells, usually makes the distinction of neonatal leukaemia from other conditions straightforward, although expert

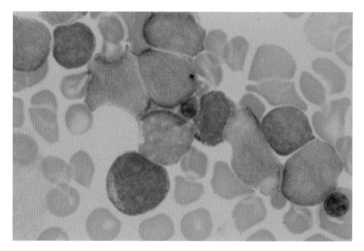

Fig. 3.26 Blood film of a newborn with congenital AML showing large numbers of myeloblasts and two normoblasts. Note the absence of neutrophils, lymphocytes and monocytes. MGG, ×100.

Fig. 3.27 'Blueberry muffin' rash due to leukaemia cutis in a neonate with congenital AML associated with *KMT2A* rearrangement. From Roberts *et al.* (2018)[119].

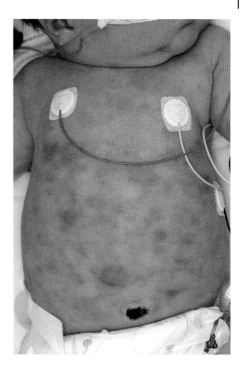

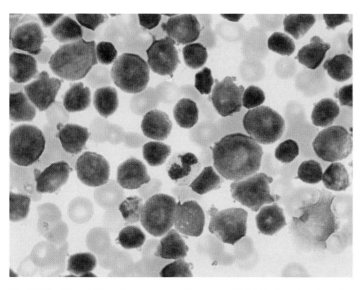

Fig. 3.28 Blood film of a neonate with congenital ALL showing hyperleukocytosis, a single neutrophil and pleomorphic blast cells. Some blast cells are large and have a diffuse chromatin pattern. Others are smaller with some chromatin condensation, a feature that is far more likely to be seen in ALL than in AML. Note also the cytoplasmic blebs, which could lead to confusion with acute megakaryoblastic leukaemia. The blast cells expressed CD19, CD34, HLA-DR and CD33 and were negative for CD10, CD15 and CD38. A *KMT2A-MLLT10* fusion was detected. MGG, ×100 (with thanks to Dr Georgina Hall for sharing this film).

immunophenotyping and genetic analysis may be required to establish the precise diagnosis, especially in MPAL cases.

Blast cells are commonly seen in preterm neonates, particularly those that are less than 26 weeks' gestation at birth (see Fig. 3.2) and especially those with infections or NEC, but they rarely exceed 8% of the total circulating white blood cells.[119] Circulating blast cells are seen in almost all neonates with Down syndrome but rarely exceed 15%. By contrast, in TAM (see earlier) the frequency of circulating blasts in neonates with Down syndrome may exceed 80% and hyperleucocytosis (white cell count $>100 \times 10^9/l$) is seen in a small proportion of cases (reviewed in reference 113). It is important to note that TAM can occur in neonates with mosaic Down syndrome who have none of the characteristic clinical features of the syndrome.

Molecular genetics

The most common molecular genetic abnormality in neonatal leukaemia is rearrangement of the *KMT2A* gene and the associated formation of an abnormal fusion gene (see Fig. 3.25). The vast majority of cases of neonatal ALL involve *KMT2A* fusion genes. Up to 120 *KMT2A* partner genes have been described in acute leukaemia.[164] In neonatal leukaemias the most common is the formation and expression of a *KMT2A-AFF1* fusion gene as a result of a t(4;11)(q21.3;q23.3) chromosomal translocation. Typically, *KMT2A-AFF1* causes early precursor or pro-B ALL in neonates and infants and AML in adults, although AML and MPAL have both been reported in neonates.[140,159] Lineage switch from a B-lineage ALL at presentation to AML at relapse is particularly associated with neonatal leukaemia due to the *KMT2A-AFF1* fusion gene and is well recognised, though uncommon.[163]

The natural history of lineage switching is consistent with a leukaemia-initiating mutation in a fetal stem or progenitor cell with lymphoid and myeloid lineage potential, although it is also possible that *KMT2A-AFF1* fusion gene is able to reactivate myeloid genes in fetal/neonatal progenitors that are already committed to the B-lineage.[165] Indeed, recent data from single-cell ribonucleic acid (RNA) sequencing studies in *KMT2A*-rearranged infant ALL suggest that 'lineage plasticity' is a specific property of fetal/neonatal haemopoietic cells.[166] It is now clear that all cases of acute leukaemia occurring within the neonatal period arise *in utero* and therefore in fetal cells. This is shown by the presence of the causative fusion genes, such as *KMT2A-AFF1*, in neonatal blood spots[167–169] and through twin studies which describe genetically identical leukaemias in monozygotic twins who present in the first month of life, indicating that leukaemia-initiating cells must have been transmitted from one twin to the other by intrauterine placental sharing.[160,170–172]

In neonatal AML, around half of the cases are caused by three specific fusion genes: *KMT2A-AFF1*, *KAT6A-CREBBP* and *RBM1-MRTFA* (previously *RBM15-MKL1*). While *KMT2A-AFF1* and *KAT6A-CREBBP* both cause predominantly monocytic/monoblastic leukaemias, the *RBM15-MRTFA* fusion gene resulting from a t(1;22)(p13.3;q13.1) translocation is always megakaryoblastic. These leukaemias are often accompanied by fibrosis in the bone marrow and/or liver.[173–176] The *KAT6A-CREBBP* fusion gene results from a translocation between chromosomes 8 and 16, t(8;16)(p11.21;p13.3), and is of particular importance because of the relatively high frequency of cases that undergo spontaneous remission.[177–184] Many of these cases subsequently relapse, but there are several well-documented cases who have remained in long-term remission.[177,179,181,182]

It is therefore very important that otherwise well neonates with AML due to the *KAT6A-CREBBP* fusion gene seen following t(8;16) translocation are carefully monitored before embarking on chemotherapy. Occasional spontaneous remissions have also been reported in neonates with *KMT2A*-associated neonatal AML,[185,186] but not in those with *KMT2A*-associated ALL. Overall, about 40% of cases of neonatal AML that appear to undergo spontaneous remission ultimately relapse (reviewed in reference 119). The mechanism of spontaneous remission of neonatal leukaemia is not clear. It seems likely that differences between the fetal and postnatal microenvironment, with the latter lacking key factors needed for the maintenance of the clone of leukaemic cells, play a role together with intrinsic properties of the transformed fetal leukaemic stem or progenitor cells.

Treatment

In neonates with symptomatic disease, expert supportive care and chemotherapy are essential as the mortality of neonatal leukaemia remains very high (up to 60% for AML and 80% for ALL).[148]

Supportive care Careful management of hyperleucocytosis, including exchange transfusion, may be needed to reduce the risk of CNS haemorrhage and leucostasis in lungs and other organs.[149,187–189] It is essential to monitor fluid balance and renal and liver function closely, especially in preterm neonates, who are more at risk of severe complications.[149,188–190] Coagulation problems are common and blood product support is often required.[140,170,174,189,190] Tumour lysis is common because of the leucocytosis and uric acid depletion with rasburicase should be used,[191] provided that glucose-6-phosphate dehydrogenase (G6PD) deficiency has been excluded, because rasburicase has been reported to trigger fatal haemolysis in G6PD deficiency;[192] allopurinol can be used where rasburicase is contraindicated.[140]

Chemotherapy and haemopoietic stem cell transplantation Neonates have been eligible for several large collaborative treatment studies in infant ALL[193,194] and AML,[195,196] although reduced doses compared with those used in older children are often employed because of treatment-related toxicity in neonates.[188,195] These studies show that a small proportion of children with neonatal leukaemia can be cured by chemotherapy.[188,197,198] For neonates with AML, combination chemotherapy is supplemented with CNS-directed therapy[119] and data from the largest study indicated comparable survival for infants aged 0–3 months compared with infants aged more than 3 months at diagnosis (51% 5-year overall survival).[198] For neonatal ALL, most cases published since 2000 have been treated with the combination chemotherapy regimens used for infant ALL.[119] Haemopoietic stem cell transplantation has been shown to cure a small number of children with relapsed neonatal leukaemia[148,159] but the number of cases is too low to properly define the role of transplantation in first or second remission.

Despite the possibility of spontaneous remission in some cases of neonatal AML, other neonates with the same molecular genetic abnormalities have an aggressive disease course[199] and therefore there is currently no clear guidance as to which children can avoid chemotherapy.[140] In addition, one series of t(8;16)-associated neonatal AML highlighted the high rate of relapse in neonates who were not treated initially because of apparent regression of their leukaemia; four of these seven neonates subsequently required chemotherapy.[183]

Juvenile myelomonocytic leukaemia and Noonan syndrome myeloproliferative disorder

Neonates with Noonan syndrome are at risk of developing either JMML or a related transient myeloproliferative disorder. JMML is a rare childhood leukaemia that usually presents in the first 5 years of life and is more common in boys.[200] It is caused by somatic or germline mutations in RAS-pathway genes, most commonly in *PTPN11*, *KRAS*, *NRAS*, *CBL* or *NF1*.[201,202] Although JMML typically presents in infancy or childhood, in Noonan syndrome it may manifest in the neonatal period when it carries a particularly bad prognosis.[203] Neonates with Noonan syndrome due to germline mutations in *PTPN11*, or occasionally *CBL*, *KRAS* or *NRAS*, can develop either JMML or a JMML-like myeloproliferative disorder often referred to as Noonan syndrome-associated myeloproliferative disorder (NS/MPD) in the first few days or weeks of life.[38,39,204] Differentiating NS/MPD from JMML is important as the prognosis is very different; this may be difficult as both have the same underlying genetic cause (Case 3.3, see page 174). A diagnosis of JMML is made in all cases that meet the internationally defined consensus criteria, which include a monocyte count more than 1×10^9/l, splenomegaly, less than 20% blasts in the blood or bone marrow and a somatic mutation in either the *PTPN11*, *KRAS* or *NRAS* genes.[205]

The clinical features of NS/MPD include splenomegaly, hepatomegaly, rash, fever and, occasionally, hydrops fetalis. The haematological features include anaemia, thrombocytopenia and leucocytosis with increased numbers of monocytes, many with dysplastic features, and increased circulating blast cells (Fig. 3.29). The percentage of blasts is usually <20%,

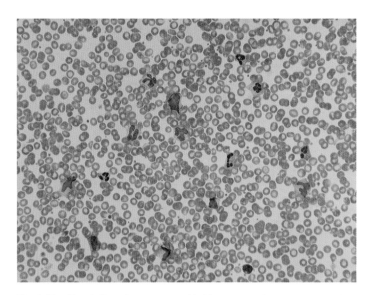

Fig. 3.29 Blood film of a neonate with Noonan syndrome-associated myeloproliferative disorder, showing large numbers of abnormal monocytes and occasional blast cells. MGG, ×20.

helping to distinguish NS/MPD from other forms of neonatal leukaemia, including many cases of TAM, and other causes of monocytosis (see Table 3.5), particularly sepsis. Where a diagnosis of Noonan syndrome is strongly suspected in a neonate, it is important that a blood count and blood film are performed and evaluated by an experienced haematologist. In any neonate where the blood film is suggestive of JMML, it is important to perform molecular analysis to identify the precise mutation and determine whether or not this is germline by analysing both peripheral blood and germline DNA (for example from a skin biopsy). Although the majority of cases of NS/MPD are not unwell and the condition undergoes spontaneous remission within a few weeks or months of birth, some germline *PTPN11* mutations and *CBL* mutations are associated with more rapidly progressive disease in the neonate.[39,203]

The mainstay of treatment for NS/MPD is good supportive care since the majority of cases resolve spontaneously and chemotherapy is rarely necessary.[206] The majority of neonates with NS/MPD will survive, in contrast to infants who are diagnosed with JMML after the neonatal period, where survival is 50–60% as the disease is refractory to chemotherapy, and the only curative treatment is haemopoietic stem cell transplantation, which is associated with a high rate of relapse.[200] It is therefore important to offer genetic counselling and molecular testing to families of patients with germline mutations. However, in contrast to TAM, neonates with NS/MPD in whom the neonatal MPD resolves do not have an increased risk of subsequent leukaemia.[38,203]

Illustrative cases

(For abbreviations used in the text of the illustrative cases, see page 176.)

Case 3.1   Pelger–Huët anomaly and infection

Case history

A term neonate was admitted to the neonatal unit with marked hypotonia and suspicion of a neuromuscular disorder. There were no other abnormalities on clinical examination. He was the first child of unrelated Caucasian parents and there was no family history of note. Routine investigations on admission included an FBC, which was normal: Hb 148 g/l, MCV 104 fl, MCH 34.5 pg, WBC 13.2×10^9/l, neutrophils no automated count, lymphocytes 5.0×10^9/l, monocytes 0.6×10^9/l, eosinophils 0.4×10^9/l and platelets 250×10^9/l. The blood film (Case 3.1, Fig. 1) showed very marked left shift with almost all neutrophil lineage cells resembling metamyelocytes or immature band cells. A diagnosis of group B streptococcal infection was suspected. However, blood cultures were negative and CRP levels were not increased.

Progress

While investigations for a possible neuromuscular disorder continued, the baby remained generally well until day 8 of life when he became irritable and developed a fever. A repeat infection screen showed an elevated CRP and *Escherichia coli* was

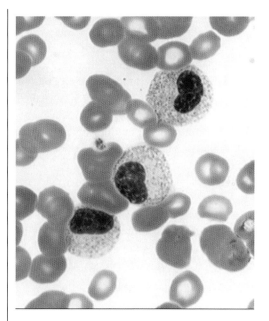

Case 3.1, Fig. 1 Blood film on first day of life. MGG, ×100 objective.

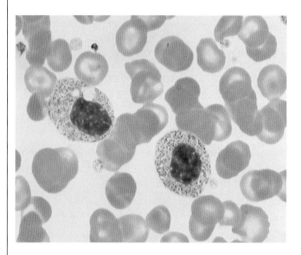

Case 3.1, Fig. 2 Blood film on day 8 of life. MGG, ×100.

isolated from blood cultures. A blood film on day 8 showed even more marked left shift with most of the neutrophil series exhibiting rounded nuclei with toxic granulation and some vacuolated forms (Case 3.1, Fig. 2). Chromosomal analysis revealed that the baby had a deletion of a segment of the long arm of chromosome 1, del(1)(q41-43), the locus containing the lamin B receptor gene (*LBR*), deletion or mutation of which causes the Pelger–Huët anomaly, thereby explaining the leucocyte abnormalities observed in this baby.[58]

Diagnostic notes

- The main differential diagnosis of the Pelger–Huët anomaly in neonates is acute bacterial infection; however, in acute bacterial infection the band forms seen in the very early stages of infection mature into segmented neutrophils within 1–2 days. Neonates with Down syndrome (as well as adults with myelodysplastic syndromes) sometimes have cells resembling those seen in Pelger–Huët anomaly (pseudo-Pelger–Huët cells).[6]
- Examination of parental blood films may be useful to confirm the diagnosis.
- Despite the abnormal morphology, these neutrophils appear to be functionally normal and individuals with Pelger–Huët anomaly are not more prone to infection.[59]

Case 3.2 Transient abnormal myelopoiesis in a neonate with Down syndrome

Case history

A baby born at 36 weeks' gestation to unrelated parents was noted at birth to have clinical features suggestive of a diagnosis of Down syndrome due to constitutional trisomy 21. The pregnancy had been uneventful and there was no family history of note. She appeared to be well but had a prominent 'blueberry muffin', vesicopapular skin rash. However, she developed rapidly worsening jaundice from day 2 of life and on examination had hepatomegaly (3 cm below the right costal margin) and splenomegaly (2 cm below the left costal margin) as well as a heart murmur. An echocardiogram revealed an atrial septal defect and she had a small pericardial effusion. A blood count sent on day 1 of life was reported to be normal and a blood film had not been requested.

Investigations

FBC: Hb 162 g/l, MCV 124 fl, MCH 40 pg, WBC 27.2 × 10^9/l, neutrophils 10.1 × 10^9/l, lymphocytes 15.0 × 10^9/l, monocytes 1.2 × 10^9/l, eosinophils 0.4 × 10^9/l, basophils 0.2 × 10^9/l, NRBC 1.2 × 10^9/l and platelets 450 × 10^9/l. Liver function tests showed hyperbilirubinaemia (425 µmol/l), which was mainly unconjugated and increased progressively from day 2 despite intensive phototherapy. Liver enzymes were normal as was a coagulation screen. Review of the blood film on day 2 of life showed increased blast cells (45% of white blood cells) as well as large numbers of giant platelets and megakaryocyte fragments with occasional circulating megakaryocytes (Case 3.2, Fig. 1). FISH analysis of peripheral blood leucocytes confirmed the presence of trisomy 21 and this, together with the blood film, allowed a presumptive diagnosis of transient abnormal myelopoiesis. This was confirmed by genomic analysis of the *GATA1* gene which showed a pathogenic mutation in exon 2.

Progress

During the second week of life, with progressively deepening jaundice, the baby developed signs of hepatic failure and disseminated intravascular coagulation. The

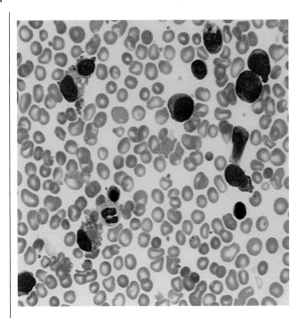

Case 3.2, Fig. 1 Blood film on day 2 of life. MGG, ×40.

leucocyte count rose to 80 × 10^9/l and the platelet count fell to 40 × 10^9/l as the coagulopathy worsened. These are considered features of life-threatening disease as outlined in the UK guidelines for management of TAM and a 5-day course of cytarabine (0.5 mg/kg once daily) was given.[126] This produced a rapid reduction in circulating blast cells within a week of commencing treatment but was also associated with marked neutropenia (nadir 0.3 × 10^9/l) and thrombocytopenia (20 × 10^9/l), which prompted platelet transfusion. She remained cytopenic for 2 weeks after the cytarabine was discontinued but her overall condition gradually improved and her liver function and coagulation returned to normal. *GATA1* mutation analysis was repeated at 6 weeks of age when the FBC had returned to normal and there were no blasts seen in her peripheral blood film. The same *GATA1* mutation was still present although at very low levels and a decision was made not to give any further treatment since she was clinically very well and the blood count and film were normal.

At 3 months of age she remained well, her FBC was normal apart from macrocytosis, no blasts were seen in her peripheral blood film and no *GATA1* mutations were detectable. Follow-up at 3 monthly intervals for the first 2 years of life was arranged. She remained well but at 12 months of age her platelet count was noted to have fallen to 120 × 10^9/l. An occasional blast cell was noted in her peripheral blood film but, as she was well, a repeat FBC in 4 weeks' time when she was 13 months old was arranged. This showed a Hb of 90 g/l, WBC 5 × 10^9/l, neutrophils 1.3 × 10^9/l, lymphocytes 2.1 × 10^9/l, monocytes 1.0 × 10^9/l, eosinophils 0.4 × 10^9/l and platelets 36 × 10^9/l. Review of her blood film showed 2% blast cells. Her mother commented that she was bruising very easily but that she was otherwise well. Repeat FBC in a further week confirmed these results and a bone marrow aspiration was performed; the marrow was very difficult to aspirate but showed clusters of blast cells. A trephine biopsy at the same time showed moderate bone marrow fibrosis and increased blast cells consistent with a diagnosis of myeloid leukaemia of Down syndrome. This diagnosis was supported by the presence of the same *GATA1* mutation as had been found in the neonatal samples. She responded very well to combination chemotherapy and remains in complete remission 4 years later.

Diagnostic notes

- Although *GATA1* mutation analysis may be useful in neonates with TAM it is not always essential. For neonates with Down syndrome and circulating blast cells of >20% during the first week of life together with megakaryocyte fragments on the blood film, these features are sufficient to make the diagnosis. However, where the percentage of blasts is <20%, particularly when assessed after the first week of life, *GATA1* mutation analysis is nearly always necessary to establish the diagnosis.[126]
- It is important to note that some neonates with TAM present at 2–6 weeks of age with prolonged and progressive unconjugated hyperbilirubinaemia due to blast cell infiltration of the liver.[126] For such cases *GATA1* mutation analysis is essential to distinguish TAM from other causes of liver disease in neonates with Down syndrome. It is important to use a sensitive method of mutation detection, such as next generation sequencing, since even small mutant clones may cause features of TAM and may later transform to ML-DS.
- Bone marrow examination is rarely helpful in TAM as the disease mainly manifests in the peripheral blood and the bone marrow findings are usually less dramatic than those seen in the blood. However, bone marrow examination is essential for the diagnosis of ML-DS.
- Immunophenotyping is often done routinely when blast cells are seen in the peripheral blood in neonates with TAM but does not usually provide useful additional information since blast cells in TAM are heterogeneous and often display similar immunophenotypes to those in neonates with Down syndrome who do not have TAM.
- Myeloid leukaemia of Down syndrome typically presents at 12–15 months of age and is usually heralded by a falling platelet count. The same *GATA1* mutation that was present in TAM is found in ML-DS; mutations in other genes, particularly cohesin genes, are required in addition to *GATA1* for ML-DS to develop.[207,208]
- Serial monitoring of *GATA1* mutations once TAM has resolved clinically and haematologically is not always sensitive to detect ML-DS at an early stage.[209]
- Macrocytosis is seen in almost all neonates and young children with Down syndrome and appears to be directly related to trisomy 21 as other causes of macrocytosis are not found in the vast majority of cases.[113]

Case 3.3   Noonan syndrome myeloproliferative disorder

Case history

A male neonate born at 37 weeks' gestation after an uneventful pregnancy was reviewed by the neonatal medicine team on the day after birth because of a low grade fever (37.7°C) and reluctance to feed. On examination, he looked generally well but was noted to have moderate hepatosplenomegaly, a heart murmur and occasional scattered petechiae on his abdomen. His birthweight was normal (3.1 kg) and he had no dysmorphic features. He was the second child of unrelated Caucasian parents and there was no family history of note. His older sister was well and neither she nor either parent had a history of neonatal problems. An FBC revealed moderate leucocytosis and thrombocytopenia and borderline anaemia. A provisional diagnosis of congenital infection was made and further investigations were arranged.

Investigations

FBC: Hb 135 g/l, MCV 103 fl, MCH 35 pg, WBC 42.1 × 10^9/l, neutrophils 16.8 × 10^9/l, lymphocytes 11.0 × 10^9/l, monocytes 5.7 × 10^9/l, eosinophils 0.35 × 10^9/l, platelets 51 × 10^9/l. His blood film confirmed the neutrophilia, monocytosis and thrombocytopenia. Platelet size appeared normal in the blood film with some larger platelets. Many of the monocytes were noted to look abnormal and occasional blasts were seen (Case 3.3, Fig. 1). Blood cultures showed no evidence of bacterial infection. In view of the marked monocytosis, an extended congenital infection screen was performed to include congenital syphilis, as well as CMV, rubella, toxoplasmosis, chickenpox and herpes simplex (SCORTCH screen),[210] but this was negative. Cardiac ultrasound showed an atrial septal

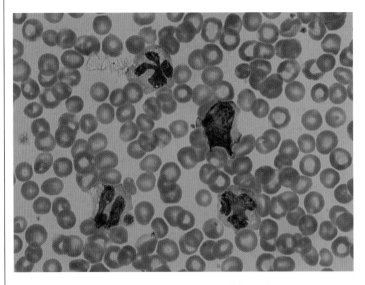

Case 3.3, Fig. 1   Blood film at presentation. MGG, ×100.

defect. The provisional diagnosis was revised to Noonan syndrome myeloproliferative disorder or Noonan syndrome JMML.

Progress

Serial FBCs showed persistence of the leucocytosis, monocytosis and thrombocytopenia over the first 5 weeks of life but the fever settled during the third week of life, the petechiae resolved and the baby remained generally well.

Age (days)	1	8	15	22	35	42
Hb (g/l)	135	132	125	120	116	112
WBC ($\times 10^9$/l)	42.1	37.1	36.2	37.4	23.4	12.2
Platelets ($\times 10^9$/l)	51	40	56	66	70	162
Monocytes ($\times 10^9$/l)	5.7	5.3	4.9	4.7	2.8	1.4
Blasts (%)	7	6	7	5	2	0

Further investigations

A peripheral blood sample was sent for next generation sequencing using a targeted gene panel containing genes known to cause JMML. This revealed a heterozygous p.Asp61Asn mutation in the *PTPN11* gene. Analysis of DNA extracted from a skin biopsy showed the same mutation, confirming the diagnosis of Noonan syndrome due to a germline mutation. As the baby was well, no treatment was given and towards the end of the first month of life the leucocytosis, monocytosis and hepatosplenomegaly began to resolve. By the age of 6 weeks the blood count was normal and blast cells could no longer be seen in the blood film, supporting a diagnosis of NS/MPD rather than JMML. The hepatosplenomegaly resolved by the age of 8 weeks and the baby had no further haematological problems.

Diagnostic notes

- Noonan syndrome MPD occurs in around 2.5% of infants with Noonan syndrome and presents usually at birth or during the first few months of life.[203]
- Neonates with Noonan syndrome may also develop true JMML, which occurs in 3% of all neonates with Noonan syndrome.[203] The diagnostic criteria for true JMML presenting in neonates are the same as in older infants.[205]
- Virtually all cases of NS/MPD resolve spontaneously within a few months and life-threatening disease is extremely unusual.
- In contrast, neonates with Noonan syndrome who develop true JMML have much more severe disease with a mortality of 50% in the first month of life.[203] As differentiating the transient myeloproliferative disorder from true JMML is largely based on the severity of the clinical features and the natural history, well neonates with a JMML-like haematological picture should initially be monitored to see whether or not the condition will resolve.

Abbreviations used in the illustrative cases

CMV	cytomegalovirus
CRP	C-reactive protein
FBC	full blood count
FISH	fluorescence *in situ* hybridisation
Hb	haemoglobin concentration
JMML	juvenile myelomonocytic leukaemia
MCH	mean cell haemoglobin
MCV	mean cell volume
MGG	May–Grünwald–Giemsa
ML-DS	myeloid leukaemia of Down syndrome
NRBC	nucleated red blood cell
NS/MPD	Noonan syndrome-associated myeloproliferative disorder
TAM	transient abnormal myelopoiesis
UK	United Kingdom
WBC	white blood cell count

References

1 Sawal M, Cohen M, Iratuzta JE, Kumar R, Kirton C and Brundler A (2009) Fulminant pertussis: a multi-center study with new insights into the clinico-pathological mechanisms. *Pediatr Pulmonol*, **44**, 970–980.

2 Torres JR, Falleiros-Arlant LH, Duenas L, Pleitez-Navarette, Salgado DM and Brea-Del Castillo J (2016) Congenital and perinatal complications of chikungunya fever: a Latin American experience. *Int J Infect Dis*, **51**, 85–88.

3 Oliveira R, Barreto F, Maia A, Gomes IP, Simiao AR and Barbosa R (2018) Maternal and infant death after probable vertical transmission of chikungunya virus in Brazil - case report. *BMC Infect Dis*, **18**, 333.

4 Dominguez-Rodriguez S, Villaverde S, Sanz-Santaeufemia FJ, Grasa C, Soriano-Arandes, Saavedra-Lozano J *et al.* (2021) A Bayesian Model to Predict COVID-19 Severity in Children. *Pediatr Infect Dis J*, **40**, e287–e293.

5 Wiedmeier SE, Henry E and Christensen RD (2008) Hematological abnormalities during the first week of life among neonates with trisomy 18 and trisomy 13: data from a multihospital healthcare system. *Am J Med Genet A*, **146A**, 312–320.

6 Roberts I, Alford K, Hall G, Juban G, Richmond H, Norton A *et al.* (2013) *GATA1*-mutant clones are frequent and often unsuspected in babies with Down syndrome: identification of a population at risk of leukemia. *Blood*, **122**, 3908–3917.

7 Meyer RE, Liu G, Gilboa SM, Ethen MK, Aylsworth AS, Powell CM *et al.*; National Birth Defects Prevention Network (2016) Survival of children with trisomy 13 and trisomy 18: A multi-state population-based study. *Am J Med Genet A*, **170A**, 825–837.

8 van de Vijver E, van den Berg TK and Kuijpers TW (2013) Leukocyte adhesion deficiencies. *Hematol Oncol Clin North Am*, **27**, 101–116, viii.

9 Dang D, Liu Y, Zhou Q, Li H, Wang Y and Wu H (2021) Identification of a novel IRF8 homozygous mutation causing neutrophilia, monocytopenia and fatal infection in a female neonate. *Infect Genet Evol*, **96**, 105121.

10 van de Vijver E, Maddalena A, Sanai O, Holland SM, Uzel G and Madkaikar M (2012) Hematologically important mutations: leukocyte adhesion deficiency (first update). *Blood Cell Mol Dis*, **48**, 53–61.

11 Wolach B, Gavrieli R, Wolach O, Stauber T, Abuzaitoun O and Kuperman A (2019) Leucocyte adhesion deficiency – A multicentre national experience. *Eur J Clin Invest*, **49**, e13047.

12 Bigley V, Maisuria S, Cytlak U, Jardine L, Care MA, Green K et al. (2018) Biallelic interferon regulatory factor 8 mutation: a complex immunodeficiency syndrome with dendritic cell deficiency, monocytopenia, and immune dysregulation. *J Allergy Clin Immunol*, **141**, 2234–2248.

13 Lambert RM, Baer VL, Wiedmeier SE, Henry E, Burnett J and Christensen RD (2009) Isolated elevated blood neutrophil concentration at altitude does not require NICU admission if appropriate reference ranges are used. *J Perinatol*, **29**, 822–825.

14 Chuang Y-Y and Huang Y-C (2019) Entoviral infection in neonates. *J Microbiol Immunol Infect*, **52**, 851–857.

15 Pesch MH, Katie Kuboushek K, McKee MM, Thome MC and Weinberg JB (2021) Congenital cytomegalovirus infection. *BMJ*, **373**, n1212. doi: 10.1136/bmj.n1212.

16 Zhang M, Wang H, Tang J, He Y, Xiong T, Li W et al. (2021) Clinical characteristics of severe neonatal enterovirus infection: a systematic review. *BMC Pediatr*, **21**, 127.

17 Kosmeri C, Koumpis E, Tsabouri S, Siomou E and Makis A (2020) Hematological manifestations of SARS-CoV-2 in children. *Pediatr Blood Cancer*, **67**, e28745.

18 Cherry JD (2016) Pertussis in young infants throughout the word. *Clin Infect Dis*, **63** (Suppl 4), S119–S122.

19 Mohan K, Omar BJ, Singh RD, Maithani AMM and Chaurasia RN (2016) Clinical and hematological features and management outcome in neonatal malaria: a nine years analysis from North India. *Curr Pediatr Rev*, **12**, 286–291.

20 Zafar R, Ver Heul A, Beigelman A, Bednarski JJ, Bayliss SJ and Dehner LP (2017) Omenn syndrome presenting with striking erythroderma and extreme lymphocytosis in a newborn. *Pediatr Dermatol*, **34**, e37–e39.

21 Le Deist F, Emile JF, Rieux-Laucat F, Benkerrou M, Roberts I, Brousse N and Fischer A (1996) Clinical, immunological, and pathological consequences of Fas-deficient conditions. *Lancet*, **348**, 719–723.

22 Chandramati J, Sidharthan N and Ponthenkandath S (2021) Neonatal autoimmune lymphoproliferative syndrome: a case report and a brief review. *J Pediatr Hematol Oncol*, **43**, e227–e229.

23 Patel L, Garvey B, Arnon S and Roberts IAG (1994) Eosinophilia in newborn infants. *Acta Paediatr*, **83**, 797–801.

24 Juul SE, Haynes JW and McPherson RJ (2005) Evaluation of eosinophilia in hospitalized preterm infants. *J Perinatol*, **25**, 182–188.

25 Yen JM, Lin CH, Yang MM, Hou ST, Lin AH and Lin YJ (2010) Eosinophilia in very low birth weight infants. *Pediatr Neonatol*, **51**, 116–123.

26 Spergel JM, Brown-Whitehorn TF, Beausoleil JL, Franciosi J, Shuker M, Verma R *et al.* (2009) 14 years of eosinophilic esophagitis: clinical features and prognosis. *J Pediatr Gastroenterol Nutr*, **48**, 30–36.

27 Asgari M, Leiferman KM, Piepkorn M and Kuechle MK (2006) Neonatal eosinophilic pustulosis. *Int J Dermatol*, **45**, 131–134.

28 Wahidi LS, Sherman J, Miller MM, Zaghouani H and Sherman MP (2015) Early persistent blood eosinophilia in necrotizing enterocolitis is a predictor of late complications. *Neonatology*, **108**, 137–142

29 Michelet M, Schluckebier D, Petit A-M and Caubet J-C (2017) Food protein-induced enterocolitis syndrome – a review of the literature with focus on clinical management. *J Asthma Allergy*, **10**, 197–207.

30 Maroz A, Stachorski L, Emmrich S, Reinhardt K, Xu J, Shao Z *et al.* (2014) GATA1s induces hyperproliferation of eosinophil precursors in Down syndrome transient leukemia. *Leukemia*, **28**, 1259–1270.

31 Minakata S, Sakata N, Wada N, Konishi Y, Marutani S, Enya T *et al.* (2016) Liver fibrosis with hypereosinophilia causing transient abnormal myelopoiesis. *Pediatr Int*, **58**, 1222–1225.

32 Wolach B, Bogger-Goren S and Whyte R (1991) Perinatal hematological profile of newborn infants with candida antenatal infections. *Biol Neonate*, **59**, 5–12.

33 Rajantie J, Siimes MA, Taskinen E, Lappalainen M and Koskiniemi M (1992) White blood cells in infants with congenital toxoplasmosis: transient appearance of cALL antigen on reactive marrow lymphocytes. *Scand J Infect Dis*, **24**, 227–232.

34 Galvis AE and Arrieta A (2020) *Congenital syphilis: a US perspective. Children (Basel)*, **7**, 203.

35 Spoulou V, Noni M, Koukou D, Kossyvakis A and Michos A (2021) Clinical characteristics of COVID-19 in neonates and young infants. *Eur J Pediatr*, **180**, 3041–3045.

36 Lai JW, Ford T, Cherian S, Campbell AJ and Blyth CC (2021) Case report: neonatal varicella acquired from maternal zoster. *Front Pediatr*, **9**, 649775.

37 Porcelijn L and de Haas M (2018) *Neonatal alloimmune neutropenia. Transfus Med Hemother*, **45**, 311–316.

38 Hasle H (2016) Myelodysplastic and myeloproliferative disorders of childhood. *Hematology Am Soc Hematol Educ Program*, **2016**, 598–604.

39 Mason-Suares H, Toledo D, Gekas J, Lafferty KA, Meeks N, Pacheco MC *et al.* (2017) Juvenile myelomonocytic leukemia-associated variants are associated with neo-natal lethal Noonan syndrome. *Eur J Hum Genet*, **25**, 509–511.

40 Pinkel D (1998) Differentiating juvenile myelomonocytic leukemia from infectious disease. *Blood*, **91**, 365–367.

41 Gupta N, Gupta R and Bakhshi S (2009) Transient myeloproliferation mimicking JMML associated with parvovirus infection of infancy. *Pediatr Blood Cancer*, **52**, 411–413.

42 Aly SA, Boyer KM, Muller BA, Marini D, Jones CH and Nguyen HH (2020) Complicated ventricular arrhythmia and hematologic myeloproliferative disorder in RIT1-associated Noonan syndrome: expanding the phenotype and review of the literature. *Mol Genet Genomic Med*, **8**, e1253.

43 Yoshimi A, Kamachi Y, Imai K, Watanabe N, Nakadate H and Kanazawa T (2013) Wiskott-Aldrich syndrome presenting with a clinical picture mimicking juvenile myelomonocytic leukemia. *Pediatr Blood Cancer*, **60**, 836–841.

44 Sano H, Kobayashi R, Suzuki D, Yasuda K, Nakanishi M, Nagashima T *et al.* (2012) Wiskott–Aldrich syndrome with unusual clinical features similar to juvenile myelomonocytic leukemia. *Int J Hematol*, **96**, 279–283.

45 Watanabe N, Yoshimi A, Kamachi Y, Kawabe T, Muramatsu H, Matsumoto K *et al.* (2007) Wiskott–Aldrich syndrome is an important differential diagnosis in male infants with juvenile myelomonocytic leukemia like features. *J Pediatr Hematol Oncol*, **29**, 836–838.

46 Rastogi S, Rastogi D, Sundaram R, Kulpa J and Parekh AJ (1999) Leukemoid reaction in extremely low birth weight infants. *Am J Perinatol*, **16**, 93–97.

47 Zanardo V, Savio V, Giacomin C, Rinaldi A, Marzari F and Chiarelli S (2002) Relationship between neonatal leukemoid reaction and bronchopulmonary dysplasia in low-birth-weight infants: a cross-sectional study. *Am J Perinatol*, **19**, 379–386.

48 Jansen E, Emmen J, Mohns T and Donker A (2013) Extreme hyperleucocytosis of the premature. *BMJ Case Rep*, **2013**, bcr2012008385.

49 Duran R, Ozbek UV, Ciftdemir NA, Acunaş B and Süt N (2010) The relationship between leukemoid reaction and perinatal morbidity, mortality, and chorioamnionitis in low birth weight infants. *Int J Infect Dis*, **14**, e998–e1001.

50 Hornik CP, Benjamin DK, Becker KC, Benjamin DK, Li J, Clark RH *et al.* (2012) Use of the complete blood cell count in early-onset neonatal sepsis. *Pediatr Infect Dis J*, **31**, 799–802.

51 Gandhi P and Kondekar S (2019) A review of the different haematological parameters and biomarkers used for diagnosis of neonatal sepsis. *EMJ Hematol*, **7**, 85–92.

52 MacQueen BJ, Christensen RD, Yoder BA, Henry E, Baer VL Bennett ST and Yaish HM (2016) Comparing automated vs manual leukocyte differential counts for quantifying the 'left shift' in the blood of neonates. *J Perinatol*, **36**, 843–848.

53 Lawn JE, Blencowe H, Oza S, You D, Lee AC, Waiswa P *et al.* (2014) Every Newborn: progress, priorities, and potential beyond survival. *Lancet*, **384**, 189–205.

54 Makkar M, Gupta C, Pathak R, Garg S and Mahajan NC (2013) Performance evaluation of hematologic scoring system in early diagnosis of neonatal sepsis. *J Clin Neonatol*, **2**, 25–29.

55 Celik IH, Hanna M, Canpolati FE and Pammi M (2022) Diagnosis of neonatal sepsis: the past, present and future. *Pediatr Res*, **91**, 337–350.

56 Wen SCH, Ezure Y, Rolley L, Spurling G, Lau CL, Riaz S *et al.* (2021) Gram-negative neonatal sepsis in low- and lower-middle-income countries and WHO empirical antibiotic recommendations: a systematic review and meta-analysis. *PLoS Med*, **18**, e1003787.

57 Mohamed IS, Wynn RJ, Cominsky K, Reynolds AM, Ryan RM, Kumar VH *et al.* (2006) White blood cell left shift in a neonate: a case of mistaken identity. *J Perinatol*, **26**, 378–380.

58 Christensen RD and Yaish HM (2012) A neonate with the Pelger-Huet anomaly, cleft lip and palate, and agenesis of the corpus callosum, with a chromosomal microdeletion involving 1q41 to 1q42.12. *J Perinatol*, **32**, 238–240.

59 Speeckaert MM, Verhelst C, Koch A, Speeckaert R and Lacquet F (2009) Pelger-Huet anomaly: a critical review of the literature. *Acta Haematol*, **121**, 202–206.

60 Rodwell RL, Leslie AL and Tudehope DI (1988) Early diagnosis of neonatal sepsis using a hematologic scoring system. *J Pediatr*, **112**, 761–767.

61 Rodwell RL, Taylor KM, Tudehope DI and Gray PH (1993) Hematologic scoring system in early diagnosis of sepsis in neutropenic newborns. *Pediatr Infect Dis J*, **12**, 372–376.

62 Hecht JL, Fichorova RN, Tang VF, Allred EN, McElrath TF and Leviton A, Elgan study investigators (2011) Relationship between neonatal blood protein concentrations and placenta histologic characteristics in extremely low GA newborns. *Pediatr Res*, **69**, 68–73.

63 Howman RA, Charles AK, Jacques A, Doherty DA, Simmer K, Strunk T *et al.* (2012) Inflammatory and haematological markers in the maternal, umbilical cord and infant circulation in histological chorioamnionitis. *PloS One*, **7**, e51836.

64 Rodwell RL, Leslie AL and Tudehope DI (1989) Evaluation of direct and buffy coat films of peripheral blood for the early detection of bacteraemia. *Aust Paediatr J*, **25**, 83–85.

65 Weimer KED, Smith PB, Puia-Dumitrescu M and Aleem S (2022) Invasive fungal infections in neonates: a review. *Pediatr Res*, **91**, 404–412.

66 Pantalone JM, Liu S, Olaloye OO, Prochaska EC, Yanowitz T, Riley MM *et al.* (2021) Gestational age-specific complete blood count signatures in necrotizing enterocolitis. *Front Pediatr*, **9**, 604899.

67 Merino A, Vlagea A, Molina A, Egri N, Laguna J, Barrera K *et al.* (2022) Atypical lymphoid cells circulating in blood in COVID-19 infection: morphology, immunophenotype and prognosis value. *J Clin Pathol*, **75**, 104–111.

68 D'Azzo A, Kolodny EH, Bonten E and Ida Annunziata I (2009) Storage diseases of the reticuloendothelial system. In: Orkin SH, Nathan DG, Ginsburg D, Look AT, Fisher DE and Lux SE (eds), *Nathan and Oski's Hematology of Infancy and Childhood*, 7th edn. Saunders, Philadelphia, pp. 1299–1376.

69 Platt FM, d'Azzo A, Davidson BL, Neufeld EF and Tifft CJ (2018) Lysosomal storage diseases. *Nat Rev Dis Primers*, **4**, 27.

70 Demaret T, Lacaille F, Wicker C, Arnoux JB, Bouchereau J, Belloche C *et al.* (2021) Sebelipase alfa enzyme replacement therapy in Wolman disease: a nationwide cohort with up to ten years of follow-up. *Orphanet J Rare Dis*, **16**, 507.

71 Strebinger G, Muller E, Feldman A and Aigner E (2019) Lysosomal acid lipase deficiency – early diagnosis is the key. *Hepat Med Evid Res*, **11**, 79–88.

72 Jones SA, Valayannopoulos V, Schneider E, Eckert S, Banikazemi M, Bialer M *et al.* (2016) Rapid progression and mortality of lysosomal acid lipase deficiency presenting in infants. *Genet Med*, **18**, 452–458.

73 Brunetti-Pierri N and Scaglia F (2008) GM1 gangliosidosis: review of clinical, molecular, and therapeutic aspects. *Mol Genet Metab*, **94**, 391–396.

74 Regier DM, Proia RL, D'Azzo A and Tifft CJ (2016) The GM1 and GM2 gangliosidoses: natural history and progress towards therapy. *Pediatr Endocrinol Rev*, **13** (Suppl 1), 663–673.

75 Rosanio FM, D'Acunzo I, Mozzillo F, Di Pinto R, Tornincasa C, Amabile S *et al.* (2021) Perinatal-lethal Gaucher disease presenting with blueberry muffin lesions. *Pediatr Dermatol*, **38**, 1357–1358.

76 Watts TL and Roberts IAG (1999) Haematological abnormalities in the growth-restricted infant. *Semin Neonatol*, **4**, 41–54.

77 Christensen RD, Yoder BA, Baer VL, Snow GL and Butler A (2015) Early-onset neutropenia in small-for-gestational-age infants. *Pediatrics*, **136**, e1259–e1267.

78 Farruggia P, Fioredda F, Puccio G, Porretti L, Lanza T, Ramenghi U *et al.* (2015) Autoimmune neutropenia of infancy: Data from the Italian neutropenia registry. *Am J Hematol*, **90**, E221–E222.

79 Flesch BK and Reil A (2018) Molecular genetics of the human neutrophil antigens. *Transfus Med Hemother*, **45**, 300–309.

80 Porcelijn L and de Haas M (2018) Neonatal alloimmune neutropenia. *Transfus Med Hemother*, **45**, 311–316.

81 Doan J, Kottayam R, Krishnamurthy MB and Malhotra A (2020) Neonatal alloimmune neutropenia: experience from an Australian paediatric health service. *J Paediatr Child Health*, **56**, 757–763.

82 van den Tooren-de Groot R, Ottink M, Huiskes E, van Rossum A, van der Voorn B, Slomp J, de Haas M and Porcelijn L (2014) Management and outcome of 35 cases with foetal/ neonatal alloimmune neutropenia. *Acta Paediatr*, **103**, e467–e474.

83 Felix JK and Calhoun DA (2000) Neonatal alloimmune neutropenia in premature monozygous twins. *Pediatrics*, **106**, 340–342.

84 Dale D (2017) How I manage children with neutropenia. *Br J Haematol*, **178**, 351–363.

85 Wiedl C and Walter AW (2010) Granulocyte Colony Stimulating Factor in neonatal alloimmune neutropenia: a possible association with induced thrombocytopenia. *Pediatr Blood Cancer*, **54**, 1014–1016

86 Latini G, Del Vecchio A, Rosati E, Borzini P, Chirico G and Rondini G (1999) Different responses to granulocyte colony-stimulating factor treatment in siblings with alloimmune neonatal neutropenia. *Acta Paediatr*, **88**, 1407–1409.

87 Maheshwari A, Christensen RD and Calhoun DA (2002) Resistance to recombinant human granulocyte colony-stimulating factor in neonatal alloimmune neutropenia associated with anti-human neutrophil antigen-2a antibodies. *Pediatrics*, **109**, e64.

88 Fung YL, Pitcher LA, Taylor K and Minchinton RM (2005) Managing passively acquired autoimmune neonatal neutropenia: a case study. *Transfus Med*, **15**, 151–155.

89 Skokowa J, Dale D, Touw IP, Zeidler C and Welte K (2017) Severe congenital neutropenias. *Nat Rev Dis Primers*, **3**, 17032.

90 Dufour C, Miano M and Fioredda F (2016) Old and new faces of neutropenia in children. *Haematologica*, **101**, 789–791.

91 Tummala H, Walne AJ, Williams M, Bockett N, Collopy L, Cardoso S *et al.* (2016) DNAJC21 mutations link a cancer-prone bone marrow failure syndrome to corruption in 60S ribosome subunit maturation. *Am J Hum Genet*, **99**, 115–124.

92 Saettini F, Cattoni A, D'Angio' M, Corti P, Maitz S, Pagni F *et al.* (2020) Intermittent granulocyte maturation arrest, hypocellular bone marrow, and episodic normal neutrophil count can be associated with SRP54 mutations causing Schwachman-Diamond-like syndrome. *Br J Haematol*, **189**, e171–e174.

93 Schmaltz-Panneau B, Pagnier A, Clauin S, Buratti J, Marty C, Fenneteau O *et al.* (2021) Identification of biallelic germline variants of *SRP68* in a sporadic case with severe congenital neutropenia. *Haematologica*, **106**, 1216–1219.

94 Donadieu J, Leblanc T, Bader Meunier B, Barkaoui M, Fenneteau O, Bertrand Y *et al.* (2005) Analysis of risk factors for myelodysplasias, leukemias and death from infection among patients with congenital neutropenia. Experience of the French Severe Chronic Neutropenia Study Group. *Haematologica*, **90**, 45–53.

95 Rosenberg PS, Zeidler C, Bolyard AA, Alter BP, Bonilla MA, Boxer LA *et al.* (2010) Stable long-term risk of leukaemia in patients with severe congenital neutropenia maintained on G-CSF therapy. *Br J Haematol*, **150**, 196–199.

96 Rosenberg PS, Alter BP, Bolyard AA., Bonilla MA., Boxer LA, Cham, B *et al.* (2006) The incidence of leukemia and mortality from sepsis in patients with severe congenital neutropenia receiving long-term G-CSF therapy. *Blood*, **107**, 4628–4635.

97 Xia J, Bolyard AA, Rodger E, Stein S, Aprikyan AA, Dale DC and Link DC (2009) Prevalence of mutations in ELANE, GFI1, HAX1, SBDS, WAS and G6PC3 in patients with severe congenital neutropenia. *Br J Haematol*, **147**, 535–542.

98 Makaryan V, Zeidler C, Bolyard AA, Kelley ML, Below JE, Bamshad MJ *et al.* (2015) The diversity of mutations and clinical outcomes for ELANE-associated neutropenia. *Curr Opin Hematol*, **22**, 3–11.

99 Kuijpers TW, Nannenberg E, Alders M, Bredius R and Hennekam RC (2004) Congenital aplastic anemia caused by mutations in the SBDS gene: a rare presentation of Shwachman–Diamond syndrome. *Pediatrics*, **114**, e387–e391.

100 Todorovic-Guid M, Krajnc O, Varda NM, Zagradisnik B, Kokalj N and Gregoric A (2006) A case of Shwachman–Diamond syndrome in a male neonate. *Acta Paediatr*, **95**, 892–893.

101 Saito-Benz M, Miller HE and Berry MJ (2015) Shwachman–Diamond syndrome (SDS) in a preterm neonate. *J Paediatr Child Health*, **51**, 1228–1231.

102 Schaballie H, Renard M, Vermylen C, Scheers I, Revencu N, Regal L *et al.* (2013) Misdiagnosis as asphyxiating thoracic dystrophy and CMV-associated haemophagocytic lymphohistiocytosis in Shwachman-Diamond syndrome. *Eur J Pediatr*, **172**, 613–622.

103 Furutani E, Liu S, Galvin A, Steltz S, Malch MM, Loveless SK *et al.* (2022) Hematologic complications with age in Shwachman-Diamond syndrome. *Blood Adv*, **6**, 297–306.

104 Visser G, de Jager W, Verhagen LP, Smit GP, Wijburg FA, Prakken BJ *et al.* (2012) Survival, but not maturation, is affected in neutrophil progenitors from GSD-1b patients. *J Inher Metab Dis*, **35**, 287–300.

105 Pinsk M, Burzynski J, Yhap M, Fraser RB, Cummings B and Ste-Marie M (2002) Acute myelogenous leukemia and glycogen storage disease 1b. *J Pediatr Hematol Oncol*, **24**, 756–758.

106 Klein C, Grudzien M, Appaswamy G, Germeshausen M, Sandrock I, Schäffer AA *et al.* (2007) HAX1 deficiency causes autosomal recessive severe congenital neutropenia (Kostmann disease). *Nat Genet*, **39**, 86–92.

107 Klein C (2017) Kostmann's disease and HCLS1-associated protein X-1 (HAX1) *J Clin Immunol*, **37**, 117–122.

108 Germeshausen M, Grudzien M, Zeidler C, Abdollahpour H, Yetgin S, Rezaei N *et al.* (2008) Novel HAX1 mutations in patients with severe congenital neutropenia reveal isoform-dependent genotype-phenotype associations. *Blood*, **111**, 4954–4957.

109 Roques G, Munzer M, Barthez MA, Beaufils S, Beaupain B, Flood T *et al.* (2014) Neurological findings and genetic alterations in patients with Kostmann syndrome and HAX1 mutations. *Pediatr Blood Cancer*, **61**, 1041–1048.

110 Lebel A, Yacobovich J, Krasnov T, Koren A, Levin C, Kaplinsky C *et al.* (2015) Genetic analysis and clinical picture of severe congenital neutropenia in Israel. *Pediatr Blood Cancer*, **62**, 103–108.

111 Kivivuori SM, Rajantie J and Siimes MA (1996) Peripheral blood cell counts in infants with Down's syndrome. *Clin Genet*, **49**, 15–19.

112 Henry E, Walker D, Wiedmeier SE and Christensen RD (2007). Hematological abnormalities during the first week of life among neonates with Down syndrome: data from a multihospital healthcare system. *Am J Med Genet A*, **143**, 42–50.

113 Roberts I and Izraeli S (2014) Haematopoietic development and leukaemia in Down syndrome. *Br J Haematol*, **167**, 587–599.

114 de Hingh YC, van der Vossen PW, Gemen EF, Mulder AB, Hop WC, Brus F and de Vries E (2005) Intrinsic abnormalities of lymphocyte counts in children with Down syndrome. *J Pediatr*, **147**, 744–747.

115 Douglas SD (2005) Down syndrome: immunologic and epidemiologic associations-enigmas remain. *J Pediatr*, **147**, 723–725.

116 Verstegen RH, Kusters MA, Gemen EF and DE Vries E (2010) Down syndrome B-lymphocyte subpopulations: intrinsic defect or decreased T-lymphocyte help. *Pediatr Res*, **67**, 557–562.

117 Bhatnagar N, Nizery L, Tunstall O, Vyas P and Roberts I (2016) Transient abnormal myelopoiesis and AML in Down syndrome: an update. *Curr Hematol Malig Rep*, **11**, 333–341.

118 Hasle H, Clemmensen IH and Mikkelsen M (2000) Risks of leukaemia and solid tumours in individuals with Down's syndrome. *Lancet*, **355**, 165–169.

119 Roberts I, Fordham N, Rao A and Bain BJ (2018) Neonatal leukaemia. *Br J Haematol*, **182**, 170–184.

120 Hasle H (2016) Myelodysplastic and myeloproliferative disorders of childhood. *Hematology Am Soc Hematol Educ Program*, **2016**, 598–604.

121 Zipursky A (2003) Transient leukaemia – a benign form of leukaemia in newborn infants with trisomy 21. *Br J Haematol*, **120**, 930–938.

122 Wechsler J, Greene M, McDevitt MA, Anastasi J, Karp JE, Le Beau MM and Crispino JD (2002) Acquired mutations in *GATA1* in the megakaryoblastic leukemia of Down syndrome. *Nat Genet*, **32**, 148–152.

123 Hitzler JK, Cheung J, Li Y, Scherer SW and Zipursky A (2003) *GATA1* mutations in transient leukemia and acute megakaryoblastic leukemia of Down syndrome. *Blood*, **101**, 4301–4304.

124 Hollanda LM, Lima CS, Cunha AF, Albuquerque DM, Vassallo J, Ozelo MC *et al.* (2006) An inherited mutation leading to production of only the short isoform of GATA-1 is associated with impaired erythropoiesis. *Nat Genet*, **38**, 807–812.

125 Klusmann JH, Creutzig U, Zimmerman M, Dworzak M, Jorch N, Langebrake C *et al.* (2008) Treatment and prognostic impact of transient leukemia in neonates with Down syndrome. *Blood*, **111**, 2991–2998.

126 Tunstall O, Bhatnagar N, James B, Norton A, O'Marcaigh AM, Watts T *et al.* (BSH Guidelines Task Force Member) On behalf of the British Society for Haematology (2018) Guidelines for the investigation and management of transient leukaemia of Down syndrome. *Br J Haematol*, **182**, 200–211.

127 Gamis AS, Alonzo TA, Gerbing RB, Hilden JM, Sorrell AD, Sharma M *et al.* (2011) Natural history of transient myeloproliferative disorder clinically diagnosed in Down syndrome neonates: a report from the Children's Oncology Group Study A2971. *Blood*, **118**, 6752–6759.

128 Kinjo T, Inoue H, Kusuda T, Fujiyoshi J, Ochiai M, Takahata Y *et al.* (2019) Chemokine levels predict progressive liver disease in Down syndrome patients with transient abnormal myelopoiesis. *Pediatr Neonatol*, **60**, 382–388.

129 Yamato G, Park M-J, Sotomatsu M, Kaburagi T, Maruyama, Kobayashi T *et al.* (2021) Clinical features of 35 Down syndrome patients with transient abnormal myelopoiesis at a single institution. *Int J Hematol*, **113**, 662–667.

130 Tamblyn JA, Norton A, Spurgeon L, Donovan V, Bedford Russell A, Bonnici J *et al.* (2016) Prenatal therapy in transient abnormal myelopoiesis: a systematic review. *Arch Dis Child Fetal Neonatal Ed*, **101**, F67–F71.

131 Heald B, Hilden JM, Zbuk K, Norton A, Vyas P, Theil KS *et al.* (2007) Severe TMD/AMKL with GATA1 mutation in a stillborn fetus with Down syndrome. *Nat Clin Pract Oncol*, **4**, 433–438.

132 Park ES, Kim SY, Yeom JS, Lim JY, Park CH and Youn HS (2008) Extreme thrombocytosis associated with transient myeloproliferative disorder with Down Syndrome with t(11;17) (q13;q21). *Pediatr Blood Cancer*, **50**, 643–644.

133 Langebrake C, Creutzig U and Reinhardt D (2005) Immunophenotype of Down syndrome acute myeloid leukemia and transient myeloproliferative disease differs significantly from other diseases with morphologically identical or similar blasts. *Klin Paediatrica*, **217**, 126–134.

134 Bozner P (2002) Transient myeloproliferative disorder with erythroid differentiation in Down syndrome. *Arch Pathol Lab Med*, **126**, 474–477.

135 Okamoto T, Nagaya K, Sugiyama T, Aoyama A, Mitsumaro N and Azuma H (2021) Two patients of trisomy 21 with transient abnormal myelopoiesis with hypereosinophilia without blasts in peripheral blood smears. *Pediatr Hematol Oncol*, **38**, 168–173.

136 Bain BJ (2016) Basophilic differentiation in transient abnormal myelopoiesis. *Am J Hematol*, **91**, 847.

137 Alford KA, Reinhardt K, Garnett C, Norton A, Bohmer K, von Neuhoff C *et al.* (2011) Analysis of GATA1 mutations in Down syndrome transient myeloproliferative disorder and myeloid leukemia. *Blood*, **118**, 2222–2238.

138 Schifferli A, Hitzler J, Bartholdi D, Heinimann K, Hoeller S, Diesch T and Kuehne T (2015) Transient myeloproliferative disorder in neonates without Down syndrome: case report and review. *Eur J Haematol*, **94**, 456–462.

139 Cruz Hernandez D, Metzner M, de Groot A, Usukhbayar B, Elliott N, Roberts I and Vyas P (2020) A sensitive, rapid diagnostic test for transient abnormal myelopoiesis and myeloid leukemia of Down syndrome. *Blood*, **136**, 1460–1465.

140 Bresters D, Reus ACW, Veerman AJP, van Wering ER, van der Does-van den Berg A and Kaspers GJL (2002) Congenital leukaemia: the Dutch experience and review of the literature. *Br J Haematol*, **117**, 513–524.

141 Yang CS, Wang J and Chang CK (2012) Congenital blastic plasmacytoid dendritic cell neoplasm. *Pediatr Blood Cancer*, **58**, 109–110.

142 Cronin DMP, George TI, Reichard KK and Sundram UN (2012) Immunophenotypic analysis of myeloperoxidase-negative leukemia cutis and blastic plasmacytoid dendritic cell neoplasm. *Am J Clin Pathol*, **137**, 367–376.

143 Ariffin E, Jones H and Bhatnagar N (2018) Congenital acute myeloid leukaemia with *KMT2A* rearrangement. *Br J Haematol*, **182**, 169.

144 Zhang IH, Zane LT, Braun BS, Maize J, Zoger S and Loh ML (2006) Congenital leukemia cutis with subsequent development of leukemia. *J Am Acad Dermatol*, **54** (Suppl.), S22–S27.

145 Lee EG, Kim TH, Yoon MS and Lee HJ (2013) Congenital leukemia cutis preceding acute myeloid leukemia with t(9;11)(p22;q23), MLL-MLLT3. *J Dermatol*, **40**, 570–571.

146 Raney RB, Mohanakumar T, Metzgar RS, Hann HW, Buck BE and Donaldson MH (1980) Acute monoblastic leukemia in two infants: clinical histochemical, and immunologic investigations. *Leuk Res*, **4**, 61–67.

147 Esmaeli M, Fischer AS, Khurana M, Gru AA, Yan AC and Rubin AI (2021) Shapiro xanthogranuloma: An essential diagnosis for dermatologists and dermatopathologists to recognize to avoid misdiagnosis of a hematopoietic malignancy in infants and neonates. *J Cutan Pathol*, **48**, 558–562.

148 Green K, Tandon S, Ahmed M, Toscano W, O'Connor D, Ancliff P *et al.* (2020) Congenital acute myeloid leukemia: challenges and lessons. A 15-year experience from the UK. *Leuk Lymphoma*, **62**, 688–695.

149 Lazure T, Beauchamp A, Croisille L, Ferlicot S, Feneux D and Fabre M (2003) Congenital anerythremic erythroleukemia presenting as hepatic failure. *Arch Pathol Lab Med*, **127**, 1362–1365.

150 Heikenheimo M, Pakkala S, Juvonen E and Saarinen UM (1994) Immuno- and cytochemical characterization of congenital leukemia: a case report. *Med Pediatr Oncol*, **22**, 279–282.

151 Ferguson EC, Talley P and Vora A (2005) Translocation (6;17)(q23;q11.2): a novel cytogenetic abnormality in congenital acute myeloid leukemia? *Cancer Genet Cytogenet*, **163**, 71–73.

152 Weis J, DeVito V, Allen L, Linder D and Magenis E (1985) Translocation X;10 in a case of congenital acute monocytic leukemia. *Cancer Genet Cytogenet*, **16**, 357–364.

153 Van Dongen JC, Dalinghaus M, Kroon AA, de Vries AC and van den Heuvel-Eibrink MM (2009) Successful treatment of congenital acute myeloid leukemia (AML-M6) in a premature infant. *J Pediatr Hematol Oncol*, **31**, 853–854.

154 Kurosawa H, Eguchi M, Sakakibara H, Takahashi H and Furukawa T (1987) Ultrastructural cytochemistry of congenital basophilic leukemia. *Am J Pediatr Hematol Oncol*, **9**, 27–32.

155 Lasson U and Goos M (1981) Congenital erythroleukemia. A case report. *Blut*, **43**, 237–241.

156 Allan RR, Wadsworth LD, Kalousek DK and Massing BG (1989) Congenital erythroleukemia: a case report with morphologic, immunophenotypic, and cytogenetic findings. *Am J Hematol*, **31**, 114–121.

157 Hadjiyannakis A, Fletcher WA, Lebrun DP, van Wylick RC and Dow KE (1998) Congenital erythroleukemia in a neonate with severe hypoxic ischemic encephalopathy. *Am J Perinatol*, **15**, 689–694.

158 Halliday GC, O'Reilly J, Kelsey C, Cole CH and Kotecha RS (2016) Successful treatment of congenital erythroleukemia with low-dose cytosine arabinoside. *Pediatr Blood Cancer*, **63**, 566–567.

159 Ishii E, Oda M, Kinugawa N, Oda T, Takimoto T, Suzuki N *et al.* (2006) Features and outcome of neonatal leukemia in Japan: experience of the Japan Infant Leukemia Study Group. *Pediatr Blood Cancer*, **47**, 268–272.

160 Bayar E, Kurczynski TW, Robinson MG, Tyrkus M and al Saadi A (1996) Monozygotic twins with congenital acute lymphoblastic leukemia (ALL) and t(4;11)(q21;q23). *Cancer Gene Cytogenet*, **89**, 177–180.

161 Bas Suarez MP, Lopez Brito J, Santana Reyes C, Gresa Munoz M, Diaz Pulido R and Lodos Rojas JC (2011) Congenital acute lymphoblastic leukemia: a two-case report and a review of the literature. *Eur J Pediatr*, **170**, 531–534.

162 Gilgenkrantz S, Benz E, Chiclet AM, Buisine J, Gregoire MJ, Olive D *et al.* (1983) Congenital acute lymphoblastic leukemia with chromosomal abnormalities including a translocation (1;4;22). *Cancer Genet Cytogenet*, **10**, 37–42.

163 Ridge SA, Cabrera ME, Ford AM, Tapia S, Risueño C, Labra S, Barriga F and Greaves MF (1995) Rapid intraclonal switch of lineage dominance in congenital leukaemia with a MLL gene rearrangement. *Leukemia*, **9**, 2023–2026.

164 Meyer C, Burmeister T, Groger D, Tsaur G, Fechina L, Renneville A *et al.* (2018) The *MLL* recombinome of acute leukemias in 2017. *Leukemia*, **32**, 273–284.

165 Rice S and Roy A (2020) MLL-rearranged infant leukemia: 'a thorn in the side' of a remarkable success story. *Biochim Biophys Acta Gene Regul Mech*, **1863**, 194564.

166 Chen C, Yu W, Alikarami F, Qiu Q, Chen CH, Flournoy J *et al.* (2022) Single-cell multiomics reveals increased plasticity, resistant populations and stem-cell-like blasts in KMT2A-rearranged leukemia. *Blood*, **139**, 2198–2211.

167 Ford AM, Ridge SA, Cabrera ME, Mahmoud H, Steel CM, Chan LC and Greaves M (1993) In utero rearrangements in the trithorax-related oncogene in infant leukaemias. *Nature*, **363**, 358–360.

168 Gale KB, Ford AM, Repp R, Borkhardt A, Keller C, Eden OB and M. F. Greaves MF (1997) Backtracking leukemia to birth: identification of clonotypic gene fusion sequences in neonatal blood spots. *Proc Natl Acad Sci U S A*, **94**, 13950–13954.

169 Hunger SP, McGavran L, Meltesen L, Parker NB, Kassenbrock CK and Bitter MA (1998) Oncogenesis in utero: fetal death due to acute myelogenous leukaemia with an *MLL* translocation. *Br J Haematol*, **103**, 539–542.

170 Greaves MF, Maia AT, Wiemels JL and Ford AM (2003) Leukemia in twins: lessons in natural history. *Blood*, **102**, 2321–2333.

171 Mahmoud HH, Ridge SA, Behm FG, Pui CH, Ford AM, Raimondi SC and Greaves MF (1995) Intrauterine monoclonal origin of neonatal concordant acute lymphoblastic leukemia in monozygotic twins. *Med Pediatr Oncol*, **24**, 77–81.

172 Park SY, Jang JJ, Kim CW, Cho HI and Chi JG (2001) Congenital monoblastic leukemia with 9;11 translocation in monozygotic twins: a case report. *J Korean Med Sci*, **16**, 366–370.

173 Lewis MS, Kaicker S and Strauchen JA (2008) Hepatic involvement in congenital acute megakaryoblastic leukemia: a case report with emphasis on the liver pathology findings. *Pediatr Develop Pathol*, **11**, 55–58.

174 Kawasaki Y, Makimoto M, Nomura K, Hoshino A, Hamashima T, Hiwatari M *et al.* (2015) Neonatal acute megakaryoblastic leukemia mimicking congenital neuroblastoma. *Clin Case Rep*, **3**, 145–149.

175 Chan WC, Carroll A, Alvarado CS, Phillips S, Gonzalez-Crussi F, Kurczynski E *et al.* (1992) Acute megakaryoblastic leukemia in infants with t(1;22)(p13;q13) abnormality. *Am J Clin Pathol*, **98**, 214–221.

176 Lion T, Haas OA, Harbott J, Bannier E, Ritterbach J, Jankovic M *et al.* (1992) The translocation t(1;22)(p13;q13) is a nonrandom marker specifically associated with acute megakaryocytic leukemia in young children. *Blood*, **79**, 3325–3330.

177 Barrett R, Morash B, Roback D, Pambrun C, Marfleet L, Ketterling RP *et al.* (2017) FISH identifies a KAT6A/CREBBP fusion caused by a cryptic insertional t(8;16) in a case of spontaneously remitting congenital acute myeloid leukemia with a normal karyotype. *Pediatr Blood Cancer*, **64**, e26450.

178 Wong KF, Yuen HL, Siu LL, Pang A and Kwong YL (2008) t(8;16)(p11;p13) predisposes to a transient but potentially recurring neonatal leukemia. *Hum Pathol*, **39**, 1702–1707.

179 Sainati L, Bolcato S, Cocito MG, Zanesco L, Basso G, Montaldi A and Piovesan AL. (1996) Transient acute monoblastic leukemia with reciprocal (8;16)(p11;p13) translocation. *Pediatr Hematol Oncol*, **13**, 151–157.

180 Dinulos JG, Hawkins DS, Clark BS, and Francis JS (1997) Spontaneous remission of congenital leukemia. *J Pediatr*, **131**, 300–303.

181 Classen CF, Behnisch W, Reinhardt D, Koenig M, Moller P and Debatin KM (2005) Spontaneous complete and sustained remission of a rearrangement CBP (16p13)-positive disseminated congenital myelosarcoma. *Ann Hematol*, **84**, 274–275.

182 Wu X, Sulavik D, Roulston D, and Lim MS (2011) Spontaneous remission of congenital acute myeloid leukemia with t(8;16)(p11;13). *Pediatr Blood Cancer*, **56**, 331–332.

183 Coenen EA, Zwaan CM, Reinhardt D, Harrison CJ, Haas OA, de Haas V *et al.* (2013) Pediatric acute myeloid leukemia with t(8;16)(p11; p13), a distinct clinical and biological entity: a collaborative study by the International-Berlin- Frankfurt-Munster AML-study group. *Blood*, **122**, 2704–2713.

184 Terui K, Sato T, Sasaki S, Kudo K, Kamio T and Ito E (2008) Two novel variants of MOZ- CBP fusion transcripts in spontaneously remitted infant leukemia with t(1;16;8) (p13;p13;p11), a new variant of t(8;16)(p11;p13). *Haematologica*, **93**, 1591–1593.

185 Bacchetta J, Douvillez B, Warin L, Girard S, Pagès MP, Rebaud P and Bertrand Y (2008) Leucémie aiguë néonatale et Blueberry Muffin syndrome: à propos d'un cas spontanément régressif. *Arch Pédiatr*, **15**, 1315−1319.

186 Jesudas R, Buck SA and Savasan S (2017) Spontaneous remission of congenital AML with skin involvement and t(1;11)(p32;q23). *Pediatr Blood Cancer*, **64**, e26269.

187 Ferguson EC, Talley P and Vora A (2005) Translocation (6;17)(q23;q11.2): a novel cytogenetic abnormality in congenital acute myeloid leukemia? *Cancer Genet Cytogenet*, **163**, 71−73.

188 Van der Linden MH, Creemers S and Pieters R (2012) Diagnosis and management of neonatal leukaemia. *Semin Fetal Neonatal Med*, **17**, 192–195.

189 Gyárfás T, Wintgens J, Biskup W, Oschlies I, Klapper W, Siebert R *et al.* (2016) Transient spontaneous remission in congenital MLL-AF10 rearranged acute myeloid leukemia presenting with cardiorespiratory failure and meconium ileus. *Mol Cell Pediatr*, **3**, 30.

190 Yarbrough CK, Bandt SK, Hurth K, Wambach JA, Rao R, Kulkarni S *et al.* (2015) Congenital acute myeloid leukemia with unique translocation t(11;19)(q23;p13.3). *Cureus*, **7**, e289

191 McNutt DM, Holdsworth MT, Wong C, Hanrahan JD and Winter SS (2006) Rasburicase for the management of tumor lysis syndrome in neonates. *Ann Pharmacother*, **40**, 1445–1450.

192 Zaramella P, De Salvia A, Zaninotto M, Baraldi M, Capovilla G, De Leo D and Chiandetti L (2013) Lethal effect of a single dose of rasburicase in a preterm newborn infant. *Pediatrics*, **131**, e309–e312.

193 Van der Linden MH, Valsecchi MG, De Lorenzo P, Möricke A, Janka G, Leblanc TM *et al.* (2009) Outcome of congenital acute lymphoblastic leukemia treated on the Interfant-999 protocol. *Blood*, **114**, 3764–3768.

194 Pui CH, Yang JJ, Hunger SP, Pieters R, Schrappe M, Biondi *et al.* (2015) Childhood acute lymphoblastic leukemia: progress through collaboration. *J Clin Oncol*, **33**, 2938–2948.

195 Creutzig U, van den Heuvel-Eibrink MM, Gibson BE, Dworzak MN, Adachi S, de Bont E *et al.*; AML Committee of the International BFM Study Group. (2012) Diagnosis and management of acute myeloid leukemia in children and adolescents: recommendations from an international expert panel. *Blood*, **120**, 3187–3205.

196 Creutzig U, Zimmermann M, Dworzak MN, Ritter J, Schellong G and Reinhardt D (2013) Development of curative treatment with AML-BFM studies. *Klin Pädiatr*, **225** (Suppl 1), S79–S86

197 Kawasaki H, Isoyama K, Eguchi M, Hibi S, Kinukawa N and Kosaka Y (2001) Superior outcome of infant acute myeloid leukemia with intensive chemotherapy: results of the Japan Infant Leukemia Study Group. *Blood*, **98**, 3589–3594.

198 Creutzig U, Zimmermann M, Bourquin J-P, Dworzak MN, Kremens B, Lehmbecher T *et al.* (2012) Favorable outcome in infants with AML after intensive first- and second-line treatment: an AML-BFM study group report. *Leukemia*, **26**, 654–661.

199 Daifu T, Kato I, Kozuki K, Umeda K, Hiramatsu H, Watanabe K *et al.* (2014) The clinical utility of genetic testing for t(8;16)(p11; p13) in congenital acute myeloid leukemia. *J Pediatr Hematol Oncol*, **36**, e325–e327.

200 Mayerhofer C, Niemeyer CM and Flotho C (2021) Current treatment of juvenile myelomonocytic leukemia. *J Clin Med*, **10**, 3084.

201 Caye A, Strullu M, Guidez F, Cassinat B, Gazal S, Fenneteau O *et al.* (2015) Juvenile myelomonocytic leukemia displays mutations in components of the RAS pathway and the PRC2 network. *Nat Genet*, **47**, 1334–1340.

202 Stieglitz E, Taylor-Weiner AN, Chang TY, Gelston LC, Wang YD, Mazor T *et al.* (2015) The genomic landscape of juvenile myelomonocytic leukemia. *Nat Genet*, **47**, 1326–1333.

203 Strullu M, Caye A, Lachenaud J, Cassinat B, Gazal S, Fenneteau O *et al.* (2014) Juvenile myelomonocytic leukaemia and Noonan syndrome. *J Med Genet*, **51**, 689–697.

204 Matsuda K, Shimada A, Yoshida N, Ogawa A, Watanabe A, Yajima S *et al.* (2007) Spontaneous improvement of hematologic abnormalities in patients having juvenile myelomonocytic leukemia with specific RAS mutations. *Blood*, **109**, 5477–5480.

205 Locatelli F and Niemeyer CM (2015) How I treat juvenile myelomonocytic leukemia. *Blood* **125**, 1083–1090.

206 Matsuda K, Taira C, Sakashita K, Saito S, Tanaka-Yanagisawa M, Yanagisawa R *et al.* (2010) Long-term survival after nonintensive chemotherapy in some juvenile myelomonocytic leukemia patients with CBL mutations, and the possible presence of healthy persons with the mutations. *Blood*, **115**, 5429–5431.

207 Yoshida K, Toki T, Okuno Y, Kanezaki R, Shiraishi Y, Sato-Otsubo A *et al.* (2013) The landscape of somatic mutations in Down syndrome-related myeloid disorders. *Nat Genet*, **45**, 1293–1299

208 Labuhn M, Perkins K, Matzk S, Varghese L, Garnett C, Papaemmanuil E *et al.* (2019) Mechanisms of progression of myeloid preleukemia to transformed myeloid leukemia in children with Down syndrome. *Cancer Cell*, **36**, 123–138

209 Flasinski M, Scheibke K, Zimmermann M, Creutzig U, Reinhardt K, Verwer F *et al.* (2018) Low-dose cytarabine to prevent myeloid leukemia in children with Down syndrome: TMD Prevention 2007 study. *Blood Adv*, **2**, 1532–1540.

210 Penner J, Hemstadt H, Burns JE, Randell P and Lyall H (2021) Stop, think SCORTCH: rethinking the traditional TORCH screen in an era of re-emerging syphilis. *Arch Dis Child*, **106**, 117–124.

4

Disorders of platelets and coagulation, thrombosis and blood transfusion

Thrombocytopenia overview

Thrombocytopenia is the commonest haematological abnormality in neonates, particularly among sick and/or very low birthweight neonates (reviewed in references 1–3). Overall, up to 5% of neonates will have platelet counts of $<150 \times 10^9$/l in the first week of life, the incidence varying depending on the population studied.[1–3] Many of these studies have analysed cord blood platelet counts, which may have over-estimated the true incidence of thrombocytopenia. The study by de Moerloose et al.[4] was also performed on cord blood samples and included samples from more than 8000 consecutive deliveries but, as all cases of thrombocytopenia were subsequently confirmed by heel-prick samples, their calculated incidence of neonatal thrombocytopenia of 0.9% probably provides the most accurate estimate. When neonates develop thrombocytopenia it is usually mild. Severe thrombocytopenia (platelet count $<50 \times 10^9$/l) is reported to occur in 0.1–0.5% of neonates, with the variation reflecting differences in the proportion of very low birthweight neonates included in the study.[5–7] For example, the incidence of thrombocytopenia is significantly higher in neonates who are admitted to neonatal intensive care units (NICUs), where thrombocytopenia occurs in approximately 40% of all babies.[6,8] Several studies have shown that the severity of thrombocytopenia worsens with prematurity and with the severity of the clinical condition; the incidence of thrombocytopenia in sick neonates requiring intensive care can be as high as 70–80%.[6,9,10]

Apparent thrombocytopenia should normally be verified by repeating the full blood count and by blood film examination, which may show platelet clumps or fibrin strands, and in addition may suggest a cause of the thrombocytopenia, such as sepsis or necrotising enterocolitis (NEC) (see Figs 1.16, 3.6 and 3.15b). The most common cause of spurious thrombocytopenia in neonates is a blood clot in the sample which may not have been detected at the time of analysis. This is a particular problem in neonates who are polycythaemic. Pseudothrombocytopenia, which is usually caused by in vitro ethylene diaminetetra-acetic acid (EDTA)-dependent platelet clumping, is not uncommon in neonatal samples. In some cases, this has been shown to be due to transplacental passage of an EDTA-dependent antibody that leads to in vitro platelet aggregation, in which case it is self-limiting.[11,12] However, severe pseudothrombocytopenia can also occur independently of EDTA and can persist for several months after birth.[13]

The vast majority of episodes of thrombocytopenia are self-limiting, occur secondary to pregnancy-related complications in the mother or to postnatally acquired infection in the baby and are accompanied by no or minor bleeding. The most common sites of minor haemorrhage in thrombocytopenic neonates are bleeding from the renal tract, from the skin or from endotracheal or nasogastric tubes.[14] Nevertheless, the risk of significant or serious haemorrhage in thrombocytopenic neonates is high,[14] particularly in extremely low birthweight neonates. The most common types of major haemorrhage in neonates are intracranial haemorrhage (ICH), which occurs in about 5% of all thrombocytopenic neonates, followed by gastrointestinal haemorrhage (1–5%), pulmonary haemorrhage (0.6–5%) and macroscopic haematuria (1–2%).[6,9,14,15]

The treatment of thrombocytopenia, particularly in the context of platelet transfusion thresholds, remains controversial, but considerable progress has been made in recent years as a result of carefully designed clinical observational and intervention trials.[16,17] In the majority of babies, thrombocytopenia resolves spontaneously with few long-term sequelae. This means that expensive and time-consuming investigations are usually not necessary provided that a clinical diagnostic algorithm, such as those shown in Figs 4.1 and 4.2 for term and preterm neonates, respectively, is followed. For preterm neonates, we have found that a practical approach is to stratify the causes of thrombocytopenia according to the postnatal age of the neonate at presentation and the gestational age, both of which can guide the clinician in making the right clinical and investigative choices.

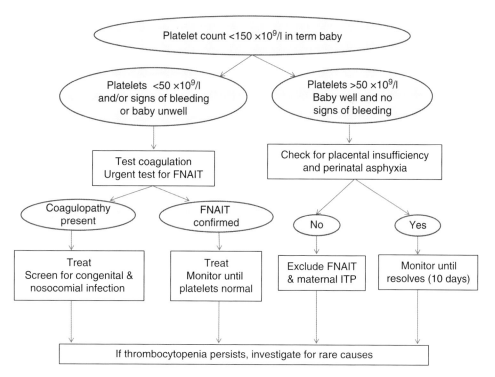

Fig. 4.1 Algorithm for the management of thrombocytopenia in a term baby. ITP, autoimmune thrombocytopenia; FNAIT, fetal/neonatal alloimmune. thrombocytopenia.

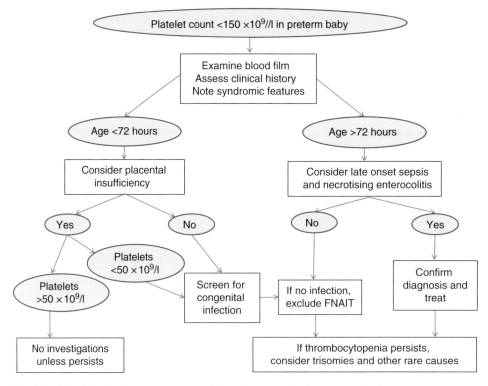

Fig. 4.2 Algorithm for the management of thrombocytopenia in a preterm baby.

Causes of neonatal thrombocytopenia: a practical classification based on age at onset

Although neonatal thrombocytopenia can have a wide variety of causes, the clinical presentation can broadly be divided into three groups depending on the age at presentation:

- fetal thrombocytopenia
- thrombocytopenia presenting at <72 hours of age
- thrombocytopenia presenting at >72 hours of age.

The main causes of thrombocytopenia presenting in fetal life are shown in Table 4.1 and include mainly constitutional abnormalities and congenital infection. Although many of these disorders may also present after birth, in practice by far the most common causes of thrombocytopenia presenting in the first 72 hours of life are related to complications of pregnancy and/or delivery (Table 4.2). In contrast, the majority of episodes of thrombocytopenia developing later than 72 hours of life are a result of a postnatally acquired bacterial infection and/or NEC (Table 4.3). This classification provides clinicians with guidance for selecting appropriate investigations and management and helps to avoid unnecessary and expensive tests in transient thrombocytopenias where prognosis can be determined by simple clinical and laboratory means alone (Figs 4.1 and 4.2).

Table 4.1 Causes of fetal thrombocytopenia

Cause	Condition
Immune	Alloimmune thrombocytopenia
	Secondary to maternal platelet autoantibodies (e.g. SLE, ITP)
Congenital infection	Cytomegalovirus
	Parvovirus B19
	Rubella
	Human immunodeficiency virus
	Toxoplasma gondii
	Malaria
Aneuploidy	Trisomy 21
	Trisomy 13
	Trisomy 18
	Triploidy
Malignancy	Transient abnormal myelopoiesis associated with Down syndrome
	Congenital leukaemia
Genetic/inherited	Congenital amegakaryocytic thrombocytopenia
	Wiskott–Aldrich syndrome
	Fas deficiency
Other	Severe Rh haemolytic disease of the newborn

ITP, autoimmune thrombocytopenia; SLE, systemic lupus erythematosus.

Table 4.2 Causes of early-onset neonatal thrombocytopenia (presenting before 72 hours)

Most common

Placental insufficiency, e.g. IUGR, secondary to maternal hypertension or maternal diabetes

Perinatal asphyxia

Perinatal bacterial infection, e.g. *Escherichia coli*, group B *Streptococcus*, *Haemophilus influenzae*

Disseminated intravascular coagulation

Alloimmune thrombocytopenia

Autoimmune thrombocytopenia, e.g. maternal ITP/SLE, neonatal lupus erythematosus

Less common or rare

Congenital infection, e.g. CMV, rubella, HIV, enteroviruses, parvovirus B19, dengue, chikungunya virus, toxoplasma, malaria

Aneuploidy, e.g. trisomy 21, trisomy 13, trisomy 18 and TAM in neonates with Down syndrome

Associated with thrombosis, e.g. HIT, TTP (congenital ADAMTS13 deficiency), renal vein thrombosis

Bone marrow replacement, e.g. congenital leukaemia, osteopetrosis, HLH

Kasabach–Merritt syndrome

Metabolic disease, e.g. propionic and methylmalonic acidaemia, Gaucher disease, subcutaneous fat necrosis of the newborn

Inherited, e.g. TAR, CAMT, type 2B VWD (see Table 4.4 and text for a more complete list)

CAMT, congenital amegakaryocytic thrombocytopenia; CMV, cytomegalovirus; HIT, heparin-induced thrombocytopenia; HIV, human immunodeficiency virus; HLH, haemophagocytic lymphohistiocytosis; ITP, autoimmune thrombocytopenia; IUGR, intrauterine growth restriction; PET, pre-eclamptic toxaemia; SLE, systemic lupus erythematosus; TAM, transient abnormal myelopoiesis; TAR, thrombocytopenia with absent radii; TTP, thrombotic thrombocytopenic purpura; VWD von Willebrand disease.

Table 4.3   Causes of late-onset neonatal thrombocytopenia (presenting after 72 hours): the most frequently occurring conditions are shown in bold

Late-onset sepsis
Necrotising enterocolitis
Congenital infection, e.g. CMV, rubella, HIV, enteroviruses, parvovirus B19, dengue, chikungunya virus, toxoplasma, malaria
Immune: maternal ITP/SLE, neonatal Kawasaki disease*
Kasabach–Merritt syndrome
Metabolic disease, e.g. propionic and methylmalonic acidaemia
Drug-induced
Inherited, e.g. TAR, CAMT (see Table 4.4 and text for a more complete list)

* Thrombocytopenia has been reported but thrombocytosis is more common.
CAMT, congenital amegakaryocytic thrombocytopenia; CMV, cytomegalovirus; HIV, human immunodeficiency virus; ITP, autoimmune thrombocytopenia; SLE, systemic lupus erythematosus; TAR, thrombocytopenia with absent radii.

Fetal thrombocytopenia

Thrombocytopenia is usually identified when fetal blood sampling is performed where there is a history of fetal haemorrhage due to a known history of inherited thrombocytopenia. Other cases are identified during the course of investigations for suspected fetal anomalies or fetal anaemia. Fetal blood sampling also remains an important tool for the diagnosis of thrombocytopenia in suspected congenital cytomegalovirus (CMV) infection[18] (discussed later) but is no longer used to monitor known fetal/neonatal alloimmune thrombocytopenia (FNAIT). The most common causes of fetal thrombocytopenia in individual centres tend to be influenced by the particular case-mix of the local fetal medicine unit but will include viral infection and thrombocytopenia secondary to severe alloimmune anaemia due to Rh antibodies.[3] The conditions presenting with thrombocytopenia in fetal life are discussed in more detail later.

Early-onset neonatal thrombocytopenia (presenting at <72 hours of age)

More than half of all episodes of thrombocytopenia in babies admitted to NICUs occur within the first 72 hours of life.[8] The majority of cases of early-onset thrombocytopenia in this setting occur in preterm neonates born following pregnancies complicated by placental insufficiency and/or chronic fetal hypoxia, secondary either to idiopathic intrauterine growth restriction (IUGR) in the fetus[19] or to maternal disease, in particular pre-eclampsia and other forms of pregnancy-induced hypertension, diabetes mellitus or HELLP syndrome (haemolysis, elevated liver enzymes and low platelets).[20]

Neonatal thrombocytopenia associated with intrauterine growth restriction and other placental insufficiency syndromes
A large retrospective study of almost 3000 neonates with IUGR (also termed 'small for gestational age' [SGA]) showed that 30% of them had early-onset thrombocytopenia compared with 10% of gestation-matched neonates of appropriate birthweight.[21] Neonates with

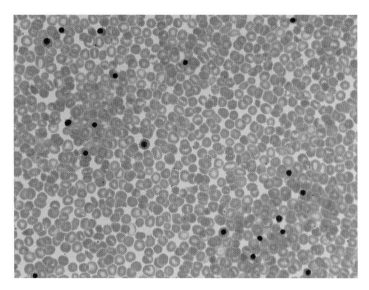

Fig. 4.3 Blood film of a preterm neonate with intrauterine growth restriction showing erythroblastosis, polychromasia, poikilocytosis and target cells. No leucocytes and only occasional platelets are seen consistent with the blood count showing neutropenia and thrombocytopenia. At least two Howell–Jolly bodies are also apparent. May–Grünwald–Giemsa (MGG), ×20 objective.

IUGR also have a number of other characteristic haematological abnormalities at birth, including increased numbers of circulating nucleated red blood cells (NRBC) (Fig. 4.3), often with an associated increased haemoglobin concentration (Hb), haematocrit and red cell count; a variable degree of neutropenia without left-shifted neutrophils or other signs of acute infection; and red cell changes on the blood film suggestive of hyposplenism, including spherocytes, target cells and Howell–Jolly bodies (see Fig. 1.10).[19] The cause of the thrombocytopenia in IUGR appears to be reduced platelet production due to impaired megakaryocytopoiesis. The numbers of megakaryocytes and their precursor and progenitor cells are severely reduced and there is no clear evidence of increased platelet consumption.[8,22,23] Similarly, the numbers of neutrophil progenitors are reduced, suggesting that the neutropenia results from reduced neutrophil production. By contrast, erythropoiesis is clearly increased, as shown by the high numbers of NRBC and the raised Hb. Furthermore, the levels of erythropoietin (EPO) are increased in fetuses and neonates with IUGR[24,25] and correlate with the severity of the haematological abnormalities.[19] These findings suggest that the underlying cause of the thrombocytopenia and other haematological abnormalities associated with IUGR is chronic fetal hypoxia. However, the mechanisms by which chronic fetal hypoxia affects platelet production as well as neutrophil and red cell production are unknown.

The natural history of this type of neonatal thrombocytopenia is characteristic. Affected neonates usually have a low normal or moderately reduced platelet count at birth ($120–200 \times 10^9/l$), which falls to a nadir of $80–100 \times 10^9/l$ at day 4–5 of life before recovering to $>150 \times 10^9/l$ by 7–10 days of age.[26] This pattern, together with the clinical history and blood film abnormalities, is sufficient to make the diagnosis[9] (see Figs 1.10 and 4.3).

Christensen *et al.* showed that neonates with this pattern of IUGR-associated early-onset thrombocytopenia had a low morbidity and mortality (2%) compared with the SGA neonates with early-onset thrombocytopenia for other reasons (65%).[21] This supports a conservative approach to management of neonatal thrombocytopenia associated with IUGR where there is no other cause for the thrombocytopenia and where the platelet count remains above 50×10^9/l and recovers with the characteristic natural history outlined above. For these neonates, no further investigations are necessary. On the other hand, if the platelet count falls below 50×10^9/l or the thrombocytopenia persists beyond the 10th day of life, additional causes for the thrombocytopenia should be sought.

Causes of severe early-onset thrombocytopenia

In contrast to the mild to moderate thrombocytopenia seen in most cases of placental insufficiency, severe early-onset thrombocytopenia ($<50 \times 10^9$/l) requires urgent investigation. The three most important causes are FNAIT, which is discussed in detail later, perinatal bacterial infection and hypoxic ischaemic encephalopathy (HIE) due to acute perinatal asphyxia/hypoxia (see Table 4.2).

Perinatal bacterial infection is commonly related to prolonged rupture of membranes and usually presents as early onset neonatal infection (present by 72 hours). Recent studies have shown that perinatal infection occurs in approximately 3.5 of 1000 births, most commonly due to group B *Streptococcus* or *Escherichia coli*.[27,28] Infections with these organisms are a relatively common cause of stillbirth and can also cause serious neonatal morbidity, with thrombocytopenia developing in about 50% of cases.[29,30] In contrast to late-onset neonatal sepsis, disseminated intravascular coagulation (DIC) appears to be an important mechanism of thrombocytopenia, probably because of the severity of the sepsis syndrome induced by the causative organisms and the fact that infection has often begun prior to delivery and therefore before effective treatment can be instituted. For this reason it is important to perform a coagulation screen in any neonate with thrombocytopenia secondary to perinatal bacterial infection.[31] Typically, the blood film will show neutrophil left shift with toxic granulation evident 1 or 2 days later (see Figs 3.3 and 3.6) and, when DIC is present, thrombocytopenia and fragmented red blood cells (schistocytes) (Fig. 4.4). Worsening thrombocytopenia and neutropenia are poor prognostic signs.

Thrombocytopenia in association with HIE is often severe and prolonged and occurs in approximately 30% of affected neonate.[32,33] In most cases, thrombocytopenia appears to result principally from DIC[31] but it is also reported in the absence of DIC when it tends to be less severe.[34] Several studies to investigate the impact of therapeutic induced hypothermia in thrombocytopenic neonates with HIE show no clinically significant effects on the platelet count.[33]

Late-onset neonatal thrombocytopenia (presenting at >72 hours of age)

Late-onset thrombocytopenia in preterm neonates in NICUs is often severe, with an acute fall in the platelet count over 24 hours, and may be prolonged. Most episodes are secondary to bacterial or fungal sepsis or NEC. Many, but not all, neonates with sepsis- or NEC-associated thrombocytopenia have evidence of DIC (see Case 3.1) and so it is important to carry out a coagulation screen, including measurement of fibrinogen levels in all neonates

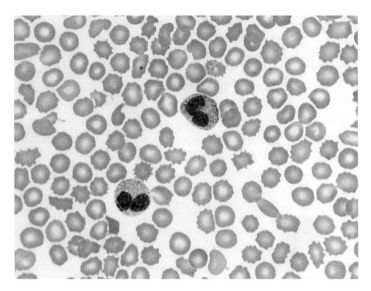

Fig. 4.4 Blood film of a preterm neonate during an acute bacterial infection showing two neutrophils with toxic granulation and some schistocytes together with thrombocytopenia consistent with disseminated intravascular coagulation. Note the large number of echinocytes consistent with the gestation at birth (24 weeks) and the Howell–Jolly body reflecting the underlying intrauterine growth restriction. MGG, ×100.

with sepsis or NEC and a rapidly falling platelet count.[35] D-dimer measurement is not usually helpful in neonates because of the high physiological levels for the first month of life and additional blood samples are also often difficult to obtain in sick neonates. Importantly, thrombocytopenia may be prolonged for several weeks beyond the onset of sepsis/NEC. Sepsis- and NEC-associated thrombocytopenias are among the commonest indications for neonatal platelet transfusion.[36] Other causes of late-onset thrombocytopenia are shown in Table 4.3 and include congenital infections, metabolic disorders, drug-induced and immune thrombocytopenias and inherited disorders, all of which are discussed later.

Conditions leading to clinically significant thrombocytopenia in the neonate

Although the majority of cases of neonatal thrombocytopenia can be diagnosed by their clinical presentation and basic laboratory parameters, there are a small number of other conditions that lead to clinically significant thrombocytopenia that require specific investigation leading to diagnosis and appropriate management.

Fetal/neonatal alloimmune thrombocytopenia

Fetal/neonatal alloimmune thrombocytopenia is the commonest cause of severe thrombocytopenia in well, term infants. It is caused by transplacental passage of maternal anti-human platelet antigen (HPA) alloantibodies directed against fetal platelet antigens that the mother lacks, leading to fetal platelet destruction and potentially also suppression of fetal megakaryopoiesis.[37] In addition to bleeding caused by the thrombocytopenia, *in vitro* and mouse studies suggest that in some cases of FNAIT bleeding may be aggravated by impaired platelet function caused by binding of anti-HPA antibodies to the receptors for fibrinogen on platelets and/or by defects in vascular integrity caused by anti-HPA antibodies binding to vitronectin receptors on endothelial cells.[38,39]

Population-based studies indicate an overall prevalence of FNAIT of 0.7 per 1000 births.[40,41] Although 41 different HPA antigens have been identified so far (Versiti HPA Database, 2020. Available from: https://www.versiti.org/hpa-gene), a recent international study found that four of these antigens were responsible for the vast majority of reported cases of FNAIT (antibodies to HPA-1, HPA-3, HPA-5 and HPA-15).[42] In Caucasian populations, HPA-1a is implicated in 80% cases and HPA-5b in 10–15%.[40,43,44] Around 10% of women who are HPA-1a-negative and carrying an HPA-1a-positive fetus have anti-HPA-1 antibodies.[45] Although the frequency of anti-HPA-5b antibodies in HPA-5b-negative women carrying an HPA-5b-positive fetus is much higher (27%), the risk of severe FNAIT-associated bleeding is lower with anti-HPA-5b than anti-HPA-1a.[46] The development of antibodies against HPA-1a in HPA-1a-negative women is very strongly associated with HLA DRB3 0101 (odds ratio 140), although the HLA DR genotype does not predict the severity of the FNAIT.[45,47] Current evidence suggests that antibodies against low-frequency antigens are rare and play little role in the morbidity of FNAIT in the Caucasian population.[41,48] In Asian and African populations FNAIT caused by anti-HPA-1a antibodies appears to be uncommon. The most frequent causes of FNAIT in the Asian population are antibodies directed against HPA-5b or anti-HPA-4b.[49] In addition, studies from a number of countries have shown that FNAIT in Asian and African populations is frequently caused by maternal anti-CD36 alloantibodies.[50–53] While CD36 deficiency is extremely rare in Caucasians, around 2% of individuals of African origin and 0.5% of individuals of Asian origin lack CD36 expression on their platelets and monocytes and are therefore at risk of developing anti-CD36 antibodies after platelet transfusion or during pregnancy.[50–53] FNAIT can also occur in the babies of women with Glanzmann thrombasthenia or Bernard–Soulier syndrome who have been immunised by platelet transfusion, developing either HLA antibodies or antibodies to the missing glycoproteins.[54]

Most neonates with FNAIT present with severe thrombocytopenia, often with a platelet count $<20 \times 10^9$/l. The most feared complication is ICH, which occurs in approximately 20% of neonates with HPA-1a-associated FNAIT and is associated with a very high risk of severe neurodevelopmental problems, including cerebral palsy.[40,55] A large international study that identified 43 cases of FNAIT-associated ICH reported that 15 (35%) neonates died within a few days of birth while another 23 (82% of the survivors) had long-term neurodevelopmental problems, including cerebral palsy.[56] A high proportion of ICH (about 80%) occurs *in utero* and FNAIT has been reported as early as 20 weeks' gestation.[56,57] Bleeding from extracranial sites, such as the gastrointestinal tract or the lungs may also occur and is occasionally fatal[58] although the overall risk of major haemorrhage due to FNAIT is fairly low (<5%).[42,59] Since FNAIT can affect first pregnancies, the diagnosis at birth is often unsuspected and the clinical presentation varies from asymptomatic thrombocytopenia or petechiae to seizures secondary to ICH. The clinical pattern of FNAIT due

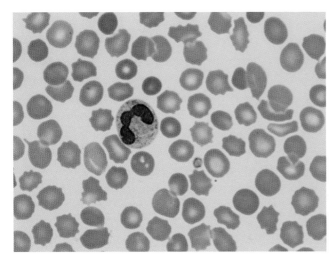

Fig. 4.5 Blood film of a neonate born at 36 weeks' gestation with severe thrombocytopenia due to fetal/neonatal alloimmune thrombocytopenia showing a single normal-sized platelet as well as a normal neutrophil and red cells. MGG, ×100.

to anti-CD36 antibodies is particularly associated with repeated early fetal loss due to miscarriage and hydrops fetalis, the antigen being also expressed on erythroid cells.[60–63]

The laboratory diagnosis of FNAIT is usually made using monoclonal antibody-specific immobilisation of platelet antigens (MAIPA) assays to detect maternal anti-HPA antibodies. Both parents, where possible, and the infant should also be genotyped for the most common HPA antigens (HPA-1a, HPA-3, HPA-5b and HPA-15) and HPA-4 and CD36 if appropriate. Because the field of platelet genotyping is advancing rapidly, an international panel of experts recently worked together to agree evidence-based guidance on the investigations of FNAIT using a systematic approach and standardised methodology.[64] There are no specific haematological features of FNAIT apart from isolated thrombocytopenia. The only finding on the blood film is thrombocytopenia and often it is the absence of additional features (such as evidence of infection) that suggests the diagnosis (Fig. 4.5).

Management of fetal/neonatal alloimmune thrombocytopenia

This diagnosis should be considered in all cases of severe early-onset neonatal thrombocytopenia (platelet count $<50 \times 10^9$/l) (see Fig. 4.1). In a retrospective analysis of 166 cases of severe thrombocytopenia where screening for FNAIT was performed, two-thirds of the neonates (110/166) were found to have FNAIT and 12 of these neonates were found to have ICH.[65] The high mortality and morbidity of FNAIT-associated ICH means that most experts recommend that all cases of suspected FNAIT should undergo cranial ultrasound scanning to exclude ICH. Most cases of FNAIT resolve within a week without long-term sequelae. Since the platelet count usually falls over the first 4–7 days of life, all thrombocytopenic neonates with FNAIT should be monitored until there is a sustained rise in the platelet count into the normal range.

There have been many changes in the recommendations for both postnatal and antenatal management of FNAIT over the last 10 years. This reflects the difficulty of conducting randomised trials in a relatively rare disease and most recommendations are based on consensus recommendations from expert groups. In well neonates with documented or suspected FNAIT who have no evidence of haemorrhage, transfusion of HPA-compatible platelets is recommended only when the platelet count is $<30 \times 10^9/l$.[41,64] In some countries, including the UK, HPA-1a-, HPA-5b-negative platelets are usually given pending a precise diagnosis. A recent systematic review confirmed that HPA-selected platelet transfusions were more effective than HPA-unselected platelets.[66] However, the same review also showed that random donor platelets were often clinically effective and could therefore be used in regions or countries where HPA-selected platelets were unavailable. In the event of major haemorrhage, including ICH, the platelet count should be maintained $>50 \times 10^9/l$ using appropriate HPA-negative platelets by preference. There is currently no clear evidence to demonstrate a benefit for administration of intravenous immunoglobulin (IVIg) in the immediate postnatal period.[66] In all cases, platelets for transfusion should be CMV-negative, single-donor apheresis units; when neonates have received intrauterine platelet transfusions the platelets should also be irradiated.[67] In some cases, thrombocytopenia persists for up to 8–12 weeks. In these cases IVIg is usually considered to be a better option than repeated platelet transfusions, although there is no evidence from clinical trials to confirm the value of IVIg for persistent thrombocytopenia.[1]

Antenatal management of fetal/neonatal alloimmune thrombocytopenia

Although the optimal approach to antenatal management of FNAIT has been controversial for many years, a recently published systematic review of the 26 most relevant studies has clearly shown that non-invasive antenatal management of FNAIT is as effective as fetal blood sampling-based approaches.[59] This is important because, as this review reported, the mortality associated with fetal blood sampling in FNAIT, is substantial (26%). This review also found that weekly maternal administration of IVIg is the most appropriate first-line antenatal treatment of FNAIT, with no consistent evidence in favour of adding corticosteroids.[59] Management of women with known HPA antibodies depends on the HPA genotype of the father and the severity of previously affected neonates. To confirm that there is a risk of FNAIT, HPA typing using non-invasive methods should be performed in any pregnancy where the father is unavailable or is known to be heterozygous for the implicated antigen.[64] Although there is some evidence that antibody titres correlate with disease severity, the single most important predictor of poor outcome is a past history of an affected infant with ICH. As a result, recent international recommendations advise that women with a previous baby with an ICH related to FNAIT should be offered IVIg infusions during subsequent affected pregnancies from 12 weeks' gestation.[64]

Neonatal thrombocytopenia due to maternal autoimmune disease

Neonates born to mothers with a history of autoimmune thrombocytopenia (ITP) or systemic lupus erythematosus (SLE) may develop thrombocytopenia as a result of transplacental passage of maternal platelet autoantibodies even if the mother had a normal platelet count during the pregnancy. Severe thrombocytopenia ($<50 \times 10^9/l$) occurs in about 10% of neonates with maternal platelet autoantibodies; about half of these have platelet counts of $<20 \times 10^9/l$.[68,69] Several studies have shown that the mortality and risk of major haemorrhage, including ICH, is very low (about 1%)[68–70] and most groups no longer recommend fetal blood sampling or caesarean delivery irrespective of the maternal platelet count.[68,71] Neonatal lupus due to transplacental passage of maternal autoantibodies to Sjögren syndrome A or B autoantigens has a distinct clinical presentation which includes total atrioventricular heart block as well as the characteristic lupus rash, hepatobiliary disease, thrombocytopenia, anaemia, neutropenia and, rarely, aplastic anaemia.[72]

The most useful factors predicting whether or not fetal or neonatal thrombocytopenia is likely to be severe are the severity of the maternal disease and/or platelet count during pregnancy, or the occurrence of severe thrombocytopenia in a previous baby.[68,69] As with FNAIT, there are no specific features in the blood film of a baby with thrombocytopenia due to maternal autoimmune disease. All neonates with a history of maternal thrombocytopenia should have their platelet count checked at birth; if it is found to be $>150 \times 10^9$/l, no further action is necessary. Thrombocytopenic neonates should have their platelet count rechecked after 2–3 days, as counts often drop to their lowest levels at this age. In addition, all neonates with severe thrombocytopenia should undergo cranial ultrasound scanning to exclude ICH. For neonates with a platelet count of $<20 \times 10^9$/l or for thrombocytopenic neonates with active bleeding, the International Consensus Report on Management of ITP recommended treatment with a single dose of IVIg (1 g/kg).[73] In most cases the thrombocytopenia resolves spontaneously by the age of 7 days. However, in a small group of neonates, thrombocytopenia persists up to the age of 12 weeks.[69] In this situation, where the thrombocytopenia is severe (platelet count $<20 \times 10^9$/l), treatment with IVIg (400 mg/kg/day for 5 days or 1 g/kg/day for 2 days, total dose 2 g/kg) may be useful.[1,69]

Thrombocytopenia due to congenital infections

The classical congenital infections associated with fetal and neonatal thrombocytopenia are often referred to as 'TORCH' organisms (toxoplasma, other infections, rubella, CMV and herpes simplex). There is an expanding range of 'other' organisms including a range of viruses, mycobacteria and protozoa. Neonatal thrombocytopenia does not appear to be a feature of transplacental infection with severe acute respiratory syndrome coronavirus-2 (SARS-CoV-2)[74] and is only rarely described in neonates with congenital human immunodeficiency virus (HIV) infection.[75] In most cases, thrombocytopenia will be present in combination with other clinical features suggestive of congenital infection, such as intracranial calcification, hepatosplenomegaly, jaundice or 'reactive' lymphocytes in the blood film (see Fig. 3.16). However, severe thrombocytopenia (platelet count $<50 \times 10^9$/l) that is present in the first days of life and persists for more than the first week is a common feature in congenital infections and may then suggest the diagnosis if other more common clinical features are absent or minimal.

Congenital cytomegalovirus infection

The best recognised, and likely commonest, cause of virus-associated neonatal thrombocytopenia is congenital CMV infection (Case 4.1, see page 227). This is also the most commonly identified congenital viral infection, affecting hundreds of thousands of neonates worldwide every year with an estimated prevalence of 0.67% overall.[76,77] Rates of congenital CMV infection are 3-fold higher in low- and middle-income countries than in high-income countries.[77] The rate of congenital CMV infection largely depends on maternal seroprevalence rates: the highest rates of congenital CMV are seen in populations with high maternal seroprevalence because the majority of affected neonates are currently born to mothers with reactivation of previously acquired CMV or reinfection with a new viral strain.[77] Maternal-to-fetal transmission of CMV is highest in the third trimester but the severity of infection is highest when transmission occurs during the first trimester.[78] Overall, primary or recrudescent maternal CMV infection during pregnancy results in intrauterine transmission of CMV in 30–40% of cases, although only 10–15% of these cases are born with clinical abnormalities.[76,79]

Around 70% of neonates with congenital CMV disease have thrombocytopenia at birth, which often manifests as a petechial rash and occasionally as a 'blueberry muffin' skin rash (see Chapter 3). CMV-associated thrombocytopenia may be severe and may persist for several months.[76,80] The diagnosis is often suggested by the combination of the petechial rash with jaundice, hepatosplenomegaly, raised transaminases, IUGR, microcephaly and/or chorioretinitis as well as the characteristic appearance of intracranial periventricular calcification.[76] Sensorineural hearing loss is an important cause of long-term morbidity.[81] The most severe cases of congenital CMV infection are detected during fetal life, usually as a result of routine ultrasound scanning. In these cases the majority of fetuses with severe neurological abnormalities are thrombocytopenic and the outlook is poor.[18]

The diagnosis of congenital CMV infection in neonates is based on the detection of CMV deoxyribonucleic acid (DNA) in urine or saliva using the polymerase chain reaction (PCR), which is quicker and more sensitive than viral culture.[82] It is important to make the diagnosis on samples collected soon after birth to differentiate congenital from nosocomially acquired CMV infection because of the implications for screening and follow-up of neonates with congenital CMV.[76,83] Although there appear to be no direct long-term haematological consequences of congenital CMV infection, the severity of fetal thrombocytopenia is likely to contribute to the considerable morbidity of this disease: up to 60% will have some form of long-term neurodevelopmental disability, three-quarters will have hearing impairment and one-third will have visual problems, including blindness.[76] Prenatal diagnosis of CMV infection is currently based on quantification of CMV DNA in amniotic fluid rather than fetal blood because of the potential risk of fetal blood sampling.[84] However, it is important to be aware that the sensitivity of CMV PCR is maximal (90%) when amniocentesis is performed after the first 20 weeks of pregnancy and at least 8 weeks after the onset of maternal infection and that a negative result therefore does not rule out CMV infection of the fetus.[84] Antiviral treatment with valganciclovir has been shown to be beneficial for hearing loss and neurodevelopmental outcome in symptomatic cases but is not recommended for asymptomatic CMV infection.[85]

Other congenital viral infections

Congenital rubella, though now very rare in countries with an active immunisation programme,[86] causes severe disease (congenital rubella syndrome) in an estimated 105 000 children per year worldwide, mostly in Southeast Asia,[87] although World Health Organization (WHO) estimates are lower than this. Occasional cases of congenital rubella syndrome still occur in high-income countries, including cases where thrombocytopenia is a prominent feature.[88] The frequency of thrombocytopenia due to rubella infection is difficult to determine because blood counts are often not reported. Estimates vary from 10% to 90%,[88–91] with the majority of studies indicating that more than 50% of cases are associated with neonatal thrombocytopenia. A review of a rubella outbreak in the USA in 1964 reported that more than 90% of neonates with congenital rubella syndrome had thrombocytopenia.[91] A retrospective study of severe cases in Japan after a rubella outbreak noted that 76% of neonates had thrombocytopenia[90] and two of the three cases reported in the USA in 2012 also had thrombocytopenia.[92] Infection results from transplacental infection due to primary infection of the mother, with the major risk occurring in the first trimester. As in many congenital infections, the diagnosis is usually suggested by the associated clinical features which, for rubella, are IUGR, sensorineural hearing loss, cardiac defects, hepatosplenomegaly, retinopathy, cataracts and, occasionally, a 'blueberry muffin' skin rash.[87] In neonates the diagnosis is confirmed by PCR for viral DNA and/or virus culture and/or positive rubella-specific immunoglobulin M (IgM) antibodies.[88] Prenatal diagnosis is made by PCR for rubella virus DNA on amniotic fluid, chorionic villus tissue or fetal blood.[93] There is no specific treatment for congenital rubella syndrome or the associated thrombocytopenia.

Congenital parvovirus B19 infection, although more usually associated with isolated fetal anaemia, also not infrequently causes fetal and neonatal thrombocytopenia in addition to anaemia.[71] As with congenital CMV and rubella infection, the likely mechanism of thrombocytopenia is reduced platelet production although the evidence for this is sparse. Thrombocytopenia secondary to congenital mumps infection is also reported but appears to be extremely rare.[94]

By contrast, in congenital herpes simplex infection, thrombocytopenia is due to the associated DIC and occurs where there is disseminated disease.[95] In addition, severe coagulopathy is an important cause of fatality in neonatal herpes simplex infection.[95] Similarly, thrombocytopenia secondary to congenital infection with enteroviruses (coxsackievirus A and B and echovirus) is due to DIC (Case 4.2, see page 230)[96,97] and is a key indicator of severe disease.[98] Importantly, neonatal enterovirus infection may also be complicated by haemophagocytic lymphohistiocytosis (HLH)[99,100] or by bone marrow failure.[101] Sporadic reports describe the successful treatment of enterovirus-associated HLH or of other severe enterovirus infection in neonates by IVIg.[98,100]

Thrombocytopenia is also reported in association with neonatal adenovirus infection, although this is relatively uncommon.[102] A review of hospitalised neonates in Dallas, Texas, USA identified 26 cases over a 17-year period of which 5 (19%) had disseminated disease and a poor outcome while all of the cases with localised respiratory tract disease survived.[102] Notably, thrombocytopenia without any evidence of coagulopathy was present in 4 of 5 neonates with disseminated disease compared with 3 of 19 with localised disease, suggesting that adenovirus infection itself may cause thrombocytopenia directly rather than in conjunction with DIC.

Congenital arbovirus infections, such as dengue, chikungunya virus and zika virus, have also all been reported to cause thrombocytopenia and occasionally to underlie the subsequent development of HLH.[103,104] In a recent series of 32 cases of neonatal dengue, almost 90% of the neonates had a petechial rash and around half had severe thrombocytopenia (platelet count $<20 \times 10^9/l$).[105] Although most cases have only mild bleeding despite severe thrombocytopenia,[105] ICH and gastrointestinal haemorrhage have been reported.[106,107] Importantly, the platelet count may be normal at birth before dropping rapidly during the febrile phase of the disease.[108] This suggests that dengue-associated thrombocytopenia is secondary to increased platelet consumption or destruction. Interestingly, in the series reported by Nguyen and colleagues,[105] just over 10% of the neonates were initially misdiagnosed as neonatal immune thrombocytopenia. Thrombocytopenia is similarly common in congenital chikungunya virus infection. In one of the largest case series, 17 of 19 neonates reported in a study from La Réunion had thrombocytopenia; this was severe in over half of the cases and associated with DIC in half of these.[109] Several of these neonates had major haemorrhage including ICH and gastrointestinal haemorrhage although none died. A recent systematic review which included 28 case reports, 14 small series and a total of 266 cases of congenital chikungunya virus infection found that thrombocytopenia was reported in around one-third of the cases and, in contrast to neonatal dengue, was often associated with major haemorrhage, including ICH, gastrointestinal and pulmonary haemorrhage.[110] This supported the findings of Gerardin *et al.*[109] Thrombocytopenia is also an occasional feature of congenital zika virus infection.[111]

Congenital parasitic infections

Congenital parasitic infection is an uncommon cause of neonatal thrombocytopenia but remains important because of the importance of prompt diagnosis and treatment to prevent further damage. Congenital toxoplasmosis affects between 1 in 2000 and 1 in 3000 newborns, depending on geographical location and dietary practices.[112–114] In contrast to many infections, the risk to the fetus increases with the gestation at which the infection occurs and can be as high as 70% in the third trimester.[115] The classical clinical features of congenital toxoplasmosis are fever, jaundice, hepatosplenomegaly, central nervous system (CNS) disease (microcephaly, intracranial calcification) and ocular disease (microphthalmia, chorioretinitis, cataracts).[116] The incidence of thrombocytopenia in affected neonates is approximately 40%,[113] which is similar to the percentage of fetuses with toxoplasmosis with platelets of less than 100×10^9/l.[117] The mechanism of toxoplasmosis-associated thrombocytopenia is likely to include a combination of reduced platelet production and increased platelet consumption as several cases of associated DIC have been reported in severely affected fetuses and neonates.[117–119] Occasional cases of 'blueberry muffin' skin rash due to congenital toxoplasmosis have also been reported.[120] The recommended treatment for congenital toxoplasmosis is prolonged (12 months) and includes pyrimethamine and sulfadiazine together with folinic acid to prevent pyrimethamine-associated haematological toxicity.[116] Follow-up during treatment should include regular full blood counts because almost half of the infants will develop treatment-related haematological toxicity, including thrombocytopenia, neutropenia and anaemia.[121]

Congenital malaria occurs with all malarial species and remains a common clinical problem in endemic areas[122] as well as an occasional cause of congenital infection in non-endemic countries, where lack of awareness may delay diagnosis.[123,124] The most frequent clinical features are anaemia, fever, hepatosplenomegaly, jaundice and thrombocytopenia, which is often severe.[123–128] The first clinical signs usually appear at 10–28 days after birth but may be delayed by up to 8 weeks.[129] Neonates born to mothers who have been successfully treated for malaria do not need to be screened for congenital malaria unless they develop signs of the disease. Where the mother has not been successfully treated, both the neonate and the placenta should be examined for malarial parasites.

Other congenital infections associated with neonatal thrombocytopenia: tuberculosis and syphilis

Although rare, both congenital tuberculosis and congenital syphilis remain clinical problems because of the high associated mortality if the diagnosis is delayed; both may cause thrombocytopenia.[130,131] In recent years the term 'perinatal' tuberculosis has largely replaced 'congenital' because it is often unclear whether the infection was acquired during the pregnancy or at delivery. While neonates with tuberculosis usually present with non-specific signs of fever, hepatomegaly and respiratory distress, thrombocytopenia in association with DIC has been reported.[132] As in congenital malaria, neonates with tuberculosis usually present at the age of 2–4 weeks and the diagnosis is often difficult, requiring microbial specimens from multiple sites, including gastric aspirates, lymph nodes, endotracheal secretions, bone marrow and/or cerebrospinal fluid.[130]

The numbers of cases of congenital syphilis remain low in many countries[131] but a recent increase in some countries, including in the USA, means that it remains a concern in view of the high morbidity and mortality.[133] Neonates with congenital syphilis typically present 3–4 weeks after birth with clinical features that include rhinitis, hepatosplenomegaly, fever, jaundice, anaemia, thrombocytopenia and a characteristic maculopapular rash on the palms and soles that becomes copper-coloured with desquamation.[134] Thrombocytopenia may be the only sign of disease.[134] However, congenital syphilis may also present with hydrops fetalis[131,134] and a study of fetal syphilis has shown that just over one-third of fetuses have thrombocytopenia.[135] The hepatosplenomegaly results from infiltration by the causative organisms (*Treponema pallidum*)[136,137] and/or extramedullary haemopoiesis and some affected neonates also have a 'blueberry muffin' rash.[131]

Neonatal thrombocytopenia associated with chromosomal abnormalities

Fetal thrombocytopenia is common in aneuploidy. Hohlfeld *et al.*[117] reported frequencies of 86% for trisomy 18, 31% for trisomy 13, 75% for triploidy and 31% for Turner syndrome at fetal diagnosis. Thrombocytopenia was rarely severe, with a platelet count of less than 50×10^9/l seen in only one of the 43 fetal cases reported. Thrombocytopenia is also common in neonates with trisomy 13 and trisomy 18. Wiedmeier and colleagues reported that thrombocytopenia was the most common haematological abnormality detected in a retrospective study of 50 neonates (22 with trisomy 13 and 28 with trisomy 18), although full blood counts were only performed in 24 of them.[138] Of the 12 neonates with trisomy 13 where a platelet count was obtained, 9 (75%) were thrombocytopenic but only 1 developed severe thrombocytopenia (platelet count less than 50×10^9/l). Similarly, of the 12 neonates with trisomy 18, thrombocytopenia was recorded in 10 (83%) and almost all the platelet counts were more than 50×10^9/l. Thrombocytopenia is also reported in neonates with partial trisomies, such as isochromosome 18q.[139] The natural history of thrombocytopenia associated with trisomy 13 or trisomy 18 is not known because the vast majority of neonates do not survive beyond the first few months of life.[140] The mechanism of the thrombocytopenia is also not known, although the pathogenesis may be similar to that seen in neonates with IUGR, given that the majority of neonates with trisomy 13 and trisomy 18 also have IUGR. However, in contrast to the high Hb and NRBC values seen in neonates with IUGR, the majority of neonates with trisomy 13 and trisomy 18 had normal Hb and NRBC values.[138]

The most common chromosomal abnormality associated with neonatal thrombocytopenia is trisomy 21 (Down syndrome). A recent large prospective study reported thrombocytopenia in 51.8% of a cohort of 200 neonates.[141] Approximately 10% of neonates with Down syndrome develop a clonal pre-leukaemic condition called transient abnormal myelopoiesis (TAM), also known as transient myeloproliferative disorder, which is characterised by increased peripheral blood myeloblasts and megakaryoblasts, abnormal megakaryocytes and variable thrombocytopenia (discussed in more detail in Chapter 3). TAM is caused by somatic mutations in the *GATA1* gene, which encodes a transcription factor essential for normal red blood cell and platelet production. An additional 15% of Down syndrome neonates have a clinically and haematologically silent disease ('silent TAM') in which the percentage of peripheral blood blasts is ≤10% and the mutant *GATA1* clone is small.[141] However, as the frequency of neonatal thrombocytopenia in Down syndrome is the same whether *GATA1* mutations are present or not, the presence of thrombocytopenia in a neonate with Down syndrome is not evidence suggestive of TAM or silent TAM.

Inherited thrombocytopenia

The number of known causes of inherited thrombocytopenia has grown very rapidly in recent years with increasing use of next generation sequencing and the formation of national and international consortia that together facilitate the identification and characterisation of previously unexplained familial thrombocytopenias.[142,143] Almost 100 bleeding, thrombotic and platelet disorder genes have now been definitively identified and validated for clinical diagnostics[144] (see also https://www.isth.org/page/GinTh_GeneLists). In neonates, inherited thrombocytopenias typically present either in the context of a more complex genetic disorder where the main features at birth are congenital anomalies (syndromic inherited thrombocytopenias) or they present with isolated thrombocytopenia, usually because of bleeding but sometimes as an incidental finding (reviewed in references 3 and 145). In the majority of cases, thrombocytopenia occurs as a result of impaired megakaryopoiesis and/or abnormal stem cell development. These include several of the disorders known collectively as inherited bone marrow failure syndromes (IBMFS), such as Fanconi anaemia and dyskeratosis congenita, which may present with thrombocytopenia even though the other haemopoietic lineages are also affected. Although the IBMFS very rarely have haematological problems in the neonatal period, the pattern of congenital anomalies present at birth may suggest the diagnosis and prompt specific investigations.[146] In the absence of congenital anomalies, a key clue to a diagnosis of inherited thrombocytopenia is thrombocytopenia that is present at birth and that persists in the absence of other causes for the thrombocytopenia, such as sepsis or NEC.

The principal inherited thrombocytopenias that present in the neonate, rather than later in childhood, are discussed here (see also Table 4.4 for disorders presenting with isolated thrombocytopenia, Table 4.5 for syndromic disorders and Table 4.6 for inherited thrombocytopenias associated with leukaemia and bone marrow failure). All of these disorders are rare. However, precise diagnosis has become more straightforward with the introduction of next generation sequencing into routine diagnosis in many countries although great care has to be taken to make sure that novel variants are fully validated.[143,144,147] Since several of these disorders include increased susceptibility to other severe haematological disorders,

Table 4.4 Inherited thrombocytopenias that may present in neonates as isolated thrombocytopenia

Disease	Gene	Comments
Bernard–Soulier syndrome	*GP1BA** *GP1BB** *GP9*	Autosomal recessive (* rare autosomal dominant forms reported) Macrothrombocytopenia Impaired platelet function
FLI1-related thrombocytopenia	*FLI1*	Autosomal recessive, autosomal dominant or contiguous gene syndrome, Macrothrombocytopenia, giant α granules Impaired platelet function
FYB-related thrombocytopenia	*FYB1*	Autosomal recessive, small platelets
Grey platelet syndrome	*NBEAL2*	Autosomal recessive Macrothrombocytopenia Impaired platelet function
ITGA2B/ITGB3-related thrombocytopenia (Glanzmann thrombasthenia variant)	*ITGA2B/ ITGB3*	Autosomal dominant and recessive forms Macrothrombocytopenia Impaired platelet function
PRKACG-related thrombocytopenia	*PRKACG*	Autosomal recessive, macrothrombocytopenia Impaired platelet function
Thrombocytopenia presenting from infancy		Mild to moderate bleeding/bruising
GFI1B-related	*GFI1B*	Autosomal dominant or recessive
PTPRJ-related	*PTPRJ*	Autosomal recessive
SLFN14-related	*SLFN14*	Autosomal dominant
Mild thrombocytopenias		All autosomal dominant
ACTN1-related	*ACTN1*	All autosomal dominant
CYCS-related	*CYCS*	
IKZF5-related	*IKZF5*	
TRPM7-related	*TRPM7*	No neonatal problems reported
TPM4-related	*TRM4*	
THPO-related	*THPO*	
TUBB1-related	*TUBB1*	

including bone marrow failure and leukaemia, it is important to establish the genetic basis for any unexplained familial thrombocytopenia whenever possible (reviewed in references 148 and 149).

Non-syndromic inherited thrombocytopenia presenting as isolated thrombocytopenia

With the exception of Bernard–Soulier syndrome (BSS), most of the inherited thrombocytopenias that present as isolated thrombocytopenia (Table 4.4) are rarely recognised in the neonatal period unless there is a family history. In all of these disorders the severity of

Table 4.5 Syndromic inherited thrombocytopenias that may present in the neonatal period

Disease	Gene	Comment
Chédiak–Higashi syndrome	*LYST*	Autosomal recessive
		Partial oculocutaneous albinism, predisposition to pyogenic infections, abnormal large granules in many cells, impaired platelet function; usually presents in infancy but bleeding in neonates has been reported
FLNA-associated thrombocytopenia	*FLNA*	X-linked, neonatal lung disease
		Otopalatodigital spectrum disorders
		Brain periventricular nodular heterotopia
		Thrombocytopenia may develop later
Jacobsen syndrome/ Paris–Trousseau thrombocytopenia	Deletions at 11q23	Autosomal dominant
		IUGR, developmental delay, craniofacial abnormalities, malformations of the heart, gastrointestinal tract, urinary tract, CNS and/or skeleton; immunodeficiency
		Impaired platelet function
MYH9-related thrombocytopenia	*MYH9*	Autosomal dominant, Macrothrombocytopenia
		Most patients develop sensorineural deafness (60%), nephropathy (30%) and/or cataracts (20%)
		Neutrophils show Döhle body-like inclusions
Stormorken syndrome/ York platelet syndrome	*STIM1*	Autosomal dominant, tubular aggregate myopathy
		Impaired platelet function
		Mild anaemia, asplenia, miosis, ichthyosis
Thrombocytopenia absent radii syndrome	*RBM8A*	Autosomal recessive, bilateral radial aplasia
		Renal, cardiac ± CNS malformations
		Cow's milk intolerance
		Platelet count may rise over time
Wiskott–Aldrich syndrome and X-linked thrombocytopenia	*WAS*	X-linked, immunodeficiency
		Small or normal sized platelets
X-linked thrombocytopenia with *GATA1* mutation	*GATA1*	X-linked, macrothrombocytopenia
		Anaemia – dyserythropoietic or thalassaemic

CNS, central nervous system; IUGR, intrauterine growth retardation.

bleeding correlates with the degree of thrombocytopenia unless there is associated platelet dysfunction as seen, for example, in BSS and the grey platelet syndrome.[150]

Bernard–Soulier syndrome Bernard–Soulier syndrome, one of the best recognised inherited platelet disorders, not infrequently presents with mild or moderate thrombocytopenia in the neonatal period. BSS is usually an autosomal recessive disorder caused by qualitative or quantitative defects of the glycoprotein (Gp)Ib-IX-V complex, a platelet receptor for von Willebrand factor (VWF), due to mutations in one of the genes

Table 4.6 Inherited thrombocytopenias associated with predisposition to leukaemia, bone marrow failure or both

Disease	Gene	Comment
Congenital amegakaryocytic thrombocytopenia	*MPL*	Autosomal recessive
	THPO (rarely)	All patients develop progressive bone marrow failure (aplastic anaemia)
Familial platelet disorder with predisposition to AML	*RUNX1*	Autosomal dominant
		Normal sized platelets
		>40% develop AML, 25% develop ALL
ANKRD26-related thrombocytopenia	*ANKRD26*	Autosomal dominant
		Normal sized platelets
		~10% develop myeloid malignancies
ETV6-related thrombocytopenia	*ETV6*	Autosomal dominant
		Normal sized platelets
		~30% develop myeloid malignancies, especially ALL
Radio-ulnar synostosis with amegakaryocytic thrombocytopenia	*HOXA11*	Autosomal dominant
		Possible evolution to aplastic anaemia
MECOM-associated syndrome	*MECOM*	Autosomal dominant
		Almost all patients develop bone marrow failure (aplastic anaemia)
Inherited bone marrow failure syndromes (trilineage)		
Fanconi anaemia	22 genes	Autosomal recessive, occasionally X-linked
Dyskeratosis congenita	16 genes	X-linked, autosomal recessive or autosomal dominant

ALL, acute lymphoblastic leukaemia; AML, acute myeloid leukaemia.

encoding components of the complex.[145] To date, bi-allelic mutations in three of these genes – *GP1BA*, *GP1BB* and *GP9* – have been described.[151] Occasional cases of autosomal dominant BSS have also been reported.[152]

Bleeding is not usually severe in the neonatal period but can occur and is typically mucocutaneous, such as bruising, purpura or bleeding associated with minor procedures.[153,154] The key diagnostic sign of BSS is the presence of macrothrombocytopenia on automated analysers and the presence of platelets that often appear larger than, or the same size as, red blood cells in the blood film.[151] The platelet count is usually in the 20–100 $\times 10^9$/l range and often fluctuates.[155] The automated platelet count may underestimate the true platelet count because of the large size of the platelets, and where there is a discrepancy with the blood film appearance, the platelet count may need to be performed manually. The other most useful initial investigation in the neonatal period is demonstration of reduced expression of the GpIb-IX-V complex by platelet flow cytometry using markers for GpIX (CD42a) and GpIbα (CD42b).[156] Treatment by platelet transfusion is effective but should be reserved for life-threatening haemorrhage since transfused patients may form alloantibodies against GpIb, GpIX or GpV.[156] Indeed, platelet alloantibodies are a cause of FNAIT in offspring of mothers with BSS.[157]

Other causes of isolated inherited thrombocytopenia presenting in the neonatal period   Around half of the known genetic causes of isolated thrombocytopenia have been known to present occasionally in neonates with a history of bleeding and/or thrombocytopenia, including *FLI1*-related thrombocytopenia,[158] *FYB*-related thrombocytopenia,[159] grey platelet syndrome due to mutations in *NBEAL2*,[160] *ITGA2B/ITGB3*-related thrombocytopenia[161] and *PRKACG*-related thrombocytopenia.[162] Mutations in the *GFI1b* and *SLFN14* genes can also present in early childhood, with at least one case of each disease reported to have had recurrent episodes of minor bleeding since infancy.[163,164] Other, usually milder, autosomal dominant forms of inherited thrombocytopenia, such as *ACTN1*-related, *CYCS*-related and *IKZF5*, *THPO*, *TRPM7*, *TPM4* and *TUBB1*-related thrombocytopenia have not yet been documented to present in the neonatal period.[145,165]

Syndromic inherited thrombocytopenias that may present in the neonatal period

A number of inherited thrombocytopenias can present with syndromic features during the neonatal period (Table 4.5). These include Wiskott–Aldrich syndrome and its variants, X-linked thrombocytopenia due to *GATA1* mutations, thrombocytopenia with absent radii (TAR) syndrome, Stormorken syndrome and *FLNA*-associated thrombocytopenia (reviewed in references 145 and 149). For other disorders, such as Chédiak–Higashi syndrome (CHS), the disease usually presents later in infancy although neonatal cases have been reported.[166,167]

Chédiak–Higashi syndrome   Chédiak–Higashi syndrome is caused by bi-allelic mutations in the lysosomal trafficking regulator (*LYST*) gene[168] and carries a high risk of progression to HLH.[167] A recent single-centre study of 14 patients found that one-third of the cases presented at or within 1 month of birth and that the median age at which clinical signs appeared was 2 months.[167] CHS is characterised by a combination of partial oculocutaneous albinism, photosensitivity and frequent bacterial infections. Often the first clinical signs are the abnormalities in skin and hair colour and 13 of 14 children in the recent study by Carneiro *et al.*[167] were noted to have silvery hair. Bleeding problems usually develop in infants rather than the newborn, although occasional cases have been reported in association with a known family history.[166] Bleeding is generally attributed to the platelet storage pool defect rather than thrombocytopenia, which may not develop until much later.[169] The diagnosis is established by the presence of giant granules within neutrophils in a peripheral blood film and is confirmed by molecular genetic testing for *LYST* mutation.

FLNA-associated thrombocytopenia   This rare X-linked disorder is caused by mutations in the *FLNA* (filamin A) gene and has been clearly shown to cause thrombocytopenia in adults.[170,171] However, *FLNA*-associated disease in neonates presents with severe interstitial lung disease together with otopalatodigital spectrum disorders, congenital heart disease and/or brain periventricular nodular heterotopia. The perinatal mortality due to these non-haematological complications is very high and the presence of thrombocytopenia is not reported in most of these cases even though it may be a feature in adult survivors.[172] The absence of a bleeding history, despite many of these affected neonates being extremely unwell, suggests that even if thrombocytopenia is present in the neonatal period it is unlikely to be clinically significant.[171,172]

Jacobsen syndrome/Paris–Trousseau thrombocytopenia The Paris–Trousseau syndrome describes the congenital platelet disorder found in more than 90% of patients with Jacobsen syndrome; the remaining 10% or so of patients having syndromic features but without the platelet abnormalities.[173] Jacobsen syndrome is caused by deletion of part of the long arm of chromosome 11 (11q23.3); this contains the *FLI1* and *ETS1* genes but their role in the pathogenesis of the condition is not clear.[158] The platelet disorder is characterised by macrothrombocytopenia with dysmegakaryopoiesis. More than 25 cases have been reported in which presentation of Jacobsen syndrome was before or shortly after birth; the majority of these were thrombocytopenic.[174,175] The severity of the clinical manifestation depends on the extent of the 11q23 deletion and can include IUGR, developmental delay, malformations of the heart, gastrointestinal tract, urinary tract and CNS, and immunodeficiency as well as thrombocytopenia.[173,176] Around 20% of patients die during the first 2 years of life either from congenital heart disease, which is often severe, or less commonly from bleeding.[176] As with several other inherited platelet disorders, in infants that survive the platelet count may spontaneously improve over the first few years of life, although the long-term outlook is unknown.[176]

MYH9-related thrombocytopenia A number of rare giant platelet syndromes caused by mutations in the *MYH9* gene can present with thrombocytopenia in the neonate or fetus.[177] The *MYH9*-related diseases include the conditions previously known as May–Hegglin anomaly, Epstein syndrome, Fechtner syndrome and Sebastian syndrome. These syndromes are autosomal dominant and characterised by macrothrombocytopenia and a high risk of developing deafness (about 60%), nephropathy (about 30%) and cataracts (about 20%) during childhood or later in life.[177] The platelet count varies from less than 20×10^9/l up to normal, but is usually $40–80 \times 10^9$/l. Although *MYH9*-related thrombocytopenia usually presents in older children, thrombocytopenia may be severe enough to cause fetal or neonatal ICH,[178,179] leading to misdiagnosis as FNAIT.[180] The diagnosis is made by observation of Döhle-like bodies in neutrophils together with giant platelets, which may cause inaccurate automated platelet counts.

Stormorken syndrome and York platelet syndrome Both Stormorken syndrome and York platelet syndrome are caused by heterozygous gain-of-function mutations in the *STIM1* gene, which encodes a calcium channel regulating protein. Both syndromes are characterised by tubular aggregate myopathy, thrombocytopenia, hyposplenism or asplenia, miosis, short stature, migraine and ichthyosis and have variable presentations in different patients. Several families in which the thrombocytopenia was present in the neonatal period have been described and where the thrombocytopenia preceded signs of myopathy both in Stormorken syndrome[181] and in York platelet syndrome.[182] In these cases the neonatal thrombocytopenia was severe and in one case was accompanied by petechiae and intraventricular haemorrhage. Electron microscopy of platelets from patients with York platelet syndrome shows characteristic ultrastructural platelet abnormalities including giant organelles and multi-layered target bodies as well as deficiency of platelet calcium storage in the delta granules.[182] Loss-of-function mutations in *STIM1* are also reported but cause a different spectrum of disease characterised by immunodeficiency, muscle hypotonia, hepatosplenomegaly, autoimmune haemolytic anaemia and intermittent, immune-related thrombocytopenia which has occasionally been reported to present within the neonatal period.[183]

Thrombocytopenia with absent radii syndrome Thrombocytopenia with absent radii (reviewed in reference 3) is characterised by bilateral absence of the radii; both thumbs are present, which may be useful in making a distinction from Fanconi anaemia. Most babies with TAR syndrome develop thrombocytopenia within the first week of life. The platelet count is usually less than 50×10^9/l and the white cell count is elevated in more than 90% of patients, sometimes exceeding 100×10^9/l and mimicking congenital leukaemia. There may be anaemia and eosinophilia. There is a high frequency of associated abnormalities, particularly cow's milk intolerance, facial dysmorphism and lower limb anomalies.[184] Although older studies have reported high infant mortality in TAR syndrome, in the study by Greenhalgh and colleagues only 2 of the 34 patients died and only 1 of these was due to major bleeding (ICH),[184] while a recent study of 26 cases of TAR documented only a single death, due to neonatal sepsis at the age of 3 weeks.[185] Those infants that survive the first year of life generally do well, because the platelet count improves spontaneously and is usually maintained at low normal levels thereafter. Inheritance of the TAR syndrome is complex. Both apparently autosomal recessive and autosomal dominant inheritance patterns occur. The majority of cases of apparently autosomal recessive disease are due to coexistence of a microdeletion (either inherited or *de novo*) of chromosome 1q21 including the *RBM8A* gene and one of two rare polymorphisms in the non-coding region of the other *RBM8A* gene, a gene which is involved in RNA processing.[185,186] However, occasional children with the same molecular abnormalities and a TAR-like phenotype but without neonatal thrombocytopenia have recently been described[187] and it is not clear how this genetic abnormality causes the thrombocytopenia and non-haematological features of TAR syndrome.

Wiskott–Aldrich syndrome and X-linked thrombocytopenia Wiskott–Aldrich syndrome and X-linked thrombocytopenia (XLT) together form a spectrum of disorders caused by mutations in the Wiskott–Aldrich syndrome protein gene (*WAS*) on the short arm of the X chromosome (Xp11-12). Over 300 different mutations have been identified.[188] The syndrome typically presents as microthrombocytopenia, eczema, recurrent infections and/ or increased susceptibility to autoimmune disorders in a male infant.[189] Although Wiskott–Aldrich syndrome typically presents in infancy, some cases do present with thrombocytopenia in the neonatal period, usually without bleeding,[190,191] although bleeding after circumcision in the neonatal period has been reported.[192] Later in infancy, the bleeding may be severe and may include gastrointestinal haemorrhage and purpura.[189] Bleeding is due both to the degree of thrombocytopenia and to abnormal platelet function. XLT causes a milder, isolated thrombocytopenia.[193]

X-linked thrombocytopenia due to GATA1 mutation In addition to contributing to TAM and acute megakaryoblastic leukaemia seen specifically in children with Down syndrome (see earlier), *GATA1* mutations also cause two different forms of inherited thrombocytopenia, which differ mainly in their associated red cell abnormalities: XLT with dyserythropoiesis and XLT with β thalassaemia (reviewed in reference 194). XLT with dyserythropoiesis, which is caused by mutations in *GATA1* that affect binding to its cofactor *FOG1*, can present either at birth, with bleeding secondary to severe thrombocytopenia, or as fetal hydrops secondary to the dyserythropoietic anaemia.[195,196] XLT with β thalassaemia is caused by mutations in the N-terminal zinc finger of *GATA1*, which affects DNA binding,[194] and presents towards the end of the first year of life rather than in the neonatal period.[197,198]

Other rare syndromic inherited platelet disorders Mutations in a number of other genes with a wide variety of clinical manifestations, including thrombocytopenia, have also been identified, including those in the *ACTB*, *ARPC1B*, *CDC42*, *GALE*, *KDSR* and *MPIG6B* genes.[149] Although thrombocytopenia during the first year of life is reported for most of these disorders, information about the presentation of these disorders, which are all very rare, in the neonatal period is sparse.

Inherited thrombocytopenias associated with predisposition to leukaemia and bone marrow failure

There is a range of inherited thrombocytopenias that are now known to predispose to other severe haematological disorders, including leukaemia, bone marrow failure (aplastic anaemia) and myelofibrosis (Table 4.6). Almost all patients with congenital amegakaryocytic thrombocytopenia (CAMT) and an unknown proportion of those with radio-ulnar synostosis with amegakaryocytic thrombocytopenia (RUSAT1) progress to bone marrow failure,[199,200] as does *MECOM*-associated syndrome.[201] All of these disorders are briefly summarised below as they typically present during the neonatal period. Several disorders that initially present as isolated thrombocytopenia have a very significant risk of subsequent evolution to acute leukaemia, particularly familial platelet disorder with propensity to acute myeloid leukaemia (FPD/AML),[202,203] *ETV6*-related thrombocytopenia[204] and *ANKRD26*-related thrombocytopenia.[177,205] These disorders more often present later in childhood unless a family history leads to specific screening tests and earlier diagnosis.

Congenital amegakaryocytic thrombocytopenia Congenital amegakaryocytic thrombocytopenia is an autosomal recessive disorder that typically presents at birth with petechiae and/or other evidence of bleeding, thrombocytopenia and morphologically normal platelets.[199] The platelet count is usually less than 20×10^9/l at birth and the bone marrow shows normal cellularity with a specific reduction in megakaryocytes. A recent series of 56 patients with CAMT found that 43 (77%) had thrombocytopenia at birth and most of the affected babies had purpura and/or petechiae.[206] However, 10% of the neonates had severe bleeding including ICH and haematemesis. Physical anomalies are present in around 50% of babies, including CNS and eye anomalies, developmental delay and craniofacial abnormalities.[206] Although the thrombocytopenia in CAMT is usually isolated, in the series described by Germeshausen and Ballmaier,[206] 4 of 56 patients (7%) were also anaemic at birth.

In the majority of patients CAMT is caused by mutation in the *MPL* gene, encoding the thrombopoietin receptor (reviewed in references 200 and 206) or, more rarely, in the thrombopoietin gene (*THPO*).[207] Diagnosis by platelet flow cytometry is feasible but unreliable and genetic confirmation is advisable both because of the risk of leukaemia and aplasia and also to identify cases with mutations in *THPO*, as these children respond to treatment with thrombopoietin mimetics.[207] Almost all CAMT patients subsequently develop aplastic anaemia and the only curative treatment is haemopoietic stem cell transplantation, which is successful in around 80% of cases.[208] Occasional cases of clonal chromosomal abnormalities have been described,[209] suggesting that these children may be at risk of developing myelodysplasia and acute myeloid leukaemia (AML) but the only case of leukaemia reported to date was a B acute lymphoblastic leukaemia (ALL).[210] Rarely, pancytopenia develops in the first month of life.[211] The only treatment for CAMT in the neonatal period is platelet transfusion for bleeding episodes.

Inherited thrombocytopenias with increased susceptibility to leukaemia (FPD/AML, ANKRD26-related thrombocytopenia and ETV6-related thrombocytopenia) This group of inherited thrombocytopenias carry a risk of subsequent development of leukaemia that varies from over 40% in FPD/AML, which is caused by mutations in the *RUNX1* transcription factor gene, to 25–30% in *ETV6*-related thrombocytopenia and 8–10% in *ANKRD26*-related thrombocytopenia.[177, 202–205] All three disorders are autosomal dominant and present with mild to moderate thrombocytopenia with little or no associated bleeding.[212] Although most cases present in adulthood, cases of persistent neonatal thrombocytopenia are reported,[213,214] the diagnosis often prompted by a family history that leads to a full blood count being performed.[215] The first comprehensive *RUNX1* germline registry has recently been established to act as a reference source to assess the clinical and prognostic significance of *RUNX1* variants, including those identified in FPD/AML cases.[216,217] The leukaemias generally present in adulthood and, in families with *ETV6*-related thrombocytopenia and FPD/AML, ALL is reported as well as AML and myelodysplastic syndromes.[204,215] As thrombocytopenia-related bleeding is usually mild or absent, the main value of making the diagnosis in the neonatal period is to put in place haematological follow-up and accurate genetic counselling.[212]

Radio-ulnar synostosis: amegakaryocytic thrombocytopenia and MECOM syndrome Patients with amegakaryocytic thrombocytopenia and radio-ulnar synostosis (ATRUS) present at birth with severe thrombocytopenia, virtually absent bone marrow megakaryocytes and characteristic skeletal abnormalities. In addition to the radio-ulnar synostosis, affected infants may have clinodactyly and shallow acetabulae. Two kindreds show that ATRUS is caused by mutation in the *HOXA11* gene that results in disruption of DNA binding.[218] A second disorder in which radio-ulnar synostosis is associated with inherited thrombocytopenia is MECOM syndrome due to mutations in *MECOM*, the gene that encodes the transcriptional regulators EVI1 and MDS1-EVI1.[201] This condition may present in the neonatal period with severe macrocytic anaemia and very severe thrombocytopenia (platelets less than 10×10^9/l).[201,219]

Other rare inherited thrombocytopenias presenting in the neonatal period   A severe form of inherited thrombocytopenia has recently been shown to be caused by mutations in the *GNE* gene that encodes an enzyme important in sialic acid biosynthesis (UDP-*N*-acetyl-glucosamine 2-epimerase/*N*-acetylmannosamine kinase).[220,221] While some families also have a congenital myopathy others have isolated thrombocytopenia without any evidence of other associated disease.[220,221] Several of the cases have presented in the neonatal period and are notable because of the severity of the thrombocytopenia (platelet count less than 10×10^9/l) and, while bleeding has been reported to be minor,[221] at least one neonate had bilateral intraventricular haemorrhages and long-term neurodevelopmental delay.[220] *DIAPH1*-related thrombocytopenia is a rare form of autosomal dominant thrombocytopenia in which, like *MYH9*-related disease, patients are at risk of developing sensorineural deafness during infancy and some also develop mild transient leucopenia.[222] Cases presenting with bleeding or thrombocytopenia in the neonatal period have not yet been reported. Although *SRC*-related thrombocytopenia is mainly recognised in adults and children and, importantly, is associated with childhood myelofibrosis,[149,223] a recent case of an affected neonate with an autosomal dominant gain-of-function mutation in the *SRC* gene has been reported where the thrombocytopenia was moderate and associated with bilateral cephalohaematomata followed, at the age of 3 months, by a stroke.[224]

Investigation of neonatal thrombocytopenia

We recommend a pragmatic approach to investigating neonatal thrombocytopenia, based on gestational age and age at presentation, to limit over-investigation of mild or self-limiting cases. Figures 4.1 and 4.2 show a practical diagnostic algorithm, which can be applied to the diagnosis and investigation of thrombocytopenia in preterm and term neonates, respectively. The sequence of diagnostic investigations differs in preterm neonates compared with term neonates because of the most frequent causes of neonatal thrombocytopenia are also different in preterm neonates from those in term neonates. For example, isolated thrombocytopenia in a term neonate should immediately raise suspicion of possible FNAIT whereas in preterm neonates FNAIT is usually considered only after other more frequent causes, such as infection, have been excluded (Case 4.3, see page 231). The cause of each episode can usually be determined by a combination of the clinical history, the timing of the onset of thrombocytopenia (Tables 4.1 and 4.2) and the blood count and film. A small proportion of term and preterm neonates (<1%) will have persistent thrombocytopenia and it is these who should have further specialised investigations performed, guided by the presence or absence of dysmorphic features or a family history. The main causes of inherited thrombocytopenia are shown in Tables 4.4–4.6 and next generation sequencing is increasingly used as a more rapid, and ultimately cost effective, way of establishing a precise diagnosis.

Management of neonatal thrombocytopenia

Overall, most episodes of thrombocytopenia are transient, self-limiting and relatively mild and therefore unlikely to have short-term or long-term consequences. Although receiving a platelet transfusion was reported in earlier studies to increase the risk of death in thrombocytopenic neonates,[225] more recent studies show that the relationship between platelet count and risk of bleeding is not straightforward.[14,16,36] The most important clinical factors that affect the frequency of major haemorrhage are low birthweight, prematurity, thrombocytopenia developing in the first 10 days of life and a diagnosis of NEC.[14] The most common site of major haemorrhage in neonates is intracranial (particularly intraventricular), which is documented in about 5% of all thrombocytopenic neonates, while gastrointestinal haemorrhage occurs in 1–5%, pulmonary haemorrhage in 0.6–5% and haematuria in 1–2% of thrombocytopenic neonates.[36] Low birthweight preterm neonates have one of the highest rates of ICH of any age group (up to 25%), and whether the aetiology of the thrombocytopenia is immune or genetic, ICH in the perinatal period is often fatal or leads to long-term neurodevelopmental disability.[5]

Indications for platelet transfusion

Platelet transfusions remain the mainstay of treatment of neonatal thrombocytopenia. The current British Committee for Standards in Haematology (BCSH) guidelines for platelet transfusion[67] employ different platelet transfusion thresholds for neonates predicted to be at 'high' or 'very high' risk of haemorrhage. 'High risk' neonates are those less than 28 weeks' gestation, or with a birthweight less than 1000 g, or who are clinically unstable, are due for planned surgery, or have minor bleeding or coagulopathy. In these children, the transfusion threshold of $25 \times 10^9/l$ is currently recommended. For 'very high risk' neonates, those with active major haemorrhage, who are considered to be at a higher risk of ICH and adverse neurodevelopmental outcome, a threshold of $50 \times 10^9/l$ is recommended (Table 4.7). Although these recommendations remain a useful guide, there have now been a number of carefully conducted studies to evaluate much more precisely the clinical signs and consequences of thrombocytopenia in neonates and to begin to define the most appropriate platelet transfusion thresholds based on more objective measures.

As discussed in detail in several recent reviews, thresholds for neonatal platelet transfusion have been controversial for many years and are likely to continue to change as data from large randomised trials become available.[16,17,226,227] As an example of the complexity of the relationship between bleeding, platelet count and platelet transfusion in neonates, the recent PlaNeT2 MATISSE Collaborators Trial involving more than 600 preterm

Table 4.7 Suggested thresholds of platelet count for neonatal platelet transfusion

Platelet count (×10⁹/l)	Indication for platelet transfusion
<25	Neonates with no bleeding (including neonates with FNAIT if no bleeding and no history of ICH in a sibling)
<50	Neonates with bleeding, current coagulopathy, before surgery, or infants with FNAIT if previously affected sibling with ICH
<100	Neonates with major bleeding or requiring major surgery (e.g. neurosurgery)

ICH, intracranial haemorrhage; FNAIT, fetal/neonatal alloimmune thrombocytopenia.
Adapted from reference 67. New *et al.* (2016) *Br J Haematol*, **175**, 784–828. John Wiley & Sons.

neonates randomised to receive platelet transfusion when their platelet count fell below a previously accepted threshold of 50×10^9/l or to be transfused only when their platelets fell below 25×10^9/l, demonstrated that platelet transfusion at the lower threshold of less than 25×10^9/l was beneficial both in reducing bleeding and the risk of death.[16] At the same time, perhaps unexpectedly, the same trial showed that transfusing platelets to neonates using the higher threshold (i.e. with platelet counts of $25-49 \times 10^9$/l) was associated with an increased risk of bleeding or death.

Platelet function disorders

The principal causes of abnormal platelet function in the neonatal period are summarised in Table 4.8. The majority of platelet function disorders in neonates are acquired and often secondary to various types of therapy. Their true incidence is unknown as they are rarely systematically sought or investigated. Secondary causes of impaired platelet function include a number of drugs, such as indomethacin, which is widely used to treat patent ductus arteriosus in preterm neonates,[228] therapeutic hypothermia, which is used to preserve cerebral function in neonates with perinatal asphyxia,[229] and extracorporeal membrane oxygenation (ECMO).[230] The inherited platelet function disorders that may present in the neonatal period are rare and many also cause thrombocytopenia, as discussed earlier. Abnormal platelet function, whether acquired or inherited, manifests with bleeding, particularly from mucocutaneous sites including the nose and mouth. More severe blood loss may occur as a result of haematuria or gastrointestinal bleeding. Assessment of platelet function in neonates has been notoriously difficult because of the large volumes of blood required for platelet aggregometry and the practical difficulties in performing and interpreting the bleeding time, especially in preterm neonates. These approaches have largely been replaced by next generation sequencing using gene panels containing known pathogenic variants responsible for inherited platelet function disorders.[143,144]

Table 4.8 Causes of abnormal neonatal platelet function

Disease	Specific causes
Acquired	
Drugs	e.g. indomethacin, prostacyclin, sodium valproate
Therapeutic procedures	e.g. ECMO, therapeutic hypothermia (for perinatal asphyxia)
Uraemia	
Inherited	
Glanzmann thrombasthenia	Bi-allelic *ITGA2B/ITGB3* mutations
Leucocyte adhesion deficiency type III	Bi-allelic *FERMT3* mutations
RASGRP2-related disease	Bi-allelic *RASGRP2* mutations

ECMO, extracorporeal membrane oxygenation.

Inherited platelet function disorders with normal platelet counts presenting in the neonate

Inherited disorders of platelet function where the platelet count is normal that may present during the neonatal period include Glanzmann thrombasthenia, leucocyte adhesion deficiency type III and *RASGRP2*-related disease. In contrast, the majority of inherited platelet function disorders present much later, in adulthood. although occasional cases of bleeding in infancy due to bi-allelic mutations in *GP6*, the gene encoding glycoprotein 6, have been reported.[231]

Glanzmann thrombasthenia is caused by bi-allelic mutations in the *ITGA2B* or the *ITGB3* gene. The disease often presents with extensive purpura at or shortly after birth.[232] Diagnosis is based on a combination of the normal platelet count and morphology despite the bleeding phenotype and platelet flow cytometry showing reduced or absent expression of glycoprotein IIb (CD41) and glycoprotein IIIa (CD61). Note that patients with qualitative defects in glycoproteins IIb/IIIa may have normal platelet glycoprotein flow cytometry profiles. Genetic analysis, preferably using a targeted next generation sequencing panel, should also be performed to confirm the diagnosis.[233] Classically, platelets from patients with Glanzmann thrombasthenia fail to aggregate *in vitro* with all agonists apart from ristocetin but in practice these tests are neither necessary nor feasible in neonates. The main differential diagnoses to consider in neonates with suspected Glanzmann thrombasthenia are leucocyte adhesion deficiency type III and *RASGRP2*-related disease, both of which cause similar defects in platelet function and also have normal platelet counts and normal platelet morphology.

Leucocyte deficiency type III is due to bi-allelic mutations in the *FERMT3* gene, which causes an activation defect of β-integrins on both platelets and leucocytes.[234] This disorder also usually presents in the neonatal period with bleeding defects very similar to those in Glanzmann thrombasthenia together with persistent neutrophilia, early-onset bacterial infection and delayed separation of the umbilical cord.[233,235] Prompt diagnosis through a combination of platelet flow cytometry and genetic testing is important because the mortality in the first 2 years of life is more than 75% and haemopoietic stem cell transplantation is curative for both the bleeding disorder and the associated immunodeficiency.[236] *RASGRP2*-related disease is caused by bi-allelic mutations in the *RASGRP2* gene and also typically presents in the neonatal period with mucocutaneous bleeding or bleeding after circumcision. The disease is very rare and in several families has been misdiagnosed as Glanzmann thrombasthenia on the basis of the clinical phenotype; the two diseases are usually distinguishable using platelet flow cytometry, when CD41 and CD61 expression will be normal in *RASGRP2*-related disease.[237]

Thrombocytosis

There is no agreed upper limit of normal for the platelet count in neonates. A large retrospective study of platelet counts retrieved from hospital records in the USA from over 47 000 neonates found that the 95th percentile upper limit was $750 \times 10^9/l$.[238] On the other hand, there is no evidence that platelet counts above this threshold cause an increase in the

Table 4.9 Causes of neonatal thrombocytosis

Conditions	Specific disorders
Acute inflammatory conditions	Kawasaki disease
	Subcutaneous fat necrosis
Infections	SARS-CoV-2
	CMV
Myeloproliferative disorders	TAM
	Familial myeloproliferative neoplasms, e.g essential thrombocythaemia due to *THPO* or *MPL* mutation
Chronic inflammation	Following surgery
	Chronic infection, e.g. osteomyelitis
In utero exposure to drugs	Methadone
	Psychopharmaceutical drugs
	Thiopurines, e.g. azathioprine, mercaptopurine
	Zidovudine

CMV, cytomegalovirus; SARS-CoV-2, severe acute respiratory syndrome coronavirus-2; TAM, transient abnormal myelopoiesis.

risk of thrombosis in neonates. Causes of neonatal thrombocytosis are shown in Table 4.9. The largest systematic study of the causes and implications of extreme thrombocytosis ($>1000 \times 10^9$/l) in neonates was reported by the same group.[239] They found 25 cases in a retrospective review of hospital records from 40 471 neonates (1 in 1600), all of which were judged to be secondary, most often in association with infection and/or surgery, and clinically insignificant. Our experience is similar. In particular, thrombocytosis is more common where there is chronic or prolonged infection, such as osteomyelitis or CMV infection and has also been reported recently after SARS-CoV-2 infection.[240] Thrombocytosis has also been reported as a complication of subcutaneous fat necrosis of the newborn, a form of panniculitis of unclear aetiology.[241]

Although more often presenting later in infancy, a number of cases of Kawasaki disease have been reported in neonates and a recent review of the literature that included 20 neonatal cases found that two-thirds of them had thrombocytosis,[242] although occasional cases of neonatal thrombocytopenia have also been reported.[243] Kawasaki disease characteristically causes acute systemic vasculitis in young children and presents with fever, rash, lymphadenopathy, bilateral conjunctivitis ('red eyes') and peripheral oedema.[242] The pathogenesis of Kawasaki disease remains poorly understood but it is believed to be triggered by viral or bacterial infection and to result from immune dysregulation, which likely drives both the vasculitis and secondary thrombocytosis in infants with an underlying genetic susceptibility. The condition is self-limiting and responds rapidly to treatment with IVIg but a high index of suspicion for the diagnosis is crucial because prompt treatment is essential to prevent long-term cardiac complication.[244]

Of note, neonates with TAM may also develop thrombocytosis,[141] perhaps indicating that the abnormal megakaryoblasts in this condition retain the ability to differentiate into megakaryocytes and platelets. Furthermore, *in utero* acquisition of the *JAK2* V617F variant associated with myeloproliferative neoplasms has been reported in children with essential thrombocythaemia or polycythaemia vera,[245] suggesting that neonates with persistent, unexplained thrombocytosis should be further investigated; however, it should be noted that although the mutation was present at the time of birth in the two reported cases, there were no data available on the platelet count in the neonatal period.[245] By contrast, familial essential thrombocythaemia due to autosomal dominant mutation in the thrombopoietin gene (*THPO*) has been shown to present in the neonatal period, as well as in older children.[246] The platelet count may be elevated at birth or may rise rapidly over the following weeks.[247] In some families the *THPO* mutation and thrombocytosis are also associated with congenital transverse limb abnormalities, such as malformations of the foot or absent digits.[246]

Finally, there have been a number of reports of neonatal thrombocytosis secondary to maternal ingestion, during pregnancy, of drugs such as methadone, psychopharmaceutical drugs, zidovudine and thiopurines, such as azathioprine and mercaptopurine.[248–251]

Abnormalities of coagulation

Neonatal coagulation disorders have been comprehensively detailed in a number of recent reviews[226,252,253] and are only briefly described here. It is important to note that although coagulation and thrombotic problems in the neonate are occasionally inherited, much more often they are secondary to intrauterine or neonatal events. In comparison with older infants and children, neonates are more at risk both of haemorrhage and of thrombosis. This partly reflects the physiologically low levels of many of the coagulation factors and of inhibitors of coagulation, particularly in preterm neonates.[226,252,254]

Developmental haemostasis

The changes in synthesis and activity of the principal coagulation proteins during fetal development were described more than 20 years ago.[255] Most of the principal proteins can be detected from the 10th week of gestation onwards and gradually rise during fetal life. As the coagulation factors do not cross the placenta, or do so only in small quantities, the fetus is reliant on its own ability to synthesise adequate amounts of these proteins. It is important to note that normal values both indicating the functional activity of the major coagulation pathways (e.g. the prothrombin time) and for the individual factors vary with postnatal age as well as gestational age.[256–259] These show that the levels of the vitamin-K-dependent factors (factors II, VII, IX and X) and of factors XI and XII are all low compared with adult values and remain so during the first month of life. Importantly, the levels of factors V and XIII and fibrinogen are similar to adult values at birth, even in preterm babies born at 30–37 weeks' gestation and levels of factor VIII and VWF are normal or increased.

Laboratory investigation of coagulation disorders in the neonate

Most significant bleeding disorders in neonates can be identified using simple screening tests, the exceptions being factor XIII deficiency and platelet function disorders. Suspicion of a coagulation defect in a neonate requires a prothrombin time (PT), activated partial thromboplastin time (APTT), thrombin time (TT), fibrinogen assay and platelet count, with results being compared with a reference range appropriate for the gestational age.[260] It may be useful to test both parents for coagulation abnormalities when an inherited disorder is suspected as there is considerable overlap between coagulation factor levels in inherited or acquired deficiency states and neonatal normal ranges, particularly in preterm neonates. D-dimer levels are not usually helpful for diagnosis because the normal neonatal values are markedly elevated at birth compared with those in older children and adults and only return to the levels seen in older children by 1 month of age.[261] The two most common practical problems in interpreting the results of coagulation screens in the newborn are: the absence of laboratory-specific reference values that reflect the normal ranges for neonates born at different gestations; the frequency of artefacts caused by partially clotted samples; incorrectly filled coagulation screen bottles with the resultant incorrect concentration of anticoagulant; and samples contaminated with heparin from indwelling intravascular catheters.

Acquired coagulation abnormalities

Causes of acquired coagulopathy in neonates include DIC, vitamin K deficiency, liver disease, metabolic disorders and giant haemangioendotheliomas (Kasabach–Merritt syndrome). Uncommonly, a coagulation abnormality in a neonate is the result of transplacental transfer of a maternal inhibitor, such as anti-VWF.[262]

Disseminated intravascular coagulation

The usual pattern of coagulation abnormalities in neonatal DIC is prolongation of the PT, APTT and TT, together with a low platelet count and fibrinogen.[35] The most common causes of DIC in the neonatal period are shown in Table 4.10. Coagulation abnormalities in the first few days of life are most often the result of perinatal hypoxia, for example due to placental abruption, especially where there is HIE. The mechanism

Table 4.10 Causes of disseminated intravascular coagulation (DIC) in neonates

Cause	Condition
Bacterial sepsis/necrotising enterocolitis	Group B *Streptococcus*
	Gram-negative infections
	Necrotising enterocolitis
Congenital infection	Enteroviruses, e.g. coxsackievirus, cytomegalovirus
Perinatal events	Hypoxic ischaemic encephalopathy
	Severe meconium aspiration
	Death of a twin *in utero*
	Twin-to-twin transfusion
	Severe fetomaternal haemorrhage/placental abruption
	Hypothermia

in such cases is DIC which is also a feature of NEC, severe sepsis and some types of congenital viral infection, such as that caused by coxsackievirus (see Case 4.2) and chikungunya virus. DIC may also complicate twin pregnancies either through retention of a dead second twin, which can trigger DIC in the surviving twin, or through hyperviscosity in the recipient twin of twin-to-twin transfusion. The vast majority of neonates with DIC are clinically very unwell and bleeding is often generalised from multiple sites, including oozing from venepuncture sites. Pulmonary haemorrhage is a major cause of death.

Vitamin K deficiency

Vitamin K deficiency remains an important cause of bleeding problems in the newborn (reviewed in references 226 and 263). Levels of vitamin K-dependent procoagulant factors (factors II, VII, IX and X), protein C and protein S are low at and after birth because of poor placental transfer of vitamin K, low vitamin K stores at birth, low vitamin K in breast milk and the lack of bacterial vitamin K synthesis in the sterile neonatal gut. Classical vitamin K-dependent bleeding (VKDB), also termed haemorrhagic disease of the newborn, typically presents with ICH or gastrointestinal bleeding 2–7 days after birth and affects babies who have not received prophylactic vitamin K at birth, especially if breastfed or with poor oral intake. The deficiency may be even more severe in neonates of mothers on anticonvulsant therapy. Late VKDB occurs between 2 and 8 weeks after birth and usually presents with ICH in an otherwise well, breastfed term baby or in babies with malabsorption or liver disease. These infants may present with prolonged or excessive bleeding after circumcision as well as ICH or gastrointestinal bleeding.

The diagnosis of vitamin K deficiency is usually straightforward. The most useful indicator is the presence of an isolated prolonged PT, which corrects following vitamin K administration. Importantly, the results of these tests need to be interpreted with reference to gestational age control values. In cases where there is any doubt, assays of the inactive form of factor II (undercarboxylated prothrombin; PIVKA-II [protein induced by vitamin K absence or antagonist]) can be used to confirm the diagnosis. Treatment of VKDB is vitamin K 1 mg intravenously or subcutaneously with fresh frozen plasma (FFP) only in the case of severe haemorrhage.

As part of an ongoing WHO project on child health care, existing recommendations for vitamin K prophylaxis in the prevention of haemorrhagic disease of the newborn were recently reviewed.[264] In the UK, the National Institute for Health and Care Excellence (NICE) recommends that, for prevention of haemorrhagic disease of the newborn, all full-term babies should receive 1 mg of intramuscular vitamin K (phytomenadione) prophylactically at or soon after birth. A lower dose is appropriate for babies of less than 36 weeks' gestation. If the mother declines intramuscular vitamin K, oral vitamin K should be offered, multiple doses then being required (e.g. 2 mg at birth, at 4–7 days and at 1 month). Incidence of deficiency has been estimated at 0.64 per 100 000 live births; around half of cases are attributable to no prophylaxis being given, mainly because parental consent has been withheld.[265] The need for administration of vitamin K is greater in breastfed infants because infant formulae are fortified. Parenteral rather than oral vitamin K is particularly important in babies with unrecognised biliary atresia[266] or other causes of malabsorption.

Inherited coagulation disorders

The most common inherited coagulation disorders presenting in the neonatal period are factor VIII deficiency (haemophilia A), which has a frequency of 1 in 5000 male births, and factor IX deficiency (haemophilia B), which occurs in 1 in 30 000 male births. Other inherited coagulation disorders that can present in the neonate include some types of von Willebrand disease, severe hypofibrinogenaemia, factor XIII deficiency and combined factor V and factor VIII deficiency. The most serious complication of these disorders is ICH (reviewed in reference 267). Other clinical presentations in the neonatal period include: cephalohaematoma; bleeding at the sites of venepuncture, heel-prick or intramuscular injections; gastrointestinal haemorrhage and bleeding following circumcision (reviewed in references 268 and 269). Up to half of babies with haemophilia A present in the first month of life.[268] The presentation of haemophilia B in the neonate is similar to that of haemophilia A.

If haemophilia A or B is suspected or has already been confirmed by antenatal diagnosis, close collaboration between obstetricians, neonatologists and haematologists to manage both the pregnancy and delivery is essential. A number of consensus national and international guidelines are available.[267,269–272] A peripheral blood or cord blood sample should be obtained for an APTT and urgent factor assay and intramuscular vitamin K should be withheld until the results of the assay are available.[65] Treatment should be with the relevant recombinant factor.

The two types of von Willebrand disease (VWD) that may present in the neonatal period are type 2B VWD and type 3 VWD. Type 3 VWD presents with similar clinical findings to haemophilia, as levels of both VWF and factor VIII are low. In contrast to haemophilia A and B, type 2B VWD is autosomal recessive and may therefore cause initial diagnostic uncertainty in male neonates. Presentation may be with cephalohaematoma, cheek haematoma (following suckling), post-venepuncture bleeding, conjunctival haemorrhage and bleeding from the umbilical stump or following circumcision.[273] The diagnosis is made by measuring VWF, factor VIII and the pattern of VWF multimers. At present, type 3 VWD is treated with a high purity VWF:factor VIII concentrate (such as Wilate). Type 2B disease is rare and typically presents with thrombocytopenia.

Factor XIII deficiency and severe hypofibrinogenaemia show a particular association with umbilical cord bleeding and delayed separation of the cord. Importantly, factor XIII deficiency is an important cause of perinatal ICH, a recent report noting that almost half of the 27 neonates in a retrospective study had CNS bleeding.[274] In addition, as for many severe inherited coagulation and platelet disorders, factor XIII deficiency may present with bleeding following circumcision.[275] The inheritance is autosomal recessive. The diagnosis of factor XIII deficiency is made using a screening test based on measuring clot solubility in 5 mol/l urea solution followed by assay of factor XIII levels; routine coagulation tests (APTT, PT and TT) are normal. The diagnosis can be confirmed using next generation sequencing to detect mutation of *F13A1* or *F13B*, the genes encoding the subunits of factor XIII. Bleeding is treated with factor XIII concentrate. A number of other rare deficiencies may also present with umbilical cord bleeding and/or delayed separation of the cord, including factor V deficiency, combined factor V and factor VIII deficiency, factor X deficiency and inherited deficiency of all vitamin K-dependent factors.[276]

Thrombosis

Neonates have an increased risk of thrombosis compared with older infants and children. This is mainly due to the physiologically low levels of many of the inhibitors of coagulation and the use of indwelling vascular catheters. Concentrations of antithrombin, heparin cofactor II and protein C are decreased at birth compared with those in older children and adults; protein S levels are also low due to the virtual absence of its binding protein (C4b-BP), but overall protein S activity is normal as it exists mainly in its free active form. Plasminogen levels at birth are only 50% of adult values so neonates have a reduced ability to generate plasmin in response to fibrinolytic agents. Neonatal thrombotic disorders have been comprehensively detailed in a number of recent reviews[277–282] and are only briefly described here. The International Pediatric Thrombosis Network is an additional source of useful and up-to-date information: https://www.isth.org/iptn.

Screening tests for thrombophilia in neonates

The only inherited deficiencies for which there is a proven role in neonatal thrombosis are deficiencies in protein C, protein S and antithrombin. Homozygous protein C deficiency and homozygous protein S deficiency can both cause purpura fulminans. Homozygous antithrombin deficiency usually presents with thrombosis much later in childhood but neonatal thrombosis has been reported.[282] Specific mutations in the factor V gene (factor V Leiden) and the prothrombin gene (*F2* G20210A) are known prothrombotic risk factors in adults but have not yet been reported to cause neonatal thrombotic problems in isolation.

Guidelines from the Haemostasis and Thrombosis Task Force of the BCSH state that congenital thrombophilia should be considered and screened for where there is a family history of neonatal purpura fulminans or in any child with clinically significant thrombosis, including spontaneous thrombotic events, unanticipated or extensive venous thrombosis, ischaemic skin lesions or purpura fulminans.[280] Importantly, thrombosis related to an intravascular catheter has been shown not to predict an underlying inherited thrombophilia and investigation is not currently recommended unless there is a family history or other risk factors suggestive of an underlying congenital deficiency.[278] Similarly, although controversial for many years, well-designed case-control studies have clearly shown that thrombophilia is not associated with a risk of perinatal stroke.[283,284]

The screening tests that should be performed in all suspected cases of neonatal thrombophilia are assays of protein C, protein S and antithrombin.[270,285] In addition, babies with thrombosis born to mothers with SLE and/or antiphospholipid syndrome should be tested for lupus anticoagulant, as antiphospholipid antibodies may cross the placenta and are a rare cause of neonatal thrombosis in such babies. The value of molecular analysis to identify the factor V Leiden and the prothrombin *F2* G20210A mutation in neonates is still unclear and such testing is not routinely recommended.[7] The relevance of serum lipoprotein a and of the *MTHFR* (methylenetetrahydrofolate reductase) genotype to neonatal management is unclear at present.

Acquired thrombotic abnormalities

The most common risk factors for neonatal thrombosis are the presence of an intravascular catheter and shock secondary to sepsis, hypoxaemia or hypovolaemia.[281,286] Catheter-related thrombosis causes more than 80% of venous thromboses and more than 90% of arterial thromboses in neonates.[278] Renal vein thrombosis, which may be bilateral, is the most common thrombotic event unrelated to the presence of a catheter, with presentation being with haematuria, proteinuria and a loin mass;[287] renal atrophy, hypertension and impaired renal function are frequent consequences.[287,288] Other sites of thrombosis include the aorta or aortic arch, cerebral vessels and intracardiac; the latter may be complicated by venous obstruction, pulmonary embolism or peripheral embolism. The diagnosis is made by Doppler ultrasound or contrast angiography.

Treatment of catheter-related thrombosis depends on the severity and extent of thrombosis and is based on prompt catheter removal as the first step.[289] If signs progress despite removal, unfractionated heparin, low molecular weight heparin or thrombolytic therapy with urokinase or tissue plasminogen activator may be used. It is important to maintain fibrinogen at levels lower than 1 g/l and the platelet count greater than 50×10^9/l in neonates receiving thrombolytic therapy. Excellent guidelines for antithrombotic therapy in neonates have been published by the American Society for Hematology[279] and the special considerations needed for preterm neonates in particular are reviewed in reference 285. Most recently, direct inhibitors of activated factor Xa or thrombin, such as rivaroxaban or bivalirudin, have been introduced as alternatives to heparin and thrombolytics, but experience in neonates is extremely limited.[285,290]

Inherited thrombotic abnormalities

Protein C deficiency occurs in 1 in 160 000–360 000 births. It is caused by bi-allelic mutations in the *PROC* gene and usually presents within hours or days of birth with purpura fulminans (defined as haemorrhagic necrosis of the skin resulting from dermal thrombosis), stroke (thrombosis or haemorrhage), ophthalmic damage and hypotension.[291,292] There is not only thrombosis but also haemorrhage as a result of DIC and thrombocytopenia may be severe. The skin lesions are caused by rapidly progressive life-threatening haemorrhagic necrosis due to dermal vessel thrombosis. The diagnosis of protein C deficiency is made from the clinical features and undetectable levels of protein C (<0.01 u/ml), together with heterozygote levels in the parents. Therapy with subcutaneous protein C concentrate (40 u/kg, aiming to maintain a plasma level >0.25 u/ml) is effective but irreversible tissue damage, leading to hemiplegia or blindness, may already have occurred, sometimes *in utero*.[291] Heterozygosity for protein C deficiency can predispose to neonatal venous thrombosis. However protein-C-deficient heterozygotes rarely present as neonates and their protein C levels can overlap with the lower limit of normal in the first few months of life, delaying diagnosis until 6 months or later. Homozygosity for protein S deficiency has a similar clinical presentation with purpura fulminans but low or undetectable levels of protein S. Treatment is with FFP (10–20 ml/kg every 12 hours) until the lesions resolve. In the long term, severe deficiency of protein C or S can be treated with oral anticoagulants.

Homozygous antithrombin deficiency is extremely rare. It may present with neonatal deep vein thrombosis and inferior vena cava thrombosis but more often manifests later in childhood. Heterozygous antithrombin deficiency may also present with arterial or venous thrombosis in the neonatal period; aortic and middle cerebral artery thrombosis, myocardial infarction, cerebral dural sinus and renal vein thrombosis have all been reported in neonates,[282] particularly following instrumental delivery[293] although presentation in the second decade of life is much more typical.

General principles of neonatal platelet and plasma component transfusion

The importance of restricting transfusions to those neonates most likely to benefit is increasingly recognised. The general principles governing this more cautious approach to transfusion in neonates have been described in detail in several recent reviews and national guidelines as well as in international consensus statements.[67,227,294–297] Red cell transfusion approaches that have proved successful include late clamping of the umbilical cord (unless resuscitation is needed) and limiting the volume of blood taken for laboratory tests to a minimum as discussed in Chapter 2.[298,299] For platelet transfusion the emphasis has been on rigorously evaluating the relevance of the platelet count to the risk of bleeding.[300]

Additional points to consider when transfusion of any blood component or blood product to a neonate is planned include the need for extra care with identification of a neonate's blood sample because of the increased risks of misidentification that arise from name changes in babies and confusion between a maternal specimen and a baby's specimen. When intrauterine transfusion has previously been employed, blood components for transfusion in a neonate should always be irradiated to avoid the risk of transfusion-associated graft-versus-host disease. Otherwise, routine irradiation of blood products for transfusion to neonates is not necessary. The principles and indications for neonatal red cell transfusion are discussed in Chapter 2 and summarised in Table 2.17.

Platelet transfusion

Platelets for use in neonates are leuco-depleted, are from CMV-negative donors and are usually obtained by apheresis of selected donors who lack high-titre anti-A and anti-B. Platelet transfusion is required for thrombocytopenic babies with bleeding; a transfusion threshold of $<50 \times 10^9/l$ is suggested.[67] The threshold for prophylactic transfusion depends on the indications and detailed guidance is available for asymptomatic babies with severe thrombocytopenia and those requiring lumbar puncture or minor or major surgery.[67] Recent data point to the value of a restrictive policy for neonatal platelet transfusion.[16]

Fresh frozen plasma

In many countries FFP for neonates and infants is pathogen-inactivated (solvent detergent or methylene blue), negative for high-titre anti-A and anti-B antibodies and sourced from male donors.[67] FFP may be required in the management of DIC and when there is bleeding in neonates with abnormal coagulation tests. Its use may be appropriate in DIC, in the presence of bleeding, when the fibrinogen concentration is less than 1.0 g/l or when the PT or

APTT is prolonged to more than 1.5 times the midpoint of an appropriate reference range.[21] FFP is required for congenital factor deficiencies and for purpura fulminans resulting from protein S or protein C deficiency when the specific concentrate is not available.[226] FFP is often over-used in NICUs for babies with abnormal laboratory tests but without bleeding or the need for invasive procedures.[67,226,301] FFP should not be used for volume replacement.

Cryoprecipitate

Cryoprecipitate contains fibrinogen, factor VIII, VWF, factor XIII and fibronectin. It is pathogen-inactivated with methylene blue and in the UK is now from male donors only.[67] Cryoprecipitate is required for severe hypofibrinogenaemia and may be required in DIC. A threshold fibrinogen concentration of 1 g/l is advised unless there is rapid consumption of fibrinogen, when a higher threshold may be advisable. Fibrinogen concentrate is licensed in the UK for congenital hypofibrinogenaemia but in the acute situation, in a neonate, cryoprecipitate is more likely to be used.

Prothrombin complex and recombinant factor VIIa

Four-factor prothrombin complex concentrate (PCC), which contains factors II, IX and X and a variable concentration of factor VII, is now the preferred product, in addition to vitamin K, for patients with bleeding due to vitamin K deficiency. Small retrospective studies and case reports have shown that PCC is effective in neonates[302] but there are no data from randomised controlled studies in this population. Similarly, a number of retrospective studies have reported good responses to recombinant factor VIIa (rFVIIa) in preterm and term neonates with intractable bleeding and severe coagulopathy.[303,304] However, there are no data available at present to identify the specific indications and safety of rFVIIa in neonates.[226]

Illustrative cases

(For abbreviations used in the text of the illustrative cases, see page 233–234.)

Case 4.1   Cytomegalovirus infection: more than one cause of thrombocytopenia

Case history

A male neonate born at 28 weeks' gestation after an uneventful pregnancy was admitted to the neonatal unit with mild tachypnoea. His birthweight was normal (1200 g) and, apart from occasional petechiae on his chest, he had no abnormal clinical findings. In particular, no congenital anomalies were noted and he had no dysmorphic features. He was the third child of unrelated Caucasian parents and there was no family history of note. Both his siblings were well and had had no neonatal problems. A routine FBC revealed isolated thrombocytopenia.

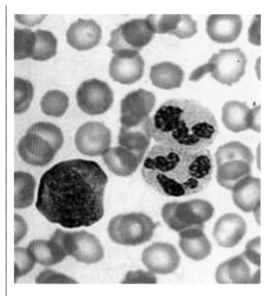

Case 4.1, Fig. 1   Blood film at presentation. MGG, ×100 objective.

Investigations

FBC: WBC 14.2 × 10^9/l, Hb 140 g/l, MCV 112 fl, MCH 37 pg, neutrophils 7.1 × 10^9/l, lymphocytes 6.0 × 10^9/l, monocytes 0.8 × 10^9/l, eosinophils 0.25 × 10^9/l, platelets 50 × 10^9/l. His blood film (Case 4.1, Fig. 1) showed atypical lymphocytes, which appeared reactive. The maternal platelet count was normal. Investigations to identify FNAIT revealed no maternal–neonatal HPA incompatibility. A TORCH screen was positive for CMV in the urine by PCR, confirming a diagnosis of congenital CMV infection.

Progress

Daily platelet counts were performed because of the thrombocytopenia and over the course of the next 2–3 days the platelet count fell progressively to 25 × 10^9/l. He was given a platelet transfusion and his blood count continue to be monitored daily through an intravenous line. Although he was clinically stable, by day 14 of life his FBC was as follows: Hb 85 g/l, WBC 9 × 10^9/l, neutrophils 5.8 × 10^9/l, lymphocytes 2 × 10^9/l, monocytes 0.8 × 10^9/l, eosinophils 0.2 × 10^9/l, platelets 148 × 10^9/l. The fall in Hb was attributed to anaemia of prematurity together with iatrogenic blood loss due to repeated phlebotomy and he was given a top-up transfusion. Two days later, on day 17 of life, he developed a low-grade fever and repeat FBC showed: Hb 125 g/l, WBC 15.8 × 10^9/l, neutrophils 11.8 × 10^9/l, lymphocytes 2 × 10^9/l, monocytes 1.4 × 10^9/l, eosinophils 0.6 × 10^9/l, platelets 70 × 10^9/l. PCR for CMV in the urine was negative and no atypical lymphocytes were seen in the blood film. However, careful review of the blood film showed neutrophil vacuolation with some vacuoles containing bacteria (Case 4.1, Fig. 2) and blood cultures collected on the same day grew *Staphylococcus epidermidis*. After removal of the intravenous line and a course of antibiotics the FBC returned to

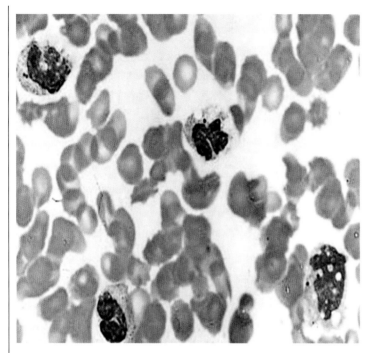

Case 4.1, Fig. 2   Blood film at day 17. MGG,×100.

normal by day 23 of life, strongly suggesting that the second episode of thrombocyto-penia in this case was caused by systemic infection with *Staphylococcus epidermidis*, especially since the urine tests for CMV were no longer positive.

Diagnostic notes

- Congenital CMV infection is common, occurring worldwide in 1 in 100 to 1 in 200 livebirths, and may be due either to primary infection of the mother during preg-nancy or to reactivation or reinfection of the mother during pregnancy.[76]
- Primary infection of the mother with CMV during pregnancy carries a risk of *in utero* transmission of CMV of 30–35%; reactivation of CMV in the mother carries a lower risk of *in utero* transmission (12%).[305]
- The majority of neonates with congenital CMV infection have no clinical findings at birth; thrombocytopenia is the most common haematological complication of CMV infection.[76]
- All cases of congenital CMV infection should be closely followed up because of the long-term risks of sensorineural hearing loss, chorioretinitis, cognitive impairment and cerebral palsy.
- Antiviral treatment is not recommended for asymptomatic CMV infection, including isolated thrombocytopenia, but has been shown to be beneficial for reducing hearing loss and improving neurodevelopmental outcome in cases with clinical signs of disease.[85]

Case 4.2   Congenital coxsackievirus infection with disseminated intravascular coagulation

---

Case history

A male neonate born at 32 weeks' gestation after an apparently uneventful pregnancy was admitted to the neonatal unit for monitoring and investigation as he was noted to have a fever, respiratory distress, tachycardia and cardiomegaly a few hours after birth. On admission he was unwell and irritable, he had mild hepatomegaly and jaundice and a petechial rash. There were no other abnormal clinical findings. He was the first child of unrelated Caucasian parents and there was no family history of note.

Preliminary investigations

FBC: WBC 11.5 × 10^9/l, Hb 140 g/l, MCV 103 fl, MCH 34 pg, neutrophils 2.1 × 10^9/l, lymphocytes 8.0 × 10^9/l, monocytes 1.0 × 10^9/l, eosinophils 0.3 × 10^9/l, platelets 6 × 10^9/l. The blood film showed a large number of schistocytes, occasional spherocytes and some echinocytes. The neutrophils were left shifted with no toxic granulation or vacuolation and there was a moderate lymphocytosis. Most of the lymphocytes were large with deeply basophilic cytoplasm (Case 4.2, Fig. 1). Few platelets were seen, consistent with the severe thrombocytopenia shown in the automated blood count. A TORCH screen for congenital infection (toxoplasmosis, rubella, CMV, herpes simplex) was performed and was negative.

Further investigations

The severe thrombocytopenia in an unwell neonate with signs suggestive of acute infection prompted the clinicians to perform coagulation studies which showed a PT of 36 seconds (normal range 12–22 seconds), an APTT of 110 seconds (normal range

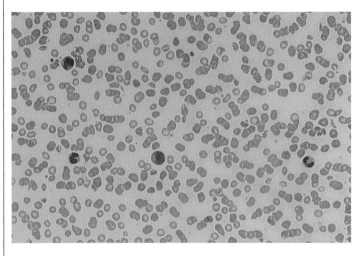

Case 4.2, Fig. 1   Blood film at presentation. MGG, ×40 objective.

36–55 seconds) and a fibrinogen of 0.3 g/l (normal range 1.5–4 g/l), consistent with a diagnosis of DIC. Liver function tests showed a moderately raised bilirubin (210 µmol/l) and aspartate aminotransferase (800 iu/l). Blood cultures were repeatedly negative. CSF examination showed a pleomorphic lymphocytosis. Investigations for maternal–neonatal HPA incompatibility excluded a diagnosis of FNAIT. Review of the maternal history confirmed that her platelet count had been normal throughout pregnancy and she had no history of autoimmune disease. However, she did recall having been unwell with a mild diarrhoeal illness a week before delivery. Maternal serology and virological investigation of the CSF sample confirmed a diagnosis of congenital coxsackievirus infection due to recent maternal infection. In view of the severity of his coagulopathy and deteriorating liver function, the baby was treated with intravenous immunoglobulin (0.5 g/kg/day total dose 2 g/kg) as well as platelet transfusion and FFP and made a full recovery.

Diagnostic notes

- In neonates with signs of acute infection and negative blood cultures, specific tests for enterovirus infection should be considered as several series have indicated that up to 40% of sepsis-like illness in neonates is due to enterovirus infection.[276]
- In addition to non-specific signs of infection (fever, lethargy, poor feeding), enterovirus infections may present with a rash, meningitis, myocarditis and/or hepatitis.[276]
- Neonatal enterovirus-mediated hepatitis may be complicated by worsening liver function and DIC and retrospective studies suggest that early administration of IVIg may improve the chance of survival in such neonates[98] but neither the dose nor indications for therapy have been established in controlled clinical trials.[97]

Case 4.3   Fetal/neonatal alloimmune thrombocytopenia in a preterm baby

Case history

A female neonate born at 30 weeks' gestation was noted to have diffuse petechiae over her chest and abdomen at birth. The pregnancy had been uneventful and, in particular, there was no history of maternal hypertension or diabetes, although the mother reported a mild upper respiratory infection a week prior to delivery. On examination, the baby looked generally well, she had no other evidence of overt bleeding and her temperature was normal. She had no hepatosplenomegaly and no dysmorphic features. Her birthweight was normal for gestation (1.4 kg). She was the first child of unrelated Caucasian parents and there was no family history of note. An FBC revealed isolated thrombocytopenia and a provisional diagnosis of congenital infection was made.

Investigations

FBC: Hb 158 g/l, MCV 102 fl, MCH 34.5 pg, WBC 17.6×10^9/l, neutrophils 11.8×10^9/l, lymphocytes 4.2×10^9/l, monocytes 1.2×10^9/l, eosinophils 0.2×10^9/l, platelets 16×10^9/l.

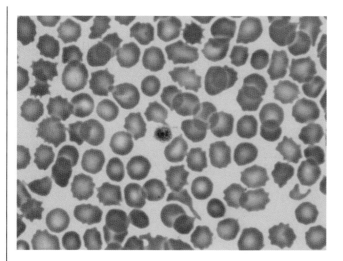

Case 4.3, Fig. 1 Blood film at presentation. MGG, ×100.

To exclude the presence of a clot in the sample, the FBC was repeated and confirmed the thrombocytopenia (12×10^9/l). Review of the blood film showed no abnormalities apart from an isolated thrombocytopenia. Platelet size and morphology appeared normal on the blood film with some larger but no giant platelets (Case 4.3, Fig. 1). A TORCH screen to identify congenital infection showed no evidence of infection with toxoplasma, rubella, CMV or herpes simplex virus. Blood and urine cultures showed no evidence of bacterial or fungal infection. While this was in progress, she was given a platelet transfusion; on the advice of the haematologist, HPA-1a- and 5b-negative platelets were given since a diagnosis of FNAIT had not been excluded. A cranial ultrasound was arranged and showed no evidence of intracranial bleeding. The mother's platelet count was also checked and found to be normal and there was no maternal history of previous ITP or other autoimmune disorders. In the absence of evidence of infection or placental insufficiency (IUGR or maternal disease) a provisional diagnosis of FNAIT was made and further investigations were arranged.

Progress

Blood samples from the baby and both parents were sent to the local reference laboratory for platelet genotyping and to test the mother's serum for anti-HPA antibodies. This showed that both the baby and her father were HPA-1a positive while the mother was HPA-1a negative and anti-HPA-1a antibodies were detected in her serum, confirming a diagnosis of FNAIT due to anti-HPA-1a. Serial FBCs were performed to monitor the platelet count and showed a good response to platelet transfusion but a subsequent fall over the ensuing week to 67×10^9/l before a rapid recovery to normal levels by 14 days of age. The parents were counselled about the likelihood of recurrence in any subsequent pregnancies and the advisability of early referral to a specialised centre for advice and management. Follow-up in the paediatric clinic at 6 and 12 months of age indicated that the baby had reached all her developmental milestones as expected.

Serial FBCs:

Age (days)	0	0 (post-platelet transfusion)	3	7	10	14
Hb (g/l)	158	160	154	148	147	143
Platelets (×10⁹/l)	16	170	80	67	89	202

Diagnostic notes

- FNAIT should be considered in any neonate with severe unexplained thrombocytopenia at birth; investigations should always include a cranial ultrasound to identify those neonates with intracranial haemorrhage as the majority of these will have long-term neurodevelopmental problems, including cerebral palsy, deadness, blindness and cognitive delay.[306]
- The absence of congenital anomalies and any signs of infection are early clues to a diagnosis of FNAIT.
- In Caucasian populations, where 95% of cases of FNAIT are caused by antibodies to HPA-1a or HPA-5b, platelet transfusions if required, should be negative for both of these antigens. The post-transfusion platelet increment is significantly less after random donor platelets compared with HPA-matched platelets,[20] but whether the type of transfusion influences the long-term outcome has not been determined.

Abbreviations used in the illustrative cases

APTT	activated partial thromboplastin time
CMV	cytomegalovirus
CSF	cerebrospinal fluid
DIC	disseminated intravascular coagulation
FBC	full blood count
FFP	fresh frozen plasma
FNAIT	fetal/neonatal alloimmune thrombocytopenia
Hb	haemoglobin concentration
HPA	human platelet antigen
ITP	autoimmune thrombocytopenic purpura
IVIg	intravenous immunoglobulin
IUGR	intrauterine growth retardation
MCH	mean cell haemoglobin
MCV	mean cell volume
MGG	May–Grünwald–Giemsa
PCR	polymerase chain reaction

234 *Neonatal Haematology: A Practical Guide*

PT   prothrombin time
TORCH toxoplasmosis, other infections, rubella, cytomegalovirus, herpes simplex
WBC   white cell count

References

1 Roberts I, Stanworth S and Murray NA (2008) Thrombocytopenia in the neonate. *Blood Rev*, **22**, 173–186.

2 Cremer M, Sallmon H, Kling PJ, Bührer C and Dame C (2016) Thrombocytopenia and platelet transfusion in the neonate. *Semin Fetal Neonatal Med*, **21**, 10–18.

3 Roberts IAG and Chakravorty S (2019) Thrombocytopenia in the newborn. In: Michelson AD (ed.), *Platelets*, 4th edn. Academic Press, New York, pp. 813–831.

4 de Moerloose P, Boehlen F, Extermann P and Hohlfeld P (1998) Neonatal thrombocytopenia: incidence and characterization of maternal antiplatelet antibodies by MAIPA assay. *Br J Haematol*, **100**, 735–740.

5 Chakravorty S and Roberts I (2012) How I manage neonatal thrombocytopenia. *Br J Haematol*, **156**, 155–162.

6 Baer VL, Lambert, DK, Henry E and Christensen RD (2009) Severe thrombocytopenia in the NICU. *Pediatrics*, **124**, e1095–e1100.

7 Rastogi S, Olmez I, Bhutada A and Rastogi D (2011) NCI classification of thrombocytopenia in extremely preterm neonates and its association with mortality and morbidity. *J Perinat Med*, **39**, 65–69.

8 Murray NA and Roberts IAG (1996) Circulating megakaryocytes and their progenitors in early thrombocytopenia preterm neonates. *Pediatr Res*, **40**, 112–119.

9 Stanworth SJ, Clarke P, Watts T, Ballard S, Choo L, Morris T *et al.* (2009) Prospective, observational study of outcomes in neonates with severe thrombocytopenia. *Paediatrics*, **124**, 826–834.

10 von Lindern JS, van den Bruele T, Lopriore E and Walther FJ (2011) Thrombocytopenia in neonates and the risk of intraventricular hemorrhage: a retrospective cohort study. *BMC Pediatr*, **11**, 16.

11 Chiurazzi F, Villa MR and Rotoli B (1999) Transplacental transmission of EDTA-dependent pseudothrombocytopenia. *Haematologica*, **84**, 664–665.

12 Ohno N, Kobayashi M, Hayakawa S, Utsonomiya A and Karakawa S (2012) Transient pseudothrombocytopenia in a neonate: transmission of a maternal EDTA-dependent anticoagulant. *Platelets*, **23**, 399–400.

13 Christensen R, Sola MC, Rimsza LM, McMahan MJ and Calhoun DA (2004) Pseudothrombocytopenia in a preterm neonate. *Pediatrics*, **114**, 273–275.

14 Muthukumar P, Venkatesh V, Curley A, Kahan BC, Choo L, Ballard S *et al.*, for the Platelets Neonatal Transfusion Study Group (2012) Severe thrombocytopenia and patterns of bleeding in neonates: results from a prospective observational study and implications for use of platelet transfusions. *Transfus Med*, **22**, 338–343.

15 Gerday E, Baer VL, Lambert DK, Paul DA, Sola-Visner MC, Pysher TJ and Christensen RD (2009) Testing platelet mass versus platelet count to guide platelet transfusions in the neonatal intensive care unit. *Transfusion*, **49**, 2034–2039.

16 Curley A, Stanworth SJ, Willoughby K, Fustolo-Gunnink SF, Venkatesh V, Hudson C *et al.*; PlaNeT2 MATISSE Collaborators (2019) Randomized trial of platelet-transfusion thresholds in neonates. *N Engl J Med*, **380**, 242–251.

17 Fustolo-Gunnink SF, Roehr CC, Lieberman L, Christensen RD, Van Der Bom JG, Dame C *et al.* (2019) Platelet and red cell transfusions for neonates: lifesavers or Trojan horses? *Expert Rev Hematol*, **12**, 797–800.

18 Hawkins-Villarreal A, Moreno-Espinos AL, Eixarcha E, Angeles Marcos M, Martinez-Portillaa RJ, Salazara L *et al.* (2019) Blood parameters in fetuses infected with cytomegalovirus according to the severity of brain damage and trimester of pregnancy at cordocentesis. *J Virol*, **119**, 37–43.

19 Watts TL and Roberts IAG (1999) Haematological abnormalities in the growth-restricted infant. *Semin Neonatol*, **4**, 41–54.

20 Perez Botero J, Reese JA, George JN and McIntosh JJ (2021) Severe thrombocytopenia and microangiopathic hemolytic anaemia in pregnancy. A guide for the consulting hematologist. *Am J Hematol*, **96**, 1655–1665.

21 Christensen RD, Baer VL, Henry E, Snow GL, Butler A and Sola-Visner MC (2015) Thrombocytopenia in small-for-gestational-age infants. *Pediatrics*, **136**, e361.

22 Murray NA, Watts TL and Roberts IAG (1998) Endogenous thrombopoietin levels and effect of recombinant human thrombopoietin on megakaryocyte precursors in term and preterm babies. *Pediatr Res*, **43**, 148–151.

23 Sola MC, Du Y, Hutson AD and Christensen RD (2000) Dose-response relationship of megakaryocyte progenitors from the bone marrow of thrombocytopenic and non-thrombocytopenic neonates to recombinant thrombopoietin. *Br J Haematol*, **110**, 449–453.

24 Teramo KA, Widness JA, Clemons GK, Voutilainen P, McKinlay S and Schwartz R (1987) Amniotic fluid erythropoietin correlates with umbilical plasma erythropoietin in normal and abnormal pregnancy. *Obstet Gynecol*, **69**, 710–716.

25 Salvesen DR, Brudenell JM, Snijders RJ, Ireland RM, and Nicolaides KH (1993) Fetal plasma erythropoietin in pregnancies complicated by maternal diabetes mellitus. *Am J Obstet Gynecol*, **168**, 88–94.

26 Watts TL, Murray NA and Roberts IAG (1999) Thrombopoietin has a primary role in the regulation of platelet production in preterm babies. *Pediatr Res*, **46**, 28–32.

27 Kuhn P, Dheu C, Bolender C, Chognot D, Keller L, Demil H *et al.* (2010) Incidence and distribution of pathogens in early-onset neonatal sepsis in the era of antenatal antibiotics. *Paediatr Perinat Epidemiol*, **24**, 479–487.

28 Puopolo KM, Benitz WE, Zaoutis TE; AAP Committee on Fetus and Newborn; AAP Committee on Infectious Diseases (2018) Management of neonates born at 35 0/7 weeks' gestation with suspected or proven early-onset bacterial sepsis. *Pediatrics*, **142**, e2018–e2894.

29 Ree IMC, Fustolo-Gunnink SF, Bekker V, Fijnvandraat KJ, Steggerda SJ and Lopriore E (2017) Thrombocytopenia in neonatal sepsis; incidence, severity and risk factors. *PLoS One*, **12**, e0185581.

30 Singh T, Barnes EH and Isaacs D; Australian Study Group for Neonatal Infections (2012) Early-onset neonatal infections in Australia and New Zealand, 2002–2012. *Arch Dis Child Fetal Neonatal Ed.*, **104**, F248–F252.

31 Veldman A, Fischer D, Nold MF and Wong FY (2010) Disseminated intravascular coagulation in term and preterm neonates. *Semin Thromb Hemost*, **36**, 419–428.

32 Jacobs S, Hunt R, Tarnow-Mordi W, Inder T and Davis P (2007) Cooling for newborns with hypoxic ischaemic encephalopathy. *Cochrane Database Syst Rev*, p. CD003311.

33 Shah PS (2010) Hypothermia: a systematic review and meta analysis of clinical trials. *Semin Fetal Neonatal Med*, **15**, 238–246.

34 Christensen R D, Baer V L and Yaish HM (2015) Thrombocytopenia in late preterm and term neonates after perinatal asphyxia. *Transfusion*, **55**, 187–196.

35 Rajagopal R, Thachil J and Monage P (2017) Disseminated intravascular coagulation in paediatrics. *Arch Dis Child*, **102**, 187–193.

36 Stanworth SJ, Clarke P, Watts T, Ballard S, Choo L, Morris T *et al.*; Platelets and Neonatal Transfusion Study Group (2009) Prospective, observational study of outcomes in neonates with severe thrombocytopenia. *Pediatrics*, **124**, e826–e834.

37 Liu ZJ, Bussel JB, Lakkaraja M, Ferrer-Marin F, Ghevaert C, Feldman HA *et al.* (2015) Suppression of in vitro megakaryopoiesis by maternal sera containing anti-HPA-1a antibodies. *Blood*, **126**, 1234–1236.

38 van Gils JM, Stutterheim J, van Duijn TJ, Zwaginga JJ, Porcelijn L, de Haas M *et al.* (2009) HPA-1a alloantibodies reduce endothelial cell spreading and monolayer integrity. *Mol Immunol*, **46**, 406–415.

39 Santoso S, Wihadmadyatami H, Bakchoul T, Werth S, Al-Fakhri N, Bein G *et al.* (2016) Antiendothelial αvβ3 antibodies are a major cause of intracranial bleeding in fetal/neonatal alloimmune thrombocytopenia. *Arterioscler Thromb Vasc Biol*, **36**, 1517–1524.

40 Kamphuis MM, Paridaans NP, Porcelijn L, Lopriore E and Oepkes D (2014) Incidence and consequences of neonatal alloimmune thrombocytopenia: a systematic review. *Pediatrics*, **133**, 715–721.

41 De Vos TW, Winkelhorst D, de Haas M, Lopriore E and Oepkes D (2020) Epidemiology and management of fetal and neonatal alloimmune thrombocytopenia. *Transfus Apher Sci*, **59**, 102704.

42 Kamphuis MM, Tiller H, van den Akker ES, Westgren M, Tiblad E and Oepkes D (2017) Fetal and neonatal alloimmune thrombocytopenia: management and outcome of a large international retrospective cohort. *Fetal Diagn Ther*, **41**, 251–257.

43 Davoren A, Curtis BR, Aster RH and McFarland JG (2004) Human platelet antigen-specific alloantibodies implicated in 1162 cases of neonatal alloimmune thrombocytopenia. *Transfusion*, **44**, 1220–1225.

44 Ghevaert C, Campbell K, Walton J, Smith GA, Allen D, Williamson LM *et al.* (2007) Management and outcome of 200 cases of fetomaternal alloimmune thrombocytopenia. *Transfusion*, **47**, 901–910.

45 Williamson LM, Hackett G, Rennie J, Palmer CR, Maciver C, Hadfield R *et al.* (1998) The natural history of fetomaternal alloimmunization to the platelet-specific antigen HPA-1a (PlA1, Zwa) as determined by antenatal screening. *Blood*, **92**, 2280–2287.

46 de Vos TW, Porcelijn L, Hofstede-van Egmond S, Pajkrt E, Oepkes D, Lopriore E *et al.* (2021) Clinical characteristics of human platelet antigen (HPA)-1a and HPA-5b alloimmunised pregnancies and the association between platelet HPA-5b antibodies and symptomatic fetal neonatal alloimmune thrombocytopenia. *Br J Haematol*, **195**, 595–603.

47 Wienzek-Lischka S, Konig IR, Papenkort EM, Hackstein H, Santoso S, Sachs UJ and Bein G (2017) HLA-DRB3*01:01 is a predictor of immunization against human platelet antigen-1a but not of the severity of fetal and neonatal alloimmune thrombocytopenia. *Transfusion*, **57**, 533–540.

48 Ghevaert C, Rankin A, Huiskes E, Porcelijn L, Javela K, Kekomaki R *et al.* (2009) Alloantibodies against low-frequency human platelet antigens do not account for a significant proportion of cases of fetomaternal alloimmune thrombocytopenia: evidence from 1054 cases. *Transfusion*, **49**, 2084–2089.

49 Ohto H, Miura S, Ariga H, Ishii T, Fujimori K and Morita S (2004) The natural history of maternal immunization against foetal platelet alloantigens. *Transfus Med*, **14**, 399–408.

50 Lee K, Godeau B, Fromont P, Plonquet A, Debili N, Bachir D *et al.* (1999) CD36 deficiency is frequent and can cause platelet immunization in Africans. *Transfusion*, **39**, 873–879.

51 Curtis BR, Ali S, Glazier AM, Ebert DD, Aitman TJ and Aster RH (2002) Isoimmunization against CD36 (glycoprotein IV): description of four cases of neonatal isoimmune thrombocytopenia and brief review of the literature. *Transfusion*, **42**, 1173–1179.

52 Masuda Y, Tamura S, Matsuno K, Nagasawa A, Hayasaka K, Shimizu C and Moriyama T (2015) Diverse CD36 expression among Japanese population: defective CD36 mutations cause platelet and monocyte CD36 reductions in not only deficient but also normal phenotype subjects. *Thromb Res*, **135**, 951–957.

53 Liu J, Shao Y, Ding H, Deng J, Xu X, Wang J *et al.* (2020) Distribution of CD36 deficiency in different Chinese ethnic groups. *Hum Immunol*, **81**, 366–371.

54 Poon MC and d'Oiron R (2018) Alloimmunization in congenital deficiencies of platelet surface glycoproteins: focus on Glanzmann's thrombasthenia and Bernard-Soulier's syndrome. *Semin Thromb Hemost*, **44**, 604–614.

55 Regan F, Lees CC, Jones B, Nicolaides KH, Wimalasundera RC, Mijovic A, on behalf of the Royal College of Obstetricians and Gynaecologists (2019) Prenatal Management of Pregnancies at Risk of Fetal Neonatal AlloimmuneThrombocytopenia (FNAIT). Scientific Impact Paper No. 61. *BJOG*, **126**, e173–185.

56 Tiller H, Kamphuis MM, Flodmark O, Papadogiannakis N, David AL, Sainio S *et al.* (2013) Fetal intracranial haemorrhages caused by fetal and neonatal alloimmune thrombocytopenia: an observational cohort study of 43 cases from an international multicentre registry. *BMJ Open*, **3**, e002490.

57 Spencer JA and Burrows RF (2001) Feto-maternal alloimmune thrombocytopenia: a literature review and statistical analysis. *Aust N Z J Obstet Gynaecol*, **41**, 45–55.

58 Winkelhorst D, Kamphuis MM, de Kloet LC, Zwaginga JJ, Oepkes D and Lopriore E (2016) Severe bleeding complications other than intracranial hemorrhage in neonatal alloimmune thrombocytopenia: a case series and review of the literature. *Transfusion*, **56**, 1230–1235.

59 Winkelhorst D, Murphy MF, Greinacher A, Shehata N, Bakchoul T, Massey E *et al.* (2017) Antenatal management in fetal and neonatal alloimmune thrombocytopenia: a systematic review. *Blood*, **129**, 1538–1547.

60 Borzini P, Riva M, Nembri P, Rossi E, Pagliaro P, Vergani P *et al.* (1997) CD36 autoantibodies and thrombotic diathesis, thrombocytopenia and repeated early fetal losses. *Vox Sang*, **73**, 46–48.

61 Okajima S, Cho K, Chiba H, Azuma H, Mochizuki T, Yamaguchi M *et al.* (2006) Two sibling cases of hydrops fetalis due to alloimmune anti-CD36 (Nak a) antibody. *Thromb Haemost*, **95**, 267–271.

62 Xu X, Li L, Xia W, Chen D, Liu J, Deng J *et al.* (2018) Successful management of a hydropic fetus with severe anemia and thrombocytopenia caused by anti-CD36 antibody. *Int J Hematol*, **107**, 251–256.

63 Wu Y, Chen D, Xu X, Mai M, Ye X, Li C *et al.* (2020) Hydrops fetalis associated with anti-CD36 antibodies in fetal and neonatal alloimmune thrombocytopenia: possible underlying mechanism. *Transfus Med*, **30**, 361–368.

64 Lieberman L, Greinacher A, Murphy MF, Bussel J, Bakchoul T, Corke S *et al.* (2019) Fetal and neonatal alloimmune thrombocytopenia: recommendations for evidence-based practice, an international approach. *Br J Haematol*, **185**, 549–562.

65 Bussel J, Zacharoulis S, Kramer K, McFarland JG, Pauliny J and Kaplan C (2005) Neonatal Alloimmune Thrombocytopenia Registry Group. Clinical and diagnostic comparison of neonatal alloimmune thrombocytopenia to non-immune cases of thrombocytopenia. *Pediatr Blood Cancer*, **45**, 176–183.

66 Baker JM, Shehata N, Bussel J, Murphy MF, Greinacher A, Bakchoul T *et al.* (2019) Postnatal intervention for the treatment of FNAIT: a systematic review. *J Perinatol*, **39**, 1329–1339.

67 New HV, Berryman J, Bolton-Maggs PHB, Cantwell C, Chalmers EA, Davies T *et al.* (2016) Guidelines on transfusion for fetuses, neonates and older children. *Br J Haematol*, **175**, 784–828.

68 Gasim T (2011) Immune thrombocytopenia in pregnancy: a reappraisal of obstetric management and outcome. *J Reprod Med*, **56**, 163–168.

69 van der Lugt NM, van Kampen A, Walther FJ, Brand A and Lopriore E (2013) Outcome and management in neonatal thrombocytopenia due to maternal idiopathic thrombocytopenic purpura. *Vox Sang*, **105**, 236–243.

70 Care A, Pavord S, Knight M and Alfirevic Z (2018) Severe primary autoimmune thrombocytopenia in pregnancy: a national cohort study. *BJOG*, **125**, 604–612.

71 Melamed N, Whittle W, Kelly EN, Windrim R, Seaward PG, Keunen J *et al.* (2015) Fetal thrombocytopenia in pregnancies with fetal human parvovirus-B19 infection. *Am J Obstet Gynecol*, **212**, 793.e1–e8.

72 Vanoni F, Lava SAG, Fossali EF, Cavalli R, Simonetti GD, Bianchetti MG *et al.* (2017) Neonatal systemic lupus erythematosus syndrome: a comprehensive review. *Clin Rev Allergy Immunol*, **53**, 469–476.

73 Provan D, Stasi R, Newland AC, Blanchette VS, Bolton-Maggs P, Bussel J *et al.* (2010) International consensus report on the investigation and management of primary immune thrombocytopenia. *Blood*, **115**, 168–186.

74 Kyle M and Dumitriou D (2021) The effect of coronavirus disease 2019 on newborns. *Curr Opin Pediatr*, **33**, 618–624.

75 Tighe P, Rimsza LM, Christensen RD, Lew J, Sola-Visner MC (2005) Severe thrombocytopenia in a neonate with congenital HIV infection. *J Pediatr*, **146**, 408–413.

76 Pesch MH, Kuboushek K, McKee MM, Thome MC and Weinberg JB (2021) Congenital cytomegalovirus infection. *BMJ*, **373**, n1212.

77 Ssentongo P, Hehnly C, Birungi P, Roach MA, Spady J, Fronterre C *et al.* (2021) Congenital cytomegalovirus infection burden and epidemiologic risk factors in countries with universal screening: a systematic review and meta-analysis. *JAMA Netw Open*, **4**, e2120736.

78 Enders G, Daiminger A, Bäder U, Exler S and Enders M (2011) Intrauterine transmission and clinical outcome of 284 pregnancies with primary cytomegalovirus infection in relation to gestational age. *J Virol*, **52**, 244–246.

79 Townsend CL, Forsgren M, Ahlfors K, Ivarsson SA, Tookey PA and Peckham CS (2013) Long-term outcomes of congenital cytomegalovirus infection in Sweden and the United Kingdom. *Clin Infect Dis*, **56**, 1232–1229.

80 Liesnard C, Donner C, Brancart F, Gosselin F, Delforge ML and Rodesch F (2000) Prenatal diagnosis of congenital cytomegalovirus infection: prospective study of 237 pregnancies at risk. *Obstet Gynecol*, **95**, 881–888.

81 Fletcher KT, Horrell EMW, Ayugi J, Irungu C, Muthoka M, Creel LM *et al.* (2018) The natural history and rehabilitative outcomes of hearing loss in congenital cytomegalovirus: a systematic review. *Otol Neurotol*, **39**, 854–864.

82 Pinniniti SG, Ross SA, Shimamura M, Novak Z, Palmer AL, Ahmed A *et al.* (2015) Comparison of saliva PCR assay versus rapid culture for detection of congenital cytomegalovirus infection. *Pediatr Infect Dis*, **34**, 536–537.

83 Luck SE, Wieringa JW, Blázquez-Gamero D, Henneke P, Schuster K, Butler K *et al.* (2017) Congenital cytomegalovirus: a European expert consensus statement on diagnosis and management. *Pediatr Infect Dis J*, **36**, 1205–1213.

84 Razonable RR, Inoue N, Pinniniti SG, Boppana SB, Lazzarotto T, Gabrielli L *et al.* (2020) Clinical diagnostic testing for human cytomegalovirus infections. *J Infect Dis*, **221** (Suppl 1), S74–S85.

85 Rawlinson WD, Boppana SB, Fowler KB, Kimberlin DW, Lazzarotto T, Alain S *et al.* (2017) Congenital cytomegalovirus infection in pregnancy and the neonate: consensus recommendations for prevention, diagnosis, and therapy. *Lancet Infect Dis*, **17**, e177–e188.

86 Tookey PA, and Peckham CS (1999) Surveillance of congenital rubella in Great Britain, 1971–96. *BMJ*, **318**, 769–770.

87 Herini ES, Triono A, Iskandar K, Prasetvo A, Nugrahanto AP and Gunadi [sic] (2021) Congenital rubella syndrome surveillance after measles rubella vaccination introduction to Yogyakarta, Indonesia. *Pediatr Infect Dis*, **40**, 1144–1150.

88 Baltimore R, Nimkin K, Sparger KA, Pierce VM and Plotkin SA (2018) Case 4-2018: A newborn with thrombocytopenia, cataracts, and hepatosplenomegaly. *N Engl J Med*, **378**, 564–572.

89 Whittembury A, Galdo J, Lugo M, Suarez-Ognio L, Ortiz A, Cabezudo E *et al.* (2011) Congenital rubella syndrome surveillance as a platform for surveillance of other congenital infections, Peru, 2004-2007. *J Infect Dis*, **204**, S706–S712.

90 Toizumi M, Motomura H, Vo HM, Takahashi K, Pham E, Nguyen HA *et al.* (2014) Mortality associated with pulmonary hypertension in congenital rubella syndrome. *Pediatrics*, **134**, e519–e526.

91 Long S (2015) 50 years ago in the Journal of Pediatrics: Congenital rubella syndrome: new clinical aspects with recovery of virus from affected infants. *J Pediatr*, **167**, 330.

92 Centers for Disease Control and Prevention (CDC) (2013) Three cases of congenital rubella syndrome in the post-elimination era- Maryland, Alabama and Illinois 2012. *MMWR Morb Mortal Wkly Rep*, **62**, 226–229.

93 Tanemura M, Suzumori K, Yagami Y and Katow S (1996) Diagnosis of fetal rubella infection with reverse transcription and nested polymerase chain reaction: a study of 34 cases diagnosed in fetuses. *Am J Obstet Gynecol*, **174**, 578–582.

94 Lacour M, Maherzi M, Vienny H and Suter S (1993) Thrombocytopenia in a case of neonatal mumps infection: evidence for further clinical presentations. *Eur J Pediatr*, **152**, 739–741.

95 Pinninti SG and Kimberlin DW (2018) Neonatal herpes simplex virus infections. *Semin Perinatol*, **42**, 168–175.

96 Chuang Y-Y and Huang Y-C (2019) Enteroviral infection in neonates. *J Microbiol Immunol Infect*, **52**, 851–857.

97 Zhang M, Wang H, Tang J, He Y, Xiong T, Li W *et al.* (2021) Clinical characteristics of severe neonatal enterovirus infection: a systematic review. *BMC Pediatr*, **21**, 127.

98 Yen MH, Huang YC, Chen MC, Liu CC, Chiu NC, Lin RY *et al.* (2015) Effect of intravenous immunoglobulin for neonates with severe enteroviral infections with emphasis on the timing of administration. *J Clin Virol*, **64**, 92–96.

99 Fukazawa M, Hoshina T, Nanishi E, Nishio H, Doi T, Ohga S and Hara T (2013) Neonatal hemophagocytic lymphohistiocytosis associated with a vertical transmission of coxsackievirus B1. *J Infect Chemother*, **19**, 1210–1213.

100 Watanabe Y, Sugiura T, Sugimoto M, Togawa Y, Kouwaki M, Koyama N *et al.* (2019) Echovirus type 7 virus-associated hemophagocytic syndrome in a neonate successfully treated with intravenous immunoglobulin therapy: a case report. *Front Pediatr*, **7**, 469.

101 Tarcan A, Ozbek N and Gurakan B (2001) Bone marrow failure with concurrent enteroviral infection in a newborn. *Pediatr Infect Dis J*, **20**, 719–721.

102 Ronchi A, Doem C, Brrock E, Pugni L and Sanchez PJ (2014) Neonatal adenoviral infection: a seventeen year experience and review of the literature. *J Pediatr*, **164**, 529–535.

103 Agrawal G, Wazir S, Sachdeva A and Kumar S (2020) Primary dengue infection triggered haemophagocytic lymphohistiocytosis in a neonate. *BMJ Case Rep*, **13**, e236881.

104 Krishnappa A, Munusamy J, Ray S, Rameshbabu M, Bhatia P, Roy PS *et al.* (2021) Neonatal dengue with HLH: perks of early diagnosis and management. *J Pediatr Hematol Oncol*, **43**, e770–e773

105 Nguyen TM, Huan VT, Reda A, Morsy S, Giang HTN and Tri VD (2021) Clinical features and outcomes of neonatal dengue at the Children's Hospital 1, Ho Chi Minh, *Vietnam*. *J Clin Virol*, **13**8, 104758.

106 Witayathawornwong P, Jirachanchai O, Kasemsut P, Mahawijit N and Srisakkwa R (2012) Severe perinatal dengue hemorrhagic fever in a low birth weight infant. *Southeast Asian J Trop Med Public Health*, **43**, 62–67.

107 Chye JK, Lim CT, Ng KB, Lim JM, George R, Lam SK *et al.* (1997) Vertical transmission of dengue. *Clin Infect Dis*, **25**, 1374–1377.

108 Yadav B, Gupta N, Gadepalli R and Nag VL (2021) Neonatal dengue: an under-diagnosed entity. *BMJ Case Rep*, **14**, e241727.

109 Gerardin P Narau G, Michault A, Bintner M, Randrianaivo H, Choker G *et al.* (2008) Multidisciplinary prospective study of mother-to-child chikungunya virus infections on the island of La Reunion. *PLoS Med*, **5**, e60.

110 Ferreira CP, da Silva AS, Recht J, Guaraldo L, Moreira ME, Siqueira AM *et al.* (2021) Vertical transmission of chikungunya virus: a systematic review. *PLoS One*, **16**, e0249166.

111 Besnard M, Dub T and Girardin P (2013) Outcomes for 2 children after peripartum acquisition of zika virus infection, French Polynesia, 2013–2014. *Emerg Infect Dis*, **23**, 1421–1423.

112 Thulliez P (1992) Screening programme for congenital toxoplasmosis in France. *Scand J Infect Dis* **84** (Suppl), 43–45.

113 McAuley J, Boyer KM, Patel D, Mets M, Swisher C, Roizen N *et al.* (1994) Early and longitudinal evaluations of treated infants and children and untreated historical patients with congenital toxoplasmosis: the Chicago Collaborative Treatment Trial. *Clin Infect Dis* **18**, 38–72.

114 McAuley JB (2014) Congenital toxoplasmosis. *J Pediatr Infect Dis Soc*, **3** (Suppl 1), S30–S35.

115 Maldonado YA and Read JS (2017) Committee on Infectious Diseases. Diagnosis, treatment, and prevention of congenital toxoplasmosis in the United States. *Pediatrics*, **139**, e20163860.

116 Saso A, Bamford A, Grewal K, Noori M, Hatcher J, D'Arco F *et al.* (2020) Fifteen-minute consultation: management of the infant born to a mother with toxoplasmosis in pregnancy. *Arch Dis Child Educ Pract Ed*, **105**, 262–269.

117 Hohlfeld P, Forestier F, Kaplan C, Tissot JD and Daffos F (1994) Fetal thrombocytopenia: a retrospective survey of 5,194 fetal blood samplings. *Blood*, **84**, 1851–1856.

118 Armstrong L, Isaacs D and Evans N (2004) Severe neonatal toxoplasmosis after third trimester maternal infection. *Pediatr Infect Dis J*, **23**, 968–969.

119 Al-Hamod D, Vauloup C, Goulet M, Zupan-Simunek V, Castel C and Boileau P (2010) Delayed onset of severe neonatal toxoplasmosis. *J Perinatol*, **30**, 231–232.

120 Fortuny LR, Cabler SS, Hunstad DA and Yarbrough ML (2021) Blueberry muffin rashbilateral cataracts, and thrombocytopenia in a neonate. *Clin Chem*, **67**, 472–475.

121 Carellos EVM, Queiroz de Andrade J, Romanelli RMC, Tiburcio JD, Januario JN, Vasconcelos-Santos DV *et al.* (2017) High frequency of bone marrow depression during congenital toxoplasmosis therapy in a cohort of children identified by neonatal screening in Minas Gerais, Brazil. *Pediatr Infect Dis*, **36**, 1169–1176.

122 Danwang C, Bigna JJ, Nzalie RNT and Robert A (2020) Epidemiology of clinical congenital and neonatal malaria in endemic settings: a systematic review and meta-analysis. *Malar J*, **19**, 312.

123 Frauchiger B, Koch D, Gaehler A, Blum J, Lura M, Kaiser D and Buettcher M (2019) Don't forget the past: a sleeping disease can be awakened. *J Pediatr Child Health*, **55**, 854–856.

124 Prior AR, Prata F, Mouzinho A and Marques JG (2012) Learning from errors. Congenital malaria in a European country. *BMJ Care Rep*, 2012: bcr2012007310.

125 Baspinar O, Bayraktaroglu Z, Karsligil T, Bayram A and Coscun Y (2006) A rare case of anemia and thrombocytopenia in a newborn: congenital malaria. *Turk J Pediatr*, **48**, 63–68.

126 Lesko CR, Arguin PM and Newman RD (2007) Congenital malaria in the United States. *Arch Pediatr Adolesc Med*, **161**, 1062–1067.

127 Voittier G, Arsac M, Farnoux C, Mariani-Kurdjian P, Baud O and Aujard Y (2008) Congenital malaria in neonates: two case report and review of literature. *Paediatrica*, **97**, 500–512.

128 Punta VD, Gulletta M, Matteeli A, Spinoni V, Regazzoli A and Castelli F (2010) Congenital Plasmodium vivax malaria mimicking neonatal sepsis: a case report. *Malar J*, **9**, 63.

129 Sanchez PJ, Patterson JC and Ahmed A (2012) Toxoplasmosis, syphilis, malaria and tuberculosis. In: Gleason CA and Devasker SU (eds), *Avery's Diseases of the Newborn*. Elsevier Saunders, Philadelphia, pp. 522–529.

130 Whittaker E and Kampmann B (2008) Perinatal tuberculosis. New challenges in the diagnosis and treatment of tuberculosis in infants and the newborn. *Early Hum Dev*, **84**, 795–799.

131 Sims I, Tookey PA, Goh BT, Lyall H, Evans B, Townsend CL *et al.* (2017) The incidence of congenital syphilis in the United Kingdom: February 2010 to January 2015. *BJOG*, **124**, 72–77

132 Klimco A, Brandt A and Bruston M-J (2020) A Case of Miliary Perinatal tuberculosis in a preterm newborn infant presenting as peritonitis. *Cureus*, **12**, e8036.

133 Bowen VB, McDonald R, Grey JA, Kimball A and Torrone EA (2021) High congenital syphilis case counts among U.S. infants born in 2020. *N Engl J Med*, **385**, 1144–1145.

134 Cooper JM and Sanchez PJ (2018) Congenital syphilis. *Semin Perinatol*, **42**, 176–184.

135 Hollier LM, Harstad TW, Sanchez PJ, Twickler DM and Wendel DG Jnr (2001) Fetal syphilis: clinical and laboratory characteristics. *Obstet Gynecol*, **97**, 947–953.

136 Wright DJM and Berry CL (1974) Liver involvement in congenital syphilis. *Br J Vener Dis*, **50**, 241.

137 Duby J, Bitnun A, Shah V, Shannon P, Shinar S and Whyte H (2019) Non-immune hydrops fetalis and hepatic dysfunction in a preterm infant with congenital syphilis. *Front Pediatr*, **7**, 508.

138 Wiedmeier SE, Henry E and Christensen RD (2008) Hematological abnormalities during the first week of life among neonates with Trisomy 18 and Trisomy 13: data from a multihospital healthcare system. *Am J Med Genet A*, **146A**, 312–320.

139 Sahoo T, Naeem R, Pham K, Chheng S, Noblin ST, Bacino C and Gambello MJ (2005) A patient with isochromosome 18q, radial-thumb aplasia, thrombocytopenia, and an unbalanced 10;18 chromosome translocation. *Am J Med Genet A*, **133A**, 93–98.

140 Meyer RE, Liu G, Gilboa S, Ethen MK, Aylsworth AS, Powell CM *et al.* (2016) Survival of children with trisomy 13 and trisomy 18: A multi-state population-based study. *Am J Med Genet A*, **170A**, 825–837.

141 Roberts, I, Alford K, Hall G, Juban G, Richmond H, Norton A *et al.* (2013) GATA1 mutant clones are frequent and often unsuspected in babies with Down syndrome: identification of a population at risk of leukemia. *Blood*, **122**, 3908–3917.

142 Nurden AT and Nurden P (2020) Inherited thrombocytopenias: history, advances and perspectives. *Haematologica*, **105**, 2004–2019.

143 Megy K, Downes K, Morel-Kopp MC, Bastida JM, Brooks S, Bury L *et al.* (2021) GoldVariants, a resource for sharing rare genetic variants detected in bleeding,

thrombotic, and platelet disorders: communication from the ISTH SSC subcommittee on genomics in thrombosis and hemostasis. *J Thromb Haemost*, **19**, 2612–2617.

144 Megy K, Downes K, Simeoni I, Bury L, Morales J, Mapeta R *et al.* (2019) Curated disease-causing genes for bleeding, thrombotic, and platelet disorders: communication from the SSC of the ISTH. *J Thromb Haemost*, **17**, 1253–1260.

145 Noris P and Pecci A (2017) Hereditary thrombocytopenias: a growing list of disorders. *Hematology Am Soc Hematol Educ Program*, **2017**, 385–399.

146 Khincha PP and Savage SA (2016) Neonatal manifestations of inherited bone marrow failure syndromes. *Semin Fetal Neonatal Med*, **21**, 57–65

147 Lentaigne C, Freson K, Laffan MA, Turro E and Ouwehand WH, BRIDGE-BPD Consortium and the ThromboGenomics Consortium (2016) Inherited platelet disorders: towards DNA-based diagnosis. *Blood*, **127**, 2814–2823.

148 Collins J, Astle WJ, Megy K, Mumford A and Vuckovic D (2021) Advances in understanding the pathogenesis of hereditary macrothrombocytopenia. *Br J Haematol*, **195**, 25–45.

149 Pecci A and Balduini CL (2021) Inherited thrombocytopenias: an updated guide for clinicians. *Blood Rev*, **48**, 100784.

150 Plutheroe FG, Di Paola J, Carcao MD and Kahr WHA (2018) NBEAL2 mutations and bleeding in patients with gray platelet syndrome. *Platelets*, **29**, 632–635.

151 Savoia A, Kunishima S, DeRocco D, Zieger B, Rand ML, Pujol-Moix *et al.* (2014) Spectrum of mutations in Bernard-Soulier syndrome. *Hum Mutat*, **35**, 1033–1045.

152 Vettore S, Scandellari R, Moro S, Lombardi AM, Scapin M, Randi ML and Fabris F (2008) Novel point mutation in a leucine-rich repeat of the GP1balpha chain of the platelet von Willebrand factor receptor, Gp1b/IX/V, resulting in an inherited dominant form of Bernard-Soulier syndrome affecting two unrelated families: the N41H variant. *Haematologica*, **93**, 1743–1747.

153 Lopez JA, Andrews RK, Afshar-Kharghan V and Berndt MC (1998) Bernard-Soulier syndrome. *Blood*, **91**, 4397–4418.

154 Boumanhi B, Kaplan C, Clabe A, Randrianaivo H and Lanza F (2011) Maternal-fetal chikungunya infection associated with Bernard-Soulier syndrome. *Arch Pediatr*, **18**, 272–275.

155 Grainger JD, Thachil J and Will A (2018) How we treat platelet glycoprotein defects: Glanzmann thrombasthenia and Bernard Soulier syndrome in children and adults. *Br J Haematol*, **182**, 621–632.

156 Alamelu J and Liesner R (2010) Modern management of severe platelet function disorders. *Br J Haematol*, **149**, 813–823.

157 Peitsidis P, Datta T, Pafilis I, Otomewo O, Tuddenham EGD and Kadir RA (2010) Bernard Soulier syndrome in pregnancy: a systematic review. *Haemophilia*, **16**, 584–591.

158 Stevenson WS, Rabbolini DJ, Beutler L, Chen Q, Gabrielli S, Mackay JP *et al.* (2015) Paris-Trousseau thrombocytopenia is phenocopied by the autosomal recessive inheritance of a DNA-binding domain mutation in FLI1. *Blood.* **126**, 2027–2030.

159 Levin C, Koren A, Pretorius E, Rosenberg N, Shenkman B, Hauschner H *et al.* (2015) Deleterious mutation in the FYB gene is associated with congenital autosomal recessive small-platelet thrombocytopenia. *J Thromb Haemost*, **13**, 1285–1292.

160 Kahr WH, Hinckley J, Li L, Schwertz H, Christensen H, Rowley JW *et al.* (2011) Mutations in NBEAL2, encoding a BEACH protein, cause gray platelet syndrome. *Nat Genet*, **43**, 738–740.

161 Nurden AT, Pillois X, Fiore M, Alessi M-C, Bonduel M, Dreyfus M *et al.* (2015) Expanding the spectrum affecting αIIbβ3 integrin in Glanzmann's thrombasthenia: screening of the ITGA2B and ITGB3 genes in a large international cohort. *Hum Mutat*, **36**, 548–561.

162 Manchev VT, Hilpert M, Berrou E, Elaib Z, Aouba R, Boukour S *et al.* (2014) A new form of macrothrombocytopenia induced by a germ-line mutation in the *PRKACG* gene. *Blood*. **124**, 2554–2563.

163 Fletcher SJ, Johnson B, Lowe GC, Bem D, Drake S, Lordkipanidzé M *et al.* (2015) UK Genotyping and Phenotyping of Platelets Study Group. SLFN14 mutations underlie thrombocytopenia with excessive bleeding and platelet secretion defects. *J Clin Invest*, **125**, 3600–3605.

164 Cheng AN, Bao EL, Fiorini C,and Sankaran VG (2019) Macrothrombocytopenia associated with a rare GFI1B missense variant confounding the presentation of immune thrombocytopenia. *Pediatr Blood Cancer*, **66**, e27874.

165 Boutroux H, David B, Guéguen P, Frange P, Vincenot A, Leverger G and Favier R (2017) ACTN1-related macrothrombocytopenia: a novel entity in the progressing field of pediatric thrombocytopenia. *J Pediatr Hematol Oncol*, **39**, e515–e518.

166 Scherber E, Beutel K, Ganschow R, Schulz A, Janka G and Stadt U (2009) Molecular analysis and clinical aspects of four patients with Chediak-Higashi syndrome (CHS). *Clin Genet*, **76**, 409–412.

167 Carneiro IM, Rodrigues A, Pinho L, Nunes-Santos CdeJ, de Barros Dorna M, Moschione Castro APB and Pastorino AC (2019) Chediak-Higashi syndrome: lessons from a single-centre case series. *Allergol Immunopathol (Madr)*, **47**, 598–603.

168 Nagle DL, Karim AM and Woolf EA (1996) Identification and mutation analysis of the complete gene for Chediak-Higashi syndrome. *Nat Genet*, **14**, 307–311.

169 Kaplan J, De Domenico I and Ward DM (2008) Chediak-Higashi syndrome. *Curr Opin Hematol*, **15**, 22–29.

170 Nurden P, Debili N, Coupry I, Bryckaert M, Youlyouz-Marfak I, Sole G *et al.* (2011) Thrombocytopenia resulting from mutations in filamin A can be expressed as an isolated syndrome. *Blood*, **118**, 5928–5937.

171 Vassallo P, Westbury SK and Mumford AD (2020) FLNA variants associated with disorders of platelet number or function. *Platelets*, **31**, 1097–1100.

172 Cannaerts A, Shukla A, Hasanhodzic M, Alaerts M, Schepers D, Van Laer L *et al.* (2018) FLNA mutations in surviving males presenting with connective tissue findings: two new case reports and review of the literature. *BMC Med Genet*, **19**, 140.

173 Favier R, Akshoomoff N, Mattson S and Grossfeld P (2015) Jacobsen syndrome: advances in our knowledge of phenotype and genotype. *Am J Med Genet C Semin Med Genet*, **169**, 239.

174 Ichimiya Y, Wada Y, Kunishima S, Tsukamoto K, Kosaki R, Sago H *et al.* (2018) 11q23 deletion syndrome (Jacobsen syndrome) with severe bleeding: a case report. *J Med Case Rep*, **12**, 3.

175 Serra G, Memo L, Antona V, Corsello G, Favero V, Lago G and Giuffre M (2021) Jacobsen syndrome and neonatal bleeding: report on two unrelated patients. *Ital J Pediatr*, **47**, 147.

176 Mattina T, Perrotta CS and Grossfeld P (2009) Jacobsen syndrome. *Orphanet J Rare Dis*, **4**, 9.

177 Balduini A, Raslova H, Di Buduo CA, Donada A, Ballmaier M, Germeshausen M and Balduini CL (2018) Clinic, pathogenic mechanisms and drug testing of two inherited thrombocytopenias, ANKRD26- and MYH9-related diseases. *Eur J Med Genet*, **61**, 715–722.

178 Takashima T, Maeda H, Koyanagi T, Nishimura J, and Nakano H (1992) Prenatal diagnosis and obstetrical management of May-Hegglin anomaly: a case report. *Fetal Diagn Ther*, **7**, 186–189.

179 Urato AC and Repke JT (1998) May-Hegglin anomaly: a case of vaginal delivery when both mother and fetus are affected. *Am J Obstet Gynecol*, **179**, 260–261.

180 Samelson-Jones BJ, Kramer PM, Chicka M, Gunning WT 3rd and Lambert MP (2018) MYH9-macrothrombocytopenia caused by a novel variant (E1421K) initially presenting as apparent neonatal alloimmune thrombocytopenia. *Pediatr Blood Cancer*, **65**, e26949.

181 Morin G, Bruechle NO, Singh AR, Knopp C, Jedraszak G, Elbracht M *et al.* (2014) Gain-of-function mutation in STIM1 (P.R304W) is associated with Stormorken syndrome. *Hum Mutat*, **35**, 1221–1232.

182 Markello T, Chen D, Kwan JY, Horkayne-Szakaly I, Morrison A, Simakova O *et al.* (2015) York platelet syndrome is a CRAC channelopathy due to gain-of-function mutations in STIM1. *Mol Genet Metab*, **114**, 474–482.

183 Picard C, McCarl CA, Papolos A, Khalil S, Luthy K, Hivroz C *et al.* (2009) STIM1 mutation associated with a syndrome of immunodeficiency and autoimmunity. *N Engl J Med*, **360**, 1971–1980.

184 Greenhalgh KL, Howell RT, Bottani A, Ancliff PJ, Brunner HG, Verschuuren-Bemelmans CC *et al.* (2002) Thrombocytopenia-absent radius syndrome: a clinical genetic study. *J Med Genet*, **39**, 876–881.

185 Boussion S, Escande F, Jourdain AS, Smol T, Brunelle P, Duhamel C *et al.* (2020) Clinical and molecular characterization of a cohort of 26 patients and description of novel noncoding variants of RBM8A. *Hum Mutat*, **41**, 1220–1225.

186 Manukjan G, Bösing H, Schmugge M, Strauß G and Schulze H (2017) Impact of genetic variants on haematopoiesis in patients with thrombocytopenia absent radii (TAR) syndrome. *Br J Haematol*, **179**, 606–617.

187 Brodie SA, Rodriguez-Auler JP, Giri N, Dai J, Steinberg M, Waterfall JP *et al.* (2019) 1q21.1 deletion and a rare functional polymorphism in siblings with thrombocytopenia-absent radius-like phenotypes. *Cold Spring Harb Mol Case Stud*, **5**, a004564.

188 Burns S, Cory GO, Vainchenker W and Thrasher AJ (2004) Mechanisms of WASp-mediated hematologic and immunologic disease. *Blood*, **104**, 3454–3462.

189 Massaad MJ, Ramesh N and Geha RS (2013) Wiskott-Aldrich syndrome: a comprehensive review. *Ann N Y Acad Sci*, **1285**, 26–43.

190 Sillers L, Van Slambrouck C and Lapping-Carr G (2015) Neonatal thrombocytopenia: etiology and diagnosis. *Pediatr Ann*, **44**, e175–e180.

191 Ochfield E, Grayer D, Sharma R, Schneiderman J, Giordano L and Makhija M (2021) A novel mutation in WAS gene causing a phenotypic presentation of Wiskott-Aldrich syndrome: a case report. *J Pediatr Hematol Oncol*, **43**, e234–e236.

192 Ochs HD, Filipovich AH, Veys P, Cowan MJ and Kapoor N (2009) Wiskott-Aldrich syndrome: diagnosis, clinical and laboratory manifestations, and treatment. *Biol Blood Marrow Transplant*, **15**, 84–90

193 Albert MA, Bittner TC, Nonyama S, Notarangelo LD, Burns S, Imai K *et al.* (2010) X-linked thrombocytopenia (XLT) due to WAS mutations: clinical characteristics, long-term outcome, and treatment options. *Blood*, **115**, 3231–3238.

194 Songdej N and Rao AK (2017) Hematopoietic transcription factor mutations: important players in inherited platelet defects. *Blood*, **129**, 2873–2881.

195 Mehaffey MG, Newton AL, Gandhi MJ, Crossley M and Drachman JG (2001) X-linked thrombocytopenia caused by a novel mutation of GATA-1. *Blood*, **98**, 2681–2688.

196 Nichols KE, Crispino JD, Poncz M, White JG, Orkin SH, Maris JM and Weiss MJ (2000) Familial dyserythropoietic anaemia and thrombocytopenia due to an inherited mutation in GATA1. *Nat Genet*, **24**, 266–270.

197 Yu C, Niakan KK, Matsushita M, Stamatoyannopoulos G, Orkin SH, Raskind WH *et al.* (2002) X-linked thrombocytopenia with thalassemia due to a mutation in the amino-finger of GATA-1 affecting DNA-binding rather than FOG-1 interaction. *Blood*, **100**, 2040–2045.

198 Balduini CL, Pecci A, Loffredo G, Izzo P, Noris P, Grosso M *et al.* (2004) Effects of the R216Q mutation of GATA-1 on erythropoiesis and megakaryocytopoiesis. *Thromb Haemost*, **91**, 129–140.

199 Geddis AE (2010) Congenital amegakaryocytic thrombocytopenia and thrombocytopenia with absent radii. *Hematol Oncol Clin North Am*, **23**, 321–331.

200 Ballmaier M and Germeshausen M (2011) Congenital amegakaryocytic thrombocytopenia: clinical presentation, diagnosis, and treatment. *Semin Thromb Hemost*, **37**, 673–681.

201 Niihori T, Ouchi-Uchiyama M, Sasahara Y, Kaeko T, Hashii Y, Irie M *et al.* (2015) Mutations in MECOM, encoding oncoprotein EVI1, cause radioulnar synostosis with amegakaryocytic thrombocytopenia. *Am J Hum Genet*, **97**, 848–854.

202 Song WJ, Sullivan MG, Legare RD, Hutchings S, Tan X, Kufrin D *et al.* (1999) Haploinsufficiency of CBFA2 causes familial thrombocytopenia with propensity to develop acute myelogenous leukaemia. *Nat Genet*, **23**, 166–175.

203 Liew E and Owen CJ (2011) Familial myelodysplastic syndromes. *Haematologica*, **96**, 1536–1542.

204 Noetzli L, Lo RW, Lee-Sherick AB, Callaghan M, Noris P, Savoia A *et al.* (2015) Germline mutations in ETV6 are associated with thrombocytopenia, red cell macrocytosis and predisposition to lymphoblastic leukemia. *Nat Genet*, **47**, 535–538.

205 Noris P, Perrotta S, Seri M, Pecci A, Gnan C, Loffredi G *et al.* (2011) Mutations in ANKRD26 are responsible for a frequent form of inherited thrombocytopenia: analysis of 78 patients from 21 families. *Blood*, **117**, 6673–6680.

206 Germeshausen M and Ballmaier M (2021) CAMT-MPL: congenital amegakaryocytic thrombocytopenia caused by MPL mutations - heterogeneity of a monogenic disorder - a comprehensive analysis of 56 patients. *Haematologica*, **106**, 2439–2448.

207 Pecci A, Ragab I, Bozzi V, De Rocco D, Barozzi S, Giangregorio T *et al.* (2018) Thrombopoietin mutation in congenital amegakaryocytic thrombocytopenia treatable with romiplostim. *EMBO Mol Med*, **10**, 63–75.

208 Cancio M, Hebert K, Kim S, Aliurf M, Olson T, Anderson E *et al.* (2022) Outcomes in hematopoietic stem cell transplantation for congenital amegakaryocytic thrombocytopenia. *Transplant Cell Ther*, **28**, 101.e1–101.e6.

209 Maserati E, Panarello C, Morerio C, Valli R, Pressato B, Patitucci F *et al.* (2008) Clonal chromosome anomalies and propensity to myeloid malignancies in congenital amegakaryocytic thrombocytopenia (OMIM 604498). *Haematologica*, **93**, 1271–1273.

210 Steinberg O, Gillad G, Dagny O, Krasnov T, Zoldan M, Laor R *et al.* (2007) Congenital amegakaryocytic thrombocytopenia-3 novel c-MPL mutations and their phenotypic correlations. *J Pediatr Hematol Oncol*, **29**, 822–825.

211 Stoddart MT, Connor P, Germeshausen M, Ballmaier M and Steward CG (2013) Congenital amegakaryocytic thrombocytopenia (CAMT) presenting as severe pancytopenia in the first month of life. *Paediatr Blood Cancer*, **60**, E94–E96.

212 Schlegelberger B and Heller PG (2017) RUNX1 deficiency (familial platelet disorder with predisposition to myeloid leukemia (FPDMM)). *Semin Hematol*, **54**, 75–80.

213 Bagla S, Regling KA, Wakeling EN, Gadgeel M, Buck S, Zaidi AU *et al.* (2021) Distinctive phenotypes in two children with novel germline *RUNX1* mutations – one with myeloid malignancy and increased fetal hemoglobin. *Pediatr Hematol Oncol*, **38**, 65–79.

214 Ouchi-Uchiyama M, Sasahara Y, Kikuchi A, Goi K, Nakane T, Ikeno M *et al.* (2015) Analyses of genetic and clinical parameters for screening patients with inherited thrombocytopenia with small or normal-sized platelets. *Pediatr Blood Cancer*, **62**, 2082–2088.

215 Melazzini F, Palombo F, Balduini A, De Rocco D, Marconi C, Noris P *et al.* (2016) Clinical and pathogenetic features of ETV6-related thrombocytopenia with predisposition to acute lymphoblastic leukemia. *Haematologica.* **101**, 1333–1342.

216 Homan CC, King-Smith SL, Lawrence DM, Arts P, Feng J and Andrews J (2021) The RUNX1 database (RUNX1db): establishment of an expert curated RUNX1 registry and genomics database as a public resource for familial platelet disorder with myeloid malignancy. *Haematologica*, **106**, 3004–3007.

217 Decker M, Lammens T, Ferster A, Erlacher M, Yoshimi A, Niemeyer CM *et al.* (2021) Functional classification of RUNX1 variants in familial platelet disorder with associated myeloid malignancies. *Leukemia*, **35**, 3304–3308.

218 Thompson AA and Nguyen LT (2000) Amegakaryocytic thrombocytopenia and radio-ulnar synostosis are associated with *HOXA11* mutation. *Nat Genet*, **26**, 397–398.

219 Niihori T, Tanoshima R, Sasahara Y, Sato A, Irie M and Saito-Nanjo Y (2022) Phenotypic heterogeneity in individuals with MECOM variants in 2 families. *Blood Adv*, bloodadvances.2020003812

220 Futterer J, Dalby A, Lowe GC, Johnson B, Simpson MA, Motwani J *et al.* (2018) Mutation in *GNE* is associated with severe congenital thrombocytopenia. *Blood*, **132**, 1855–1858.

221 Xin L, Li Y, Lei M, Tian J, Yang Z, Kuang S, Tan Y and Bo T (2020) Congenital thrombocytopenia associated with GNE mutations in twin sisters: a case report and literature review. *BMC Med Genet*, **21**, 224.

222 Stritt S, Nurden P, Turro E, Greene D, Jansen SB, Westbuty SK *et al.* (2016) BRIDGE-BPD Consortium. A gain-of-function variant in DIAPH1 causes dominant macrothrombocytopenia and hearing loss. *Blood*, **127**, 2903–2914.

223 Turro E, Greene D, Wijgaerts A, Thys C, Lentaigne C, Bariani T *et al.*; BRIDGE-BPD Consortium (2015) A dominant gain-of-function mutation in universal tyrosine kinase

SRC causes thrombocytopenia, myelofibrosis, bleeding, and bone pathologies. *Sci Transl Med*, **8**, 328ra30.

224 Barozzi S, Di Buduo CA, Marconi C, Bozzi V, Seri M, Romano F *et al.* (2021) Pathogenetic and clinical study of a patient with thrombocytopenia due to the p.E527K gain-of-function variant of *SRC*. *Haematologica*, **106**, 918–922.

225 Baer VL, Lambert DK, Henry E, Snow GL, Sola-Visner MC and Christensen RD (2007) Do platelet transfusions in the NICU adversely affect survival? Analysis of 1600 thrombocytopenic neonates in a multihospital healthcare system. *J Perinatol*, **27**, 790–796.

226 Davenport P and Sola-Visner M (2021) *Hemostatic challenges in neonates. Front Pediatr*, **9**, 627715.

227 Fustolo-Gunnink SF, Huisman EJ, van der Bom JG, van Hout FMA, Makineli S, Lopriore E and Fijnvandraat K (2019) Are thrombocytopenia and platelet transfusions associated with major bleeding in preterm neonates? A systematic review. *Blood Rev*, **36**, 1–9.

228 Chen YJ, Chu WY, Yu WH, Chen CJ, Chia ST, Wang JN *et al.* (2021) Massive gastric hemorrhage after indomethacin therapy: a rare presentation and critical management in an extremely preterm neonate. *Children (Basel)*, **8**, 545.

229 Christensen RD, Sheffield MJ, Lambert DK and Baer VL (2012) Effect of therapeutic hypothermia in neonates with hypoxic-ischemic encephalopathy on platelet function. *Neonatology*, **101**, 91–94.

230 Van den Helm S, Yaw HP, Letunica N, Barton R, Weaver A and Newall F (2022) Platelet phenotype and function changes with increasing duration of extracorporeal membrane oxygenation. *Crit Care Med*, Jan 12, doi: 10.1097/CCM.0000000000005435

231 Nurden P, Stritt S, Favier R and Nurden AT (2021) Inherited platelet diseases with normal platelet count: phenotypes, genotypes and diagnostic strategy. *Haematologica*, **106**, 337–350.

232 George JJ, Caen JP and Nurden AT (1990) Glanzmann's thrombasthenia: the spectrum of clinical disease. *Blood*, **75**, 1383–1395.

233 Harris ES, Smith TL, Sprigett GM, Weyrich AS and Zimmerman GA (2012) Leukocyte adhesion deficiency-I variant syndrome (LAD-Iv, LAD-III): molecular characterization of the defect in an index family. *Am J Hematol*, **87**, 311–313.

234 Wolach B, Gavrieli R, Wolach O, Stauber T, Abuzaitoun O and Kuperman A (2019) Leucocyte adhesion deficiency – a multicentre national experience. *Eur J Clin Invest*, **49**, e13047.

235 Perez Botero J, Lee K, Branchford BR, Bray PF, Freson K, Lambert MP *et al.* (2020) Glanzmann thrombasthenia: genetic basis and clinical correlates. *Haematologica*, **105**, 888–894.

236 Bakhtiar S, Salzmann-Manrique E, Blok H-J, Eikema D-J, Hazelaar S, Ayas M *et al.* (2021) Allogeneic hematopoietic stem cell transplantation in leukocyte adhesion deficiency type I and III. *Blood Adv*, **5**, 262–273.

237 Rosenberg N, Dardika R, Hauschner H, Nakavd S and Barel O (2021) Mutations in *RASGRP2* gene identified in patients misdiagnosed as Glanzmann thrombasthenia patients. *Blood Cells Mol Dis*, **89**, 102560.

238 Wiedmeier SE, Henry E, Sola-Visner MC and Christensen RD (2008) Platelet reference ranges for neonates, defined using data from over 47,000 patients in a multihospital healthcare system. *J Perinatol*, **29**, 130–136.

239 Wiedmeier SE, Henry E, Burnett J, Anderson T and Christensen RD (2010) Thrombocytosis in neonates and young infants: a report of 25 patients with platelet counts of ≥1 000 000 μl^{-1}. *J Perinatol*, **30**, 222–226.

240 Ng KF, Bandi S, Bird PW and Wei-Tze Tang J (2020) COVID-19 in neonates and infants: progression and recovery. *Pediatr Infect Dis J*, **39**, e140–e142.

241 Sahni M, Patel P and Muthukumar A (2020) Severe thrombocytosis in a newborn with subcutaneous fat necrosis and maternal chorioamnionitis. *Case Rep Hematol*, **2020**, 5742394.

242 Li C, Du Y, Wang H, Wu G and Zhu X (2021) Neonatal Kawasaki disease: case report and literature review. *Medicine (Baltimore)*, **100**, e24624.

243 Thapa R, Pramanik S, Dhar S and Kundu R (2007) Neonatal Kawasaki disease with multiple coronary aneurysms and thrombocytopenia. *Pediatr Dermatol*, **24**, 662–663.

244 Lo J, Gauvreau K, Baker AL, de Ferranti SD, Friedman KG, Lo MS *et al.* (2021) Multiple emergency department visits for a diagnosis of Kawasaki disease: an examination of risk factors and outcomes. *J Pediatr*, **232**, 127–132.e3.

245 Langabeer SE, Haslam K and McMahon C (2013) A prenatal origin of childhood essential thrombocythaemia. *Br J Haematol*, **173**, 674–647.

246 Graziano C, Carone S, Panza E, Marino F, Magini P, Romeo P *et al.* (2009) Association of hereditary thrombocythemia and distal limb defects with a thrombopoietin gene mutation. *Blood*, **114**, 1655–1657.

247 Jung N, Kim DH, Ha JS and Shim YJ (2020) Thrombocythemia 1 with *THPO* variant (c.13+1G>A) diagnosed using targeted exome sequencing: first case in Korea. *Ann Lab Med*, **40**, 341–344.

248 Sutor AH (1995)Thrombocytosis in childhood. *Semin Thromb Hemost*, **21**, 330–339.

249 Bruel H, Chabrolle JP, el Khoury E, Poinsot J, el Forzi N, Amusini, P and Col JY (2001) Thrombocytosis and cholestasis in a newborn treated with zidovudine. *Arch Pediatr*, **8**, 893–894.

250 Nako Y, Tachibana A, Fujiu T, Tomomasa T and Morikawa A (2001) Neonatal thrombocytosis resulting from the maternal use of non-narcotic antischizophrenic drugs during pregnancy. *Arch Dis Child*, **84**, F198–F200.

251 Flanagan E, Wright EK, Hardikar W, Sparrow MP, Connell WR, Kamm MA, de Cruz P *et al.* (2021) Maternal thiopurine metabolism during pregnancy in inflammatory bowel disease and clearance of thiopurine metabolites and outcomes in exposed neonates. *Aliment Pharmacol Ther*, **53**, 810–820.

252 Kenet G, Barg AA and Nowak-Göttl U (2018) Hemostasis in the very young. *Semin Thromb Hemost*, **44**, 617–623.

253 Eberl W (2020) Diagnostic challenges in newborns and infants with coagulation disorders. *Hamostaseologie*, **40**, 84–87.

254 Monagle P, Cuello, CA, Augustine, C, Bonduel M, Brandão LR, Capman T *et al.* (2018) American Society of Hematology 2018 guidelines for management of venous thromboembolism: treatment of pediatric venous thromboembolism. *Blood Adv*, **2**, 3292–3316.

255 Reverdiau-Moalic P, Delahousse B, Body G, Bardos P, Leroy J and Gruel Y (1996) Evolution of blood coagulation activators and inhibitors in the healthy human fetus. *Blood*, **88**, 900–906.

256 Andrew M, Paes M, Milner R, Johnston M, Mitchel L, Tollefsen DM *et al.* (1987) Development of the human coagulation system in the full-term infant. *Blood*, **70**, 165–172.

257 Andrew M, Paes B, Milner R, Johnston M, Mitchell L, Tollefsen DM *et al.* (1988) Development of the human coagulation system in the healthy premature infant. *Blood*, **72**, 1651–1657.

258 Poralla C, Traut C, Hertfelder H-J, Oldenberg J, Bartmann P and Heep A (2012) The coagulation system of extremely preterm infants: influence of perinatal risk factors on coagulation. *J Perinatol*, **32**, 869–873.

259 Will A (2015) Neonatal haemostasis and the management of neonatal thrombosis. *Br J Haematol*, **169**, 324–332.

260 Pal S, Curley A and Stanworth SJ (2015) Interpretation of clotting tests in the neonate. *Arch Dis Child Fetal Neonatal Ed*, **100**, F270–F274.

261 Monagle P, Barnes C, Ignjatovic V, Furmedge J, Newall F, Chan A *et al.* (2006) Developmental haemostasis. Impact for clinical haemostasis laboratories. *Thromb Haemost*, **95**, 362–372.

262 Rao AAN, Rodriguez V, Long ME, Winters JL, Nichols WL and Pruthi RK (2009) Transient neonatal acquired von Willebrand syndrome due to transplacental transfer of maternal monoclonal antibodies. *Pediatr Blood Cancer*, **53**, 655–657.

263 McNinch A (2010) Vitamin K dependent bleeding: early history and recent trends in the United Kingdom. *Early Hum Dev*, **86** (Suppl 1), 63–65.

264 Jullien S (2021) Vitamin K prophylaxis in newborns. *BMC Paediatr*, **21** (Suppl 1), 350.

265 Busfield A, Samuel R, McNinch A and Tripp JH (2013) Vitamin K deficiency bleeding after NICE guidance and withdrawal of Konakion. Neonatal: British Paediatric Surveillance Unit study, 2006–2008. *Arch Dis Child*, **98**, 41–47.

266 van Hasselt PM, de Koning TJ, Kvist N, de Vries E, Lundin CD, Berger R *et al.* (2008) Prevention of vitamin K deficiency bleeding in breastfed infants: lessons from the Dutch and Danish biliary atresia registries. *Pediatrics*, **121**, e857–e863.

267 Chalmers EA, Alamelu J, Collins PW, Mathias M, Payne J, Richards M *et al.*; Paediatric & Rare Disorders Working Parties of the UK Haemophilia Doctors Organization (2018) Intracranial haemorrhage in children with inherited bleeding disorders in the UK 2003–2015: a national cohort study. *Haemophilia*, **24**, 641–647.

268 Kulkarni R and Lusher J (2001) Perinatal management of newborns with haemophilia. *Br J Haematol*, **112**, 264–274.

269 Punt MC, Waning ML, Mauser-Bunschoten EP, Kruip MJHA, Eikenboom J, Nieuwenhuizen L *et al.* (2021) Maternal and neonatal bleeding complications in relation to peripartum management in hemophilia carriers. *Blood Rev*, **49**, 100826.

270 Chalmers E, Williams M, Brennand J, Liesner R, Collins P and Richards M; Paediatric Working Party of United Kingdom Haemophilia Doctors' Organization (2011) Guideline on the management of haemophilia in the fetus and neonate. *Br J Haematol*, **154**, 208–215.

271 Andersson NG, Chalmers EA, Kenet G, Ljung R, Mäkipernaa A and Chambost H; PedNet Haemophilia Research Foundation (2019) Mode of delivery in hemophilia: vaginal delivery and Cesarean section carry very similar risks for intracranial hemorrhages and other major bleeds. *Haematologica*, **104**, 2100–2106.

272 Streif W and Knoepfler R (2020) Perinatal management of hemophilia. *Hamostaseologie*, **40**, 226–232.

273 Sanders YV, Fijnvandraat K, Boender J, Mauser-Bunschoten EP, van der Bom JG, de Meris J *et al.*; WiN study group (2015) Bleeding spectrum in children with moderate or severe von Willebrand disease: Relevance of pediatric-specific bleeding. *Am J Hematol*, **90**, 1142–1148.

274 Naderi M, Cohan N, Shahramian I, Miri-Aliabad G, Haghpanah S and Imani M (2019) A retrospective study on clinical manifestations of neonates with FXIII-A deficiency. *Blood Cells Mol Dis*, **77**, 78–81.

275 Cohen EL, Millikan SE, Morocco PC and de Jong JLO (2021) Hemorrhagic shock after neonatal circumcision: severe congenital factor XIII deficiency. *Case Rep Pediatr*, **2021**, 5550199.

276 Palla R, Peyvandi F and Shapiro AD (2015) Rare bleeding disorders: diagnosis and treatment. *Blood*, **125**, 2052–2061.

277 Haley KM (2017) *Neonatal venous thromboembolism. Front Pediatr*, **5**, 136.

278 van Ommen CH and Nowak-Gottl U (2017) Inherited thrombophilia in pediatric venous thromboembolic disease: why and who to test. *Front Pediatr*, **5**, 50.

279 Monagle P and Newell F (2018) American Society of Hematology 2018 Guidelines for management of venous thromboembolism: treatment of pediatric venous thromboembolism. *Blood Adv*, **2**, 3292–3316.

280 Chalmers E, Ganesen V, Liesner R, Maroo S, Nokes T, Saunders D *et al.* (2011) Guideline on the investigation, management and prevention of venous thrombosis in children. *Br J Haematol*, **154**, 196–207.

281 Robinson V, Achey MA, Nag UP, Reed CR, Pahl KS, Greenberg RG *et al.* (2021) Thrombosis in infants in the neonatal intensive care unit: analysis of a large national database. *Thromb Haemost*, **19**, 400–407.

282 Smith N, Warren BB, Smith J, Jacobson L, Armstrong J, Kim J *et al.* (2021) Antithrombin deficiency: a pediatric disorder. *Thromb Res*, **202**, 45–51.

283 Curtis C, Mineyko A, Massicotte P, Leaker M, Jiang XY, Floer A, Kirton A (2017) Thrombophilia risk is not increased in children after perinatal stroke. *Blood*, **129**, 2793–2800.

284 Lehman LL, Beaute K, Kapur K, Danehy AR, Bernson-Leung ME, Malkin H *et al.* (2017) Workup for perinatal stroke does not predict recurrence. *Stroke*, **48**, 2078–2083.

285 Bhat R and Monagle P (2020) Anticoagulation in preterm and term neonates: why are they special? *Thromb Res*, **187**, 113–121.

286 Bhat R, Kumar R, Kwon S, Murthy K and Liem RI (2018) Risk factors for neonatal venous and arterial thromboembolism in the Neonatal Intensive Care Unit – a case control study. *J Pediatr*, **195**, 28–32.

287 Kosch A, Kuwertz-Bröking E, Heller C, Kurnik K, Schobess R and Nowak-Göttl U (2004) Renal venous thrombosis in neonates: prothrombotic risk factors and long-term follow-up. *Blood*, **104**, 1356–1360.

288 Lau KK, Stoffman JM, Williams S, McCusker P, Brandão L, Patel S and Chan AKC (2007) Neonatal renal vein thrombosis: review of the English-language literature between 1992 and 2006. *Pediatrics*, **120**, e1278–e1284.

289 Cohen CT, Anderson V, Desai SB, Arunachalam A, Ahmed M and Diaz R (2021) Patient characteristics and treatment outcomes of symptomatic catheter-related arterial thrombosis in infants: a retrospective cohort study. *J Pediatr*, **231**, 215–222.

290 Letunica N, Busuttil-Crellin X, Cowley J, Monagle P and Ignjatovic V (2020) Age-specific differences in the in vitro anticoagulant effect of Bivalirudin in healthy neonates and children compared to adults. *Thromb Res*, **192**, 167–173.

291 Minford A, Behnisch W, Brons P, David M, Gomez G, Hertfelder H-J *et al.* (2014) Subcutaneous protein C concentrate in the management of severe protein C deficiency – experience in 12 centres. *Br J Haematol*, **164**, 414–421.

292 Inoue H, Terachi SI, Uchiumi T, Sato T, Urata M, Ishimura M *et al.* (2017) The clinical presentation and genotype of protein C deficiency with double mutations of the protein C gene. *Pediatr Blood Cancer*, **64**, e26404.

293 Chaireti R, Tronnhagen I, Bremme K and Ranta S (2020) Management and outcomes of newborns at risk for inherited antithrombin deficiency. *J Thromb Haemost*, **18**, 2582–2589.

294 Carson JL, Guyatt G, Heddle NM, Grossman BJ, Cohn CS, Fung MK *et al.* (2016) Clinical practice guidelines from the AABB: red blood cell transfusion thresholds and storage. *JAMA*, **316**, 2025–2035.

295 Howarth C, Bannerjee J and Aladangady N (2018) Red blood cell transfusion in preterm infants: current evidence and controversies. *Neonatology*, **114**, 7–16.

296 Keir AK, New H, Robitaille N, Crighton GL, Wood EM and Stanworth SJ (2019) Approaches to understanding and interpreting the risks of red blood cell transfusion in neonates. *Transfus Med*, **29**, 231–238.

297 Goel R and Josephson CD (2018) Recent advances in transfusions in neonates/infants. *F1000Res*, **7**, F1000 Faculty Rev-609.

298 Widness JA, Madan A, Grindeanu LA, Zimmerman MB, Wong DK and Stevenson DK (2005) Reduction in red cell transfusions among preterm infants: results of a randomized trial with an in-line blood gas and chemistry monitor. *Pediatrics*, **115**, 1299–1306.

299 Ballin A, Livshiz V, Mimouni FB, Dollberg S, Kohelet D, Oren A *et al.* (2009) Reducing blood transfusion requirements in preterm infants by a new device: a pilot study. *Acta Paediatr*, **98**, 247–250.

300 Fustolo-Gunnink SF, Fijnvandraat K, van Klaveren D, Stanworth SJ, Curley A, Onland W *et al.*; PlaNeT2 and MATISSE collaborators (2019) Preterm neonates benefit from low prophylactic platelet transfusion threshold despite varying risk of bleeding or death. *Blood*, **134**, 2354–2360.

301 Motta M, Del Vecchio A and Chirico G (2015) Fresh frozen plasma administration in the neonatal intensive care unit: evidence-based guidelines. *Clin Perinatol*, **42**, 639–650.

302 Mitsiakos G, Karametou M, Gkampeta A, Karali C, Papathanasiou AE, Papacharalambous E *et al.* (2019) Effectiveness and safety of 4-factor prothrombin complex concentrate (4PCC) in neonates with intractable bleeding or severe coagulation disturbances: a retrospective study of 37 cases. *J Pediatric Hematol Oncol*, **41**, e135–e140.

303 Young G, Wicklund B, Neff P, Johnson C and Nugent DJ (2009) Off-label use of rFVIIa in children with excessive bleeding: a consecutive study of 153 off-label uses in 139 children. *Pediatr Blood Cancer*, **53**, 1074–1078.

304 Gkiougki E, Mitsiakos G, Chatziioannidis E, Papadakis E and Nikolaidis N (2013) Predicting response to rFVIIa in neonates with intractable bleeding or severe coagulation disturbances. *J Pediatr Hematol Oncol*, **35**, 221–226.

305 Coppola T, Mangold JF, Cantrell S and Permar SR (2019) Impact of maternal immunity on congenital cytomegalovirus birth prevalence and infant outcomes: a systematic review. *Vaccines (Basel)*, **7**, 129.

306 Winkelhorst D, Kamphuis MM, Steggerda SJ, Rijken M, Oepkes D, Lopriore E and van Klink JMM (2019) Perinatal outcome and long-term neurodevelopment after intracranial haemorrhage due to fetal and neonatal alloimmune thrombocytopenia. *Fetal Diagn Ther*, **45**, 184–191.

Index

Note:
All index entries relate to neonates, unless otherwise described (e.g. fetal).
Page numbers in *italics* refer to figures; those in **bold** refer to tables.

Neonatal Haematology: A Practical Guide, First Edition. Irene Roberts and Barbara J. Bain.
© 2022 John Wiley & Sons Ltd. Published 2022 by John Wiley & Sons Ltd.